"Detailed narrative accounts are essential for learning lessons from the global tragedy of COVID-19. Sweden's approach – which became famous for all the wrong reasons – is meticulously documented here. It should be essential reading for those involved in planning for future public health emergencies."

– Professor Trisha Greenhalgh, GP and Public Health academic, University of Oxford, UK

"For many reasons this book is a unique and special contribution to public health coming at a unique time. There are many reasons why 'herd immunity' is not applicable in a pandemic. This book will tell why. There are more reasons why government as medical scientific leader is also not applicable. The COVID-19 pandemic proved that, and this book tells why. Which government should we follow (many differed one from another)? Why should we limit expertise where we know it is limited or even lacking?"

– Robert Gallo, MD, Gudelsky Professor of Medicine and Microbiology/Immunology and Founding Director, Institute of Human Virology, University of Maryland School of Medicine, Baltimore, Md., and Co-Founder and Chair of the International Scientific Committee of the Global Virus Network

"From the earliest months of the coronavirus pandemic, international observers have been taken aback by Sweden's policy choices in responding to COVID-19. Countering its long history of leadership in public health, the Swedish state has advanced a laissez-faire approach in which the population is allowed to be exposed to the virus in a manner that experts believed would remain controlled. To date, it has remained difficult for outsiders to understand Sweden's permissive attitude towards the pandemic, the unwillingness of national leaders to revisit counterproductive policies, the state's controversial trafficking in misinformation, and ultimately a lack of reflection on highly disparate rates of infection and death.

Sweden's Pandemic Experiment resolves these puzzles by offering a rich account of the context informing Sweden's COVID-19 response. Its interdisciplinary contributors illuminate a wide array of inputs – sociological, historical, cultural, and political – to the so-called 'Swedish way.' As they show, Sweden's pandemic failures have drawn on a constellation of institutional failures: in media, in crisis management, in health care, in public health, and in national scientific research institutes.

Presented without fear or favor, *Sweden's Pandemic Experiment* should prompt a reckoning in Swedish society. This meticulously documented account will also be a model for researchers elsewhere, inspiring comparative analysis of pandemic strategies that have underperformed in other global settings."

– Martha Lincoln, Assistant Professor of Anthropology at San Francisco State University and author of *Epidemic Politics in Vietnam: Public Health and the State* (Bloomsbury Academic, 2021)

"This volume is one of the first to provide an interdisciplinary critical assessment of the Swedish response to the pandemic of COVID-19. This is a timely and welcome contribution to study the interplay of scientific, political, and public discussion about a 'Swedish puzzle' that has triggered essential moral questions while deeply affecting the social compact."

– Yohann Aucante, Associate Professor at the School of Advanced Studies in the Social Sciences (EHESS), Paris; author of *The Swedish Experiment. The COVID-19 Response and Its Controversies* (Bristol University Press, 2022)

"Different national states launched different medical-political strategies to combat the Covid pandemic. If nations are willing to learn from each other how to cope with such an unusual situation that, however, may repeat with another infectious disease, such strategies must be comprehensibly assessed and evaluated according to ethical standards. Bergmann and Lindström present such critical assessment for the specific Swedish case. I see this interdisciplinary volume as paradigm case for a holistic survey which is of interest far beyond the Swedish case as such. It is a 'must read' for all persons and organizations worldwide even if it may remind doubtful whether there are final 'lessons learned.'"

– Konrad Ott, Professor of Philosophy and Ethics of the Environment at Kiel University

SWEDEN'S PANDEMIC EXPERIMENT

This book considers Sweden's pandemic management which differed so significantly from much of the rest of the world: it provoked intense and wide-reaching interest, curiosity and criticism. Transdisciplinary Swedish authors from the humanities, life sciences, social sciences and cultural studies use a variety of tools to mine deeper into some of the central elements and dimensions in their country's pandemic management such as understandings of freedom, the execution of power, denialism, exceptionalism, patriotism, the role of expertise and trust in the national state to give a deeper understanding of Sweden's decisions, failures, successes and the lessons to be learned.

Aimed at readers with interest in global health and politics, it will also be of interest in disciplines such as virology, epidemiology, history, cultural studies, ethics, media studies, medicine and economics.

Sigurd Bergmann is Emeritus Professor of Religious Studies at the Norwegian University of Science and Technology, Trondheim; Visiting Researcher at the Faculty of Theology, Uppsala University; and Fellow at the Rachel Carson Center at Munich University. His research covers religion and the environment, and religion, arts and architecture, and among his multiple books and articles are *Weather, Religion and Climate Change* (2020), *Religion, Space and the Environment* (2014), *In the Beginning Is the Icon* (2009) and *God in Context* (2003).

Martin Lindström is Professor of Social Medicine at the Medical Faculty, Lund University, Sweden. He holds a PhD in Social Medicine (2000) and a second PhD in Economic History (Historical Demography) (2015). Lindström is a Fellow of the Center for Economic Demography (CED) and EpiHealth, both at Lund University. His research covers social capital and health, socioeconomic differences in health, life course epidemiology and historical demography (including epidemics in the 18th and 19th centuries). Lindström has authored many international research articles and chapter contributions in edited books.

The Politics of Pandemics

Understanding the Politics of Pandemic Emergencies in the time of COVID-19
An Introduction to Global Politosomatics
Mika Aaltola

Pandemic Response and the Cost of Lockdowns
Global Debates from Humanities and Social Sciences
Edited by Peter Sutoris, Sinéad Murphy, Aleida Mendes Borges and Yossi Nehushtan

The COVID-19 Pandemic in the Middle East and North Africa
Public Policy Responses
Edited by Anis Ben Brik

Sweden's Pandemic Experiment
Edited by Sigurd Bergmann and Martin Lindström

For more information see www.routledge.com/The-Politics-of-Pandemics/book-series/TPOP

SWEDEN'S PANDEMIC EXPERIMENT

Edited by Sigurd Bergmann
and Martin Lindström

Routledge
Taylor & Francis Group
LONDON AND NEW YORK

First published 2023
by Routledge
4 Park Square, Milton Park, Abingdon, Oxon OX14 4RN

and by Routledge
605 Third Avenue, New York, NY 10158

Routledge is an imprint of the Taylor & Francis Group, an informa business

British Library Cataloguing-in-Publication Data
A catalogue record for this book is available from the British Library

ISBN: 978-1-032-26670-1 (hbk)
ISBN: 978-1-032-26671-8 (pbk)
ISBN: 978-1-003-28936-4 (ebk)

DOI: 10.4324/9781003289364

Typeset in Bembo
by Apex CoVantage, LLC

CONTENTS

FIGURES

TABLES

CONTRIBUTORS

Peter Baldwin is Professor of History at UCLA and Global Distinguished Professor at NYU. Among other works, he has written three books on the comparative history of public health in which Sweden figures prominently: *Contagion and the State in Europe, 1830–1930* (Cambridge, 1999); *Disease and Democracy: The Industrialized World Faces AIDS* (California, 2005); and most recently, *Fighting the First Wave: Why the Coronavirus Was Tackled so Differently across the Globe* (Cambridge, 2021).

Emil J. Bergholtz is Professor of Theoretical Physics at the Department of Physics, Stockholm University. His research comprises theoretical physics, topological quantum phenomena and when needed theoretical epidemiology. He has worked as Fellow at the Max Planck Institute for the Physics of Complex Systems in Dresden and as Emmy Noether Group Leader at the Free University of Berlin. In 2022 he was awarded the "Göran Gustafsson Prize in Physics" by the Royal Swedish Academy of Sciences.

Sigurd Bergmann is Emeritus Professor in Religious Studies at the Norwegian University of Science and Technology in Trondheim; Visiting Researcher at the Faculty of Theology, Uppsala University; Docent in Systematic Theology at Lund University; and Fellow at the Rachel Carson Center for Environment and Society, Munich University. His previous studies have investigated the relationship between the image of God and the view of nature in late antiquity, the methodology of contextual theology, visual arts in the indigenous Arctic and Australia, as well as visual arts, architecture and religion, and religion in climate change. He has initiated the European Forum for the Study of Religion and the Environment, and among his many publications are *God in Context* (2003), *Creation Set Free* (2005), *In the Beginning Is the Icon* (2009), *Raum und Geist* (2010), *Religion, Space and the Environment* (2014), *Theology in Built Environments* (2009), *Religion in Global Environmental and*

Climate Change (2011), *Religion in the Anthropocene* (2017), *Arts, Religion and the Environment: Exploring Nature's Texture* (2018) and *Weather, Religion and Climate Change* (2020).

Nele Brusselaers is a medical doctor and clinical epidemiologist currently working as Associate Professor of Clinical Epidemiology (Docent) and Senior Researcher at the Karolinska Institutet in Stockholm and as Visiting Professor at Antwerp University in Belgium. She has followed the development of the pandemic closely in Sweden, Belgium and internationally and became part of Vetenskapsforum Covid-19 during Spring 2020. She is an advocate of solid and transparent research methodology and likes to work with research questions close to clinics.

Rodney Edvinsson is Professor in Economic History at Stockholm University. His main study areas are long-term economic growth, monetary history and historical demographics. He has, for example, reconstructed vital rates for Sweden for the pre-census era, and studied the impact of macroeconomic fluctuations on mortality levels.

Johanna Höög is Associate Professor at the Department of Chemistry & Molecular Biology, Gothenburg University. She holds a PhD from Heidelberg, Germany and continued her training as a postdoc in Oxford (UK), Boulder (USA) and Dresden (Germany). Her research in cell biology investigates the cell's interior by reconstructing it in 3D using cryo-electron microscopy. Johanna Höög's experience of giving birth in the pandemic context in March 2022 has led her to follow the knowledge creation in science about children and Covid-19. She wrote her first debate article in a national newspaper on the topic in October 2020, focused on the asymptomatic spread that is common amongst children, and has been an engaged science communicator since then.

Kajsa Klein is media researcher, writer and democracy activist. She teaches Journalism and Media and Communication Science at Jönköping University. Her research explores strategies of resistance, hate on the internet, election campaigns and issues of democracy and communication.

Lapo Lappin is a philosopher and cultural writer, with degrees from Uppsala University and Università degli Studi di Siena. He runs the podcast *Metafysiska laboratoriet* (https://metafysiskalaboratoriet.wordpress.com/) and has edited, with Åke Gavelin, *Filosofi och pandemi* (Skellefteå: Artos & Norma, 2021).

Martin Lindström is Professor of Social Medicine at the Department of Clinical Sciences in Malmö (IKVM), Lund University, and the Center for Primary Health Care Research, Lund University and Region Skåne. He is affiliated with the Center for Economic Demography (CED), Lund School of Economics, and EpiHealth: Epidemiology for Health, both at Lund University. His research mainly concerns social capital and its effects on health, health-related behaviours, access to health care and amenities and crime. Important aspects of social capital include social participation, generalized trust in other people and trust in institutions. Lindström conducts studies with cross-sectional as well as longitudinal (mainly prospective cohort studies) study designs based on individual-level and multilevel data. These studies explore social participation, trust in others, and institutional trust in relation to self-reported general and psychological health, health-related behaviours (tobacco smoking, physical activity, diet, alcohol, cannabis), total and diagnosis specific mortality, access to health care, sense of security in the neighbourhood and violence and threat of violence. Lindström has published more than 180 articles, and enriched the debates on Sweden's pandemic management with several significant contributions.

Gunnar Steineck, MD, PhD, is Senior Professor in clinical cancer epidemiology at the Department of Oncology, Gothenburg University, and Researcher at Karolinska Institute, Stockholm. His research intends at learning how to cure cancer patients at the same time as they can recover their physical and mental health afterward. Steineck draws on epidemiologic methodology, and has authored more than 350 science articles.

Jens Stilhoff Sörensen is Associate Professor in the School of Global Studies, University of Gothenburg, Sweden. He has worked for the Swedish Government, Ministry of Foreign Affairs and for international organizations like the OSCE. His publications include *Splitting Europe: The EU, Russia and the West* (Lanham: Rowman & Littlefield, 2021).

Anders Vahlne, MD, PhD, Professor Emeritus, is the former chair of the Division of Clinical Virology at the Karolinska Institute in Stockholm, Sweden. He was also chief physician of the Clinical Virology Laboratory at the Karolinska Hospital. Vahlne serves as the director for the Karolinska Center of Excellence of the Global Virus Network (GVN) and is the co-chair of the GVN's Taskforce on Long Covid-19. He obtained his medical doctoral degree and license to practice medicine from the Gothenburg University in 1973 and his PhD from the same University in 1978. He is a certified specialist in Clinical Virology since 1978. In 1982–83 he spent a sabbatical at Scripps Clinic and Research Foundation in La Jolla, CA, on a Fogarty Fellowship. From 1972 to 1986 his research focused on the neuro-pathogenesis of herpes simplex virus infections. He thereafter switched to mainly work on human retroviruses, in particular HIV. Vahlne was on the President's Advisory Board for the Irish National Virus Reference Laboratory at the University College Dublin from 2010 to 2021.

ACKNOWLEDGEMENTS

I would like to thank cordially my co-authors for our fruitful cooperation, in a valuable, intense, constructive and mutually supportive solidarity of communicating, writing, reading, commenting, and re-writing. I am likewise grateful to my co-editor Martin Lindström for our long and deep continuity of exchange about the numerous challenges of the pandemic and our editing process. Thanks, Martin, for your commitment, open-mindedness and constancy.

I would also personally like to embrace the opportunity to give thanks to all those with whom I corresponded about the pain and hope in our common pandemic emergency. Sharing the plaguing varied experiences of the virus's spread and the political and cultural responses with so many old and new friends, committed citizens, scholars, journalists, artists, writers all over the Earth our home – from Melbourne to Berlin, Helsinki, New York, Oslo, Cape Town, and even as far as to Stockholm and many other places – has opened for me a kind of God-given, undiscovered land where hope, comfort, morality and communitarian power could again flourish. I am especially grateful to the scholars and members in our Science Forum Covid-19 – and the countervailing power that we have developed together – in the research group of the international ESCAPE project, and to Christoph Stückelberger, Zurich; Hans Günter Heimbrock, Frankfurt/M.; Alf Hornborg, Yxnevik; Gina Gustavsson, Uppsala; Konrad Ott, Greifswald; Volker Küster, Mainz; Nicholas Aylott, Stockholm; and Lars Johan Materstvedt, Trondheim. Without Ingela Bergmann at home, and our at times heated daily trials to mutually understand what was going on, including her apropos political cartoons, life in socio-pandemic asceticism, and also working on this book, would have been most unbearable.

In addition I would like to thank those who have resourcefully assisted the emergence of some of the book's pieces: Andrew Ewing, David Steadson, Marilyn Burton, Galina Esther Shubina, Kathleen Myrestam, Reed Curtis, Emma

Wikberg, Per O. Widlund, Sofia Breland, and Maria Thorlund for their skilled and dedicated work of commenting on and language editing of chapters. Thanks also to the Faculty of Arts at the Norwegian University of Science and Technology in Trondheim for providing a subsidy for the language editing of my chapter. Martin Lindström and I are moreover grateful to Lund University Library's generous fund that allows us to offer the book to a worldwide audience as Open Access. Finally I want to thank Robert Sorsby and Aneta Byzdra for professional and fluent support with and production of the work in the promising new book series.

Sigurd Bergmann
Lund in April 2022

SWEDEN STUMBLES ALONG THE THIRD WAY

Peter Baldwin

"What, me worry?" was the slogan of Alfred E. Neuman, avatar of *Mad Magazine*. Sweden took it to heart during the Covid pandemic. The country was commonly regarded as efficiently run and competently administered. Exhaustive government investigations preceded policy changes, and its politicians were steeped in a culture devoted to the science and technology that fuelled its export economy. Yet this nation now decided instead to channel its inner libertarian and let its freak flag fly.

The Covid pandemic provided plenty of surprises. Nations that were thought to be well prepared in public health terms, such as the US and UK, stumbled badly during the phase before vaccines arrived. Others sought to make a virtue of doing nothing, such as Brazil and Belarus. China touted its prowess in clamping down and admirably managed to keep infection at bay through rigorous measures. When its own vaccine proved ineffective against later variants, it found itself painted into a locked-down corner with no exit strategy. Despite their swagger as rugged, individualistic Crocodile Dundees, Australians meekly accepted one of the democratic world's most drastic and prolonged shutdowns. In this bestiary of different responses to a disease that brandished much the same threat worldwide, the anomaly of the Swedish approach still stands out. Why?

Alone in Europe, even more so in Scandinavia, the Swedes decided neither to shut down nor impose more than mild restrictions. With some distancing measures in place, secondary schools, stores, restaurants, amusements, and most of normal life remained open. Masking was not required, and Swedes were assumed to take individual precautions on their own without needing the authorities' mandate. Only once deaths started soaring at the end of 2020 did they finally clamp down a bit, passing a new contagious disease law that gave the government extra powers.

With its laissez-faire approach, Sweden showed the way for self-styled anti-authoritarians worldwide. They bristled against public health impositions, whether

DOI: 10.4324/9781003289364-1

lockdowns, travel restrictions, masking, or eventually vaccination. Basking in publicity, Swedish public health authorities preened themselves in the unexpected glow of attention. Once the poster boy of social democracy, Sweden was now an exemplar for the libertarian lunatic fringe.

Why this fall from grace? This book's chapters explore the causes of Sweden's *Sonderweg*. They show that incompetence and a national narcissism bordering on arrogance stand out among the most general sources. The Swedish public health authorities ignored the science as it developed, deliberately failed to implement most useful preventive strategies, and hooked their wagon to a quixotic hope for "natural" herd immunity achieved via unchecked infection. Massaging the numbers, they waited in vain for the protection that would supposedly result as disease spread widely. Most striking about the chapters here is their relentless drumbeat of examples of how wilfully ignorant, misleading, and inept the public health authorities were, above all Tegnell and Giesecke.

Aggravating their technical shortcomings, they were also utilitarian to the point of moral obtuseness. No nation outside Asia did well in protecting the old, but few authorities elsewhere – backed by their court ethicists – dared speculate openly, as did the Swedes, that the elderly were less worth protecting than the young. Indeed, they went so far as to triage some elderly, practicing involuntary euthanasia by providing end-of-life palliative care rather than treating Covid symptoms.

Even as such shortcomings became painfully evident, the public health authorities were allowed to continue. Critical experts from outside the bureaucracy were shunned, international experience and opinion ignored. Klein's chapter gives details. The politicians from a weak coalition government used the fig leaf of the Swedish administrative system's supposed autonomy to abdicate responsibility for taking the reins. No one dared call out the authorities in their bubble. Many journalists and much of the public cheered them on as exemplifying the best Sweden has to offer.

These chapters also show that, besides squandering a once-deserved national reputation for competence and moral rectitude, the Swedish approach helped undermine basic trust in government and authority. The first two qualities matter for Sweden's standing in the world. Trust, in contrast, is a problem for its own citizens. Though their approach assumed that citizens could be entrusted with their own protection, the authorities shunned the restrictions common elsewhere because they did not expect Swedes willingly to follow them. Swedes were not to be counted on, after all.

Conversely, as Bergmann asks, how does a system reliant on mutual trust between citizens and government regain its equilibrium once the authorities are revealed to have dissimulated, manipulated, and fallen short? Why trust the untrustworthy? Worse, if no one – whether citizens or leaders – trusts science, how does the nation re-emerge from its collective rabbit hole? Either way, can a system whose unelected authorities routinely obfuscated their intentions and denied the existence of basic documentation such as the minutes of government deliberations be considered democratic – a question raised in Sörensen's chapter.

Sweden prides itself on technocratic expertise. The relevant data and know-how inform policy-making. Experts, not politicians, make the decisions. In public health especially, political interference is restricted on the assumption that expertise reigns. Their unique approach to Covid, the Swedes liked to think, was the outcome of allowing professionals to decide, untainted by political expediency. They were following a venerable tradition of bowing to trained, not popular, opinion. Other nations, including neighbouring Denmark and Norway, instead responded to populist cries for security and therefore locked down.[1]

Yet, if the experts got it wrong, there was no one to rein them in. Cobbled together to restrain the resurgent ethno-nationalist Sweden Democrats, a feeble coalition government provided only lacklustre leadership. That left decisions to a narrow, self-perpetuating cadre of public health authorities whose judgement was never challenged. In other nations, politicians took the ultimate responsibility, second-guessing and counterweighting the technocrats. Experts ought to be on tap, not on top, was the principle. In March 2020, Danish public health advisors recommended a laissez-faire approach. But their political masters overruled them, imposing strict measures against the pandemic. Not in Sweden. The nation was left to the mercies of unelected technocrats, responsible to no one.

Worse, their expertise proved unimpressive. On several crucial matters, the public health experts got the science wrong. They ignored asymptomatic spreaders, children as vectors, the aerosolized spread of Covid, and the effectivity of masking. Vahlne and Lindström give examples in their chapters. Of course, knowledge developed only gradually as the epidemic spread, and it took time for such insights to emerge. Yet the cumulation of these particular blind spots and their tendency to dovetail with the authorities' evident political preference for a hands-off approach suggests they were tendentious. Everyone makes mistakes. But when errors conveniently align with prior political choices, they cease being innocent.

Denying that asymptomatic Covid victims could spread infection, the authorities refused to forbid, isolate, or later test incoming travellers, require or even supply protective gear for caretakers in old age homes, or ask the public to mask. Acknowledging the role of asymptomatic carriers would have undermined their hopes of a voluntary approach. However well intentioned, those who did not know they were infectious could not do what was necessary to avoid transmission. Ignoring the threat that children might spread disease allowed the authorities to keep schools and day-care centres open, as Höög shows in her chapter. Without their childcare function, the economy would have been hobbled. Inexplicably, the experts also rejected the usefulness of masking. They ignored the evidence that Covid spread through aerosolized exhalations, not just coughing and sneezing. Here their arguments bordered on the ludicrous. Sweden was a land of wide-open spaces. No need then to mask. Even in public transport, they insisted, the distances among passengers sufficed to make masking pointless.[2]

More generally, the authorities prayed for herd immunity. Brusselaers and Lappin show how an experiment in mass immunity was conducted on the Swedish people without their knowledge. Bergholtz details the mendacity of the authorities and their media lickspittles as they denied what was up. Why were they so wedded to an approach widely regarded elsewhere as immoral, ineffectual, and scientifically illiterate? Herd immunity was the necessary corollary of the public health authorities' voluntarist strategy of mitigating, not suppressing, the pandemic. If allowing disease to run slowly through the population delivered broad natural immunity, then life could soon return to normal – for those who survived. In the pandemic's early stages, before a vaccine or cure, herd immunity was the only exit strategy available to nations that sought to mitigate.

Of course, those countries seeking to suppress the pandemic faced the same dilemma. But they made no bones about it. Rejecting herd immunity, suppression was a gamble on vaccination. They sought to spare as many lives as possible in hopes that a medical solution would soon arrive. Mitigation, in contrast, deliberately accepted the cost of higher immediate mortality for the expected payoff of broader – herd-like – immunity regardless of a vaccine. The assumptions were that suppression could not work and that a vaccine was unlikely soon. Natural immunity was the only solution.

Herd immunity was therefore crucial for the voluntarist Swedish approach. Without that as an achievable goal, why not clamp down more firmly, suppressing the epidemic? Why let more people die, as they would without a lockdown, if the aim were not to achieve broad infection-based immunity? The calculus was openly utilitarian. Herd immunity as an exit strategy meant letting more people die now so that, over the pandemic's lifespan, fewer – or at least no more – would perish. One Swedish medical professor said, "Much better to have high mortality today if that brings us closer to herd immunity." His proviso, that, in the long run, overall mortality would be lower, was only a pious wish.[3]

Herd immunity was bad science when first proposed. It has remained so even with the arrival of vaccines. None of the vaccines developed so far are sterilizing. They do not prevent infected vaccinees from spreading Covid, except in the indirect sense of temporarily lowering their overall viral load, thus making them less dangerous. Yet, the Swedish authorities were desperate for herd immunity. A necessary consequence of their slapdash voluntary approach, widespread infectivity would then conveniently also justify it. So keen on having Covid spread broadly were they that they gamed the numbers of the infected, fiddling them to fit their hopes for a widespread immunity that never arrived. Edvinsson's chapter details how. Refusing to countenance extensive lockdown, the authorities grasped herd immunity as their get-out-of-jail card.

To the authorities' incompetence then came a vainglorious epidemiological nationalism persuading them that Sweden's uniqueness allowed it to sidestep the dilemmas faced elsewhere. "We are the heroes of our times," the Swedish crooner Måns Zelmerlöw sang to win the Eurovision contest in 2015. That was certainly the opinion of the country's public health authorities. Other nations whose citizens were not schooled in correct thinking and acting might need the lash of mandates – those whose politicians bowed to the easy certainties of populist demands for lockdown. Not the Swedes. They were sufficiently self-controlled and disciplined to do voluntarily what elsewhere required compulsion. The Swedish *Sonderweg* was motivated by a view of the nation's political uniqueness, with citizens and government trusting each other so that enforcing public health strictures was unnecessary.[4]

Like citizens elsewhere, Swedes sensibly restricted their movements, working from home and avoiding crowds, even without that being required. But not as much as where behaviour was regulated. Nor enough to prevent the inevitable outcome of allowing the pandemic free rein. As of this writing, in April 2022, 18,000 Swedes have succumbed to coronavirus. In comparison, 2500 Norwegians have died. Norway has half Sweden's population but is otherwise indistinguishable in terms of size, location, coastline, and so forth. Adjusting for size, more than 13,000 Swedes would thus still be alive had the Norwegians run Sweden's public health system. Much the same holds elsewhere in Scandinavia. Finland has about 30% the Swedish per capita mortality rate, Iceland 16%. Much more densely populated and closer to the main currents of travel and transmission in Western Europe, Denmark achieved only the feat of holding death rates to half the Swedish. The WHO's figures for excess deaths due to Covid were equally harrowing. The mean Swedish figures for 2020–21 were about twice the Danish and Finnish ones, while Norway and Iceland actually had lower than normal mortality during the pandemic.[5] In comparison with their Nordic neighbours, the Swedish approach was toxic.

Reason to celebrate? One would have thought not. Yet, a book by a Swedish journalist Johan Anderberg, *Flocken* (*The Herd*), sought to pull victory from the ashes. It proclaimed 2020 the year of Swedish freedom. While the rest of the world cowered at home, the Swedes were out and about, almost as normal. As long, of course, as you did not belong to that 20% of the population considered old or at-risk, who were admonished to stay at home so the rest could swan about. Or to that other 20% of frontline workers who operated the restaurants, shops, transport, and delivery services so that others could enjoy themselves – many more put at risk than if the economy had shut down. Freedom, it turns out, meant shopping and drinking in public for the younger and better-off. That seems an odd priority for a nation that regularly trumpets the virtues of its solidaristic instincts. Yet, on that altar, 13,000 Swedes were sacrificed. Not for nothing is "journalistic" a pejorative term.

Sweden has long been a darling of the moderate left, avatar of the supposed Third Way between communism and capitalism. It has enjoyed a comfortable position on the global sidelines, whence it has scourged larger and more powerful nations for their shortcomings. Swedes imagine their country as the apex of many developments – the most modern, egalitarian, democratic, and environmentally conscious of anyone. They deal poorly with failure, unaccustomed to having become international pariahs. Yet, despite much defensive bluster, even they understand the magnitude of their mistake. Bergmann's chapter explores the effects of this sense of shame. It is implicitly acknowledged in the public health apologists' desperate search for the most forgiving comparators. If they can find nations whose performance was even worse, the quicker the stench of Sweden's failure will dissipate.

Unsurprisingly, high death rates were the outcome of Sweden's off-piste approach. But high compared to whom? Yes, some nations did worse than Sweden and many equally badly. As of this writing, Sweden hovers in the 50s in the world rankings of per capita mortality. It has done better than Peru and Bulgaria, Brazil, the UK, and the US. But worse than Austria, Switzerland, Germany, the Netherlands, Ireland, worse than the overall global average, and – more to the point – far worse than any of its Nordic neighbours. By the standards of Slovenia, they have done brilliantly. But abysmally compared to New Zealand, another small, culturally homogenous, remote, topographically isolated nation. Much hangs on the choice of the comparator.

Apologists for the Swedish approach prefer comparison with nations in the heart of Europe, not their Nordic neighbours.[6] For this implausible choice, they advance various arguments. Sweden's cities are larger and denser than its neighbours'. They house more immigrants. Swedes travel more than other Scandinavians. Indeed, the nation has more skiers, the sort of tourists responsible for the first seeding of disease in the north as they returned from the Austrian and Swiss slopes. Some such arguments are self-contradictory, others just plain wrong. Blaming both immigrants and travellers points in two different directions since the Somalis of Stockholm were not the ones returning infected from après-ski in Ischgl.

Such apologists claim that Sweden is a normal European country with normal European infection and mortality rates. But that is nonsense. It is a vast and thinly populated territory with few travel connections, on the continent's distant periphery. It could and should have withstood the pandemic much better, following the lead of its fellow Scandinavians. Sweden is not a dense, throbbing, metropolitan Hong Kong of the north, at the epicentre of global peregrination. It is a sparse Nordic wilderness, the end station of most itineraries. Compared to Oslo and Copenhagen, Stockholm airport has per capita fewer than half as many air passengers annually and but a tiny fraction of Amsterdam or London. Stockholm is less densely populated than Oslo and 70% less than London. The Netherlands are 50 times as thickly settled as Sweden.[7] The apologists eagerly search for large, structural reasons to explain the awfulness of Sweden's mortality. But in reality, decisions taken by the public health authorities, and not vetoed by their political masters, explain the misfortune. They could have had Norwegian outcomes but chose Belgian ones.

And for what? Another argument in favour of offering thousands of fellow Swedes on the altar of "freedom" was to keep the economy open and flourishing. Had Sweden been on its own planet, perhaps? But since its export-oriented economy relies on its trading partners, it shares their fates. GDP was up in Sweden only as much as in Denmark (2.1%) during the pandemic, less than in Norway (3.5%).[8] Sweden's unemployment rate remained consistently above its Nordic neighbours' in 2020 and 2021. Children in Sweden's open schools fell even further behind than their British remote-learning peers, as Höög reports. In other words, regardless of the morality of such calculations, the return on high mortality was zero.

The Swedish approach to Covid was incoherent. Even worse than unpalatable death rates was the inherent contradiction at its heart. The authorities claimed that Swedes were well socialized enough to prevent transmission voluntarily, even though not required to. But at the same time, they were intent on achieving herd immunity. Covid should therefore spread through the population, prompting widespread immunity even before a vaccine. Voluntary compliance and herd immunity were at odds. The Swedes could have voluntary compliance, or they could have herd immunity, but not both. Aiming for herd immunity meant assuming that voluntary compliance would not hold. The Swedish authorities, in fact, did not trust their citizens to do the right thing. They specifically counted on them not to, thus spreading the virus and achieving herd immunity.

Their approach was a categorical mistake, applying the wrong tools to the problem. Voluntary measures may work for chronic lifestyle diseases, seeking to convince people to smoke, drink, and eat less, exercise more. But faced with an exponentially multiplying pandemic, consensus, confidence building, and self-motivated compliance are unlikely to be useful in the brief moments left to act. As herd immunity failed to arrive and deaths multiplied, it became clear that the Swedish emperor was wearing no clothes.

Notes

1 Details may be found in Baldwin, Peter. *Fighting the First Wave: Why the Coronavirus Was Tackled so Differently across the Globe*, Cambridge: Cambridge University Press, 2021.
2 "Tegnell om WHO:s råd om munskydd: Inget för Sverige", *Svenska Dagbladet*, 5 June 2020; Johanna Cederblad. "Tegnell: 'Ute efter enkla lösningar'", *Svenska Dagbladet*, 7 June 2020.
3 Kulldorff, Martin. "Hög dödlighet i dag kan ge färre döda på sikt", *Dagens Nyheter*, 4 May 2020.
4 The implicit nationalism of Swedish public health is the subject of the brilliant book, Gustavsson, Gina. *Du stolta, du fria: Om svenskarna, Sverigebilden och folkhälsopatriotismen*, Stockholm: Kaunitz-Olsson, 2021.
5 WHO. "Global Excess Deaths Associated with COVID-19 (Modelled Estimates)", 5 May 2022, www.who.int/data/sets/global-excess-deaths-associated-with-covid-19-modelled-estimates .
6 An example of such cherry-picking tendentiousness in Anderberg, Johan. "How Sweden Swerved Covid Disaster", *Unherd*, 8 November 2021, https://unherd.com/2021/11/how-sweden-swerved-covid-disaster/ .
7 Baldwin. *Fighting the First Wave*, 127.
8 "Which Economies Have Done Best and Worst during the Pandemic?" *Economist*, 1 January 2022.

1

IN THE RUPTURE BETWEEN THIS AND ANOTHER WORLD TO COME

Introductory remarks on pandemic emergency and Sweden's response

Sigurd Bergmann and Martin Lindström

Entering the pandemic century

Since the first cases of human infection with the SARS-CoV-2 virus were reported and the outbreak of the pandemic started between December 2019 and January 2020 in Wuhan, China,[1] the world's inhabitants, nations, and institutions have been extensively challenged in all areas of social life. Arundhati Roy aptly described the pandemic as "a portal, a transition between this and the world to come".[2] Scientists have for a long time explicitly warned about the risks of dangerous zoonoses, which are pathogens that can pass between species, for example "jumping" from a non-human animal to the human. Societies were obviously not prepared; although we know from the origins of HIV, Ebola, and Salmonella about such spill overs we should have raised our awareness about the significance of human-animal relations and livelihoods in the context of accelerating dangerous environmental-and-climatic-change. Continuous logging of tropical rain forests and human population growth constantly reduce the habitats of wild animals, forcing them to move closer to humans, thereby increasing the risk for further zoonotic diseases and pandemics.[3] Viewed from this perspective it is clear that it is the human species itself that is responsible for causing the pandemic. Accordingly, the solution and further precautionary measures are an explicitly human undertaking. As infection expert Björn Olsen stated: "We are now entering the pandemic century".[4] Without doubt we will remember the years of 2020–21 as a "rupture" and a time of "transition of life world".[5] They will not simply be remembered as "a crisis that fades past" but as an "era".[6]

Striding through this pandemic portal, and into this new era, therefore requires us to reconsider how global and individual health are interconnected in the context of the changing natural climate. Drawing from Goethe's wisdom about how intimately tied a human's understanding of their self is to their knowledge of

DOI: 10.4324/9781003289364-2

the world around them, where he wrote that the human being can only by and through her knowledge of the world become aware of herself,[7] we can use the SARS-CoV-2 pandemic as an opportunity to learn how we can become aware of ourselves through the anthropogenic and pandemic changes in the Anthropocene.[8] Contagious diseases can, as Mika Aaltola aptly states, be regarded as complex open-ended phenomena and cannot be reduced to biology; they are "politosomatic".[9] Our book reflects this perspective by approaching the pandemic emergency in a variety of academic fields. Though the following reflections are specifically about Sweden's experience with SARS-CoV-2 pandemic management, it is valuable to consider the surrounding global and environmental context, as well as the Swedish experience's place within the worldwide challenge to cooperate "as one humanity"[10] across all kinds of borders, and with the renewed focus towards "One world – one health".[11] Can the pandemic experiences teach us how to deepen our skills of local and trans-local solidarity and synergy?[12] Following Ivan Krastev, a pandemic rarely transforms the society, but it offers us the potential to open "our eyes to the world we have been living in".[13] This book intends to contribute through opening our eyes to the Swedish context and discussing ways to understand it. The authors hope to provide, while nations in the post-Covid world are turning against globalization, some valuable perspectives on the new cosmopolitanism that Covid has "infected the world with"[14] in this pandemic century.

Although the SARS-CoV-2 pandemic health crisis was caused by one *single* virus – in the context of anthropogenic environmental degradation – and although the life sciences through an impressing international research process have investigated and analyzed the infection in one common understanding, the nations' responses have taken highly differentiated courses. Within the wide range of differing pandemic management styles (between strong and soft measures, general lockdowns/particular lockdowns/no-lockdowns, attempts to eradicate the virus, or simply mitigate and allegedly control its spread), Sweden's pandemic management strategy has differed significantly from other nations' responses, and it has provoked an intense and wide-reaching interest from scientists and international media. This book's overarching intention therefore is to contribute to the global discourse on what Ivan Krastev calls "paradoxes of the pandemic" with reflections on what one could learn from the failures in Sweden's pandemic management. How did Sweden respond to the pandemic as *Totalereignis*?[15] This book will not provide a full explanation of Sweden's choice of pandemic management strategy and the history of it, but it will explore a range of central themes that appear to be contained within it. The themes in this book, which were selected by the authors due to their relevance, are explored in order to gain a deeper understanding of Sweden's path for pandemic management, which has been interpreted by many people as a "disaster".[16] The authors, whose disciplines vary from life sciences and humanities to social sciences, use transdisciplinary perspectives and a variety of tools from their respective disciplines in order to help us learn from the Swedish path for managing SARS-CoV-2.

With regard to these introductory remarks we would like to make clear from the beginning that our intention with such a sharp critical discussion of the Swedish experience that follows is not to question the national structure and achievements of the Swedish society and state in general (even if the pandemic revealed several systemic shortcomings). Rather, this book aims to provide a critical, sometimes necessarily harsh analysis through a constructive perspective. It is our hope that this book will encourage others to contribute by fostering a learning environment with the aim of achieving the best common future for us all. Following Kant's "categorical imperative"[17] can be useful for us. Consider the following: criticism as reason's self-criticism should never become its own end in itself but serve as a constructive tool for the self-adjustment of knowledge. Used within our context this means: it is important to self-critically explore the lessons taught for this and other countries' constructive handling for the next forthcoming pandemic.

Sweden's attracted attention as "the world's cautionary tale"

With regard to the Swedish Public Health Agency's (Folkhälsomyndigheten/FHM) passive line, which attempted to avoid any strict measures and focused mainly encouraging individual responsibility by recommendations, German media coined the term *Sonderweg* to describe Sweden's specific path.[18] In July 2020 the *New York Times* reported that the Swedish Agency had begun a pandemiological "open air experiment" without including the people in this decision; in this article, Sweden was pictured as "the world's cautionary tale".[19] *Science Magazine* highlighted Sweden's refusal of facemasks, how its approach to the coronavirus pandemic was "out of step with much of the world", and how critics of the country's lax pandemic policies faced "fierce backlash".[20] *The Lancet* published several articles discussing the "futile and cynical" presuppositions of the Swedish ideology,[21] the Swedish "enigma", and the failure of the Covid-19 strategy.[22] German national television channel ZDF had a widespread, long broadcast where popular moderator Markus Lanz concluded that the Swedish pandemic management choices signalled "the end of Sweden as a global moral superpower".[23] Gina Gustavsson compared in a column the Swedish Corona strategy with the fiasco that occurred when the proud but misconstrued warship *Vasa* sunk in its central harbour in Stockholm during the middle of the Swedish empire in 1628.[24] A political cartoon played with the nautical metaphor with the undeterred PM presiding on the *M/S Strategia Suedecia* as it runs into ruin, while chief epidemiologist Anders Tegnell is searching for herd immunity and the scientists jump ship.

Only a few examples of the numerous sources that monitored and explored Sweden's strategy can be mentioned here, but both defenders and supporters of the strategy were able to speak their opinions. Former Swedish State epidemiologist, Anders Tegnell, has been celebrated in other countries as "the icon of freedom".[25] As the waves of SARS-CoV-2 swept through Sweden, leaving death tolls immensely higher than in the other Nordic countries, voices of those critical of the

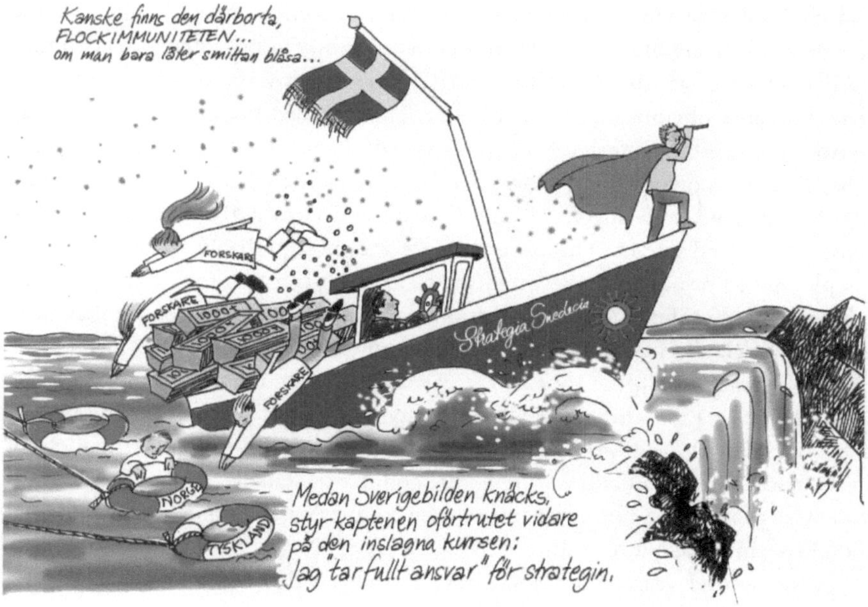

FIGURE 1.1 Ingela Bergmann, *M/S Strategia Suedecia*, Picture-Letter to the Editor, *Dagens Nyheter*

Source: Ingela Bergmann, 21 January 2021, ["Maybe it exists over there: HERD IMMUNITY, and one can let the infection blow . . ."/"While the image of Sweden is broken the captain unwaveringly stays the fixed course: 'I take the full responsibility' for the strategy."], by courtesy of the artist.

Swedish Strategy began to appear more often, and supporters of the Swedish strategy, nationally as well as internationally, began to quiet. Nevertheless the debate in the summer and autumn of 2021 provided intense attempts of historical revisionism and imperatives about learning to "live with the virus".[26] Minister of Social Affairs Lena Hallengren concluded, "we have survived the crisis pretty well",[27] a mind-boggling statement after there at that time had been more than 15,000 deaths from Covid and still in September 2021 Sweden had higher death tolls than its neighbouring countries. Who are "we" here, and who has survived what?

After the first nine months of dominant conformism around the Public Health Agency's concept of reality, aptly described as "bunker mentality" by Göran K. Hanson, The Royal Swedish Academy of Sciences' secretary, and distinguished economist Lars Calmfors,[28] level of trust in the Agency and Government's strategy decreased from more than 80% to roughly 50% at the end of 2020. Ethnographers have characterized the strong support as "public health nationalism" which was fuelled by the daily press conferences from the FHM. In August–October 2021 support fell even further to 35%.[29] The obvious repeat of the same lax measures as in the spring caused Sweden to see a repeat of deaths and suffering in autumn 2020 – meaningless and "undignified deaths".[30] The lack of honouring the dead and commemorating their suffering was obvious among the responsible Government leaders and civil servants, which was embarrassing and uncompassionate.[31] The Swedish media, unlike many media outlets in other countries, did not attempt to continuously commemorate the deaths from SARS-CoV-2.[32] It was around autumn 2020 that it became obvious that there were people who had not got better relatively shortly after getting infected with SARS-CoV-2, but rather were dealing with what is now known as long-Covid. Today it is estimated that there are around 200 000 patients suffering from long-Covid[33] and circa 300 000 who lost their sense of taste and smell.[34] This pandemic can and most probably will disable many people due to possible long term effects of Covid, similar to the "history lesson" from influenza, polio, and other infection waves. One must wonder if policymakers, in Sweden and in other countries, will ignore or learn from this.[35]

In November 2020 the tone of the Swedish media columnists appeared to be changing, after a long period of alleged safety in a mix of suppression and exceptionalism. King Carl XVI Gustaf summarized the Swedish situation concisely in his Christmas broadcast and declared, "the country has failed".[36] His statement was widely acknowledged but unfortunately the country's responsible decision-makers did not seem to take it to heart.

In the second year of this pandemic, a circle of debaters and scientists who were signatories and supporters of the *Great Barrington Declaration* (GBD) began to appear in Swedish media. The signatories of the GBD,[37] demanded that society should let the SARS-CoV-2 virus spread throughout the population and focus only on protecting the weaker groups of society, especially the elderly and immunocompromised (which has proven to be impossible). Martin Kulldorf, a Swedish-born bio-statistician and GBD initiator, had a prominent role among the GBD supporters in Sweden.[38] In 2021 Kulldorf retired from Harvard University. Much of the GBD movement is financed by the well-known Koch brothers, who economically support the US movement of climate sceptics and deny on-going climate change.[39] Influential paediatrician Jonas Ludvigsson, professor of epidemiology at the Karolinska Institute, signed and propagated the statements from the GBD and appears to have influenced Swedish decision-makers to disregard the threat to children and to keep schools open.[40] Ludvigsson was also accused of scholarly misconduct after completing his article for NEJM with correct data, first after being contacted by a *Science Magazine* journalist who questioned why he had not mentioned the data given to support his argument.[41]

There were a few other alleged experts who participated eagerly in the public debate. Agnes Wold, Professor of Clinical Bacteriology, was featured regularly in the mainstream Swedish media outlets. She spread non-committal advice, disinformation as well as dangerous messages, such as that smoking reduces the risk of Covid and that immigrants played a central role in the spread of the virus.[42] Emma Frans, doctor of epidemiology, had a contract with the Swedish Public Broadcasting network, SVT, where she presented mostly cherry-picked, not necessarily relevant information that was always in line with the FHM's messages. Her book "All Are Washing Hands"[43] was an attempt to enter the public scene of prominent debaters but it did not offer any proof of self-critical reflection on her own role in the Swedish media's fatal patriotism where, in her own words, "Tegnell's voluminous phallus should verify his objectivity".[44] With regard to the author's ambition to contribute to history, her writing offers a revisionist story rather than a balanced history. Mathematician Tom Britton produced several calculations for the FHM in order to support the belief in quickly achieving herd immunity. All of them failed substantially. Britton nevertheless tried again and again, and he almost could admit that he went wrong.[45] In stark contrast to the European values and human rights, in which the life of every human is equal, Swedish paediatrician Johnny Ludvigsson along with philosopher Torbjörn Tännsjö contributed to the debate with dubious biopolitical thoughts, including suggesting ranking the lives of children higher than the elderly.[46] Their points attempted to defend the nation's loss of many elderly lives to Covid-19. Ordinary people aptly understood their reasoning as meaning: *so what – they would have died anyway*. Did Sweden practice ageism? A columnist reminded of a popular older song written by Beppe Wolgers for a revue in 1968, titled: "Bundle them and kill them" (*Bunta ihop dom och slå ihjäl dem*), a saying that became common after that.[47]

Most decision-makers in the world, though, seemed to follow the suggestions from the *John Snow Memorandum*,[48] striving for the best possible minimizing of the infection spread, in a spectrum between those who demand a zero-Covid strategy for elimination and others arguing for a no-Covid strategy for least possible infection within the virus's endemicity with some diffuse hope to control it. In autumn 2021 Sweden was still following their original strategy, although in a modified form; that is, they did not attempt to minimize the spread of SARS-CoV-2 as much as possible. In addition, the Swedish officials in charge of the strategy continued to deny aerosol spread, effectiveness of facemasks, asymptomatic transmission, and denied children's role in the spread of the contagion.[49] The Government's decision-making capabilities were minimized, and the FHM was given the ability to make decisions, without having to engage with the outside scientific community. Unilateral delivery of crisis information to the public continued, and the Government and Agency refused to admit any fault in their strategy, because they were "always implementing the right measures at the right time" (as Minister Hallengren has phrased it).[50] If one goes by Government statements, it actually is a bit unclear if Sweden ever had a real "strategy", as Minister Hallengren, when being questioned by the constitutional committee, denied that there was a strategy by stating that the Swedish strategy was to not have a strategy and instead to implement the right measures at the right time. In other words, the Swedish strategy was to do everything correctly. However, it should be noted that PM Stefan Löfven had in April 2020 already pointed there being a clear strategy which was explained in six points on the Government's website.[51]

To summarize: It was not easy to be a critical thinker living in Sweden during the SARS-CoV-2 pandemic. The Swedish Public Health Agency and the Government made it clear that they were not to be questioned, and that they were not open to listening to outside opinions. This attitude from the decision-makers left those who were critical thinkers, who wanted only to help achieve the best possible outcome through proper pandemic management, with only two options; either they could quiet themselves and blindly trust the state, leaving their fate to the gods or they could search for reliable information, often internationally, in order to design their own personal strategy. With these options in mind, many immigrants chose to follow the policies of their home country; others chose to leave Sweden in despair. Those born in traditionally more religious countries have been especially concerned and complained over the lack of compassion and solidarity in the Swedish choice of pandemic management strategy. This has led to the image of Sweden that other countries had held, being damaged for what might be a long time.[52] We hope that the reflections and discussions in this book, can, to some extent, help pave the way for a national process of healing and reconciliation.

The state of knowledge

The majority of Sweden's pandemic history has been documented in the media, both nationally and internationally. Professional writers, science journalists, and columnists have raised critical questions about Sweden's pandemic response which diverged from those that most of the world's nations followed. Several poignant documentary films have been produced and broadcasted in Australia, Germany, and other countries.[53] Scientists were initially careful not to judge Sweden's choice of pandemic management, but eventually, international scientific journals such as *The Lancet* and *Science* published critical analyses. There have been some excellent studies conducted investigating the Swedish pandemic response. One study conducted by an interdisciplinary group from Munich University used reliable mathematic tools and empirical data to investigate what would have happened if Sweden would have executed a lockdown as part of their pandemic management strategy, like many other countries.[54] The study concluded that a lockdown in Sweden could have saved 38% of the lives that were lost, and could have prevented 75% of serious infections from SARS-CoV-2. Other studies came to similar conclusions. Others made the conclusion that one, by comparing Norway and Sweden (two countries very similar to each other on most parameters), could have saved circa 92% of lost lives in the first wave.[55] Applying the same logic to the first four waves of the virus, one can estimate that circa 10,000–12,000 lives, of the more than 18,500 that have been lost as of 13 April 2022, could have been saved, if Sweden simply had taken the same actions as in Norway. Sweden's original strategy and parts of the later modified strategy have endangered the lives of Swedish citizens and residents, and jeopardized their health.[56] Professor of medicine Ola Stenqvist was able to elegantly describe the ethical problem that arises from the Swedish strategy with the following question: "In what decent country would a Government and Agency be allowed to appraise more than 10,000 human lives less valuable than the rest of the population's rights of freedom?"[57] This is even more unbelievable for a population that for decades have been used to maximum of trust and safety, protected by the state's authorities. Nevertheless former General Director (GD) for the FHM, Johan Carlson, denied the facts in November 2021, by stating in the media "no countries can know which measures are most efficient".[58] The cost of the "freedom" that the Swedish pandemic management strategy offered came in the number of residents and citizens who became sick or died. It would appear that the Swedish decision-makers weighed individual freedom against the suffering and potential death of those infected, which is an ethical choice that can only be defended using a rough utilitarian perspective.[59]

The rationale behind this national strategy, which appeared to be focused on achieving herd immunity in the quickest way possible, is the reason why we have chosen to describe the pandemic response as Sweden's pandemic *experiment*. This focus on herd immunity could be seen from the actions of the FHM in the early days of the pandemic; one such example could be the subsidizing of antibody tests by the public health system. The Swedish, mostly abdicated, Government had, by placing their trust solely in the hands of the FHM, given the Agency a type of absolute power. The Agency was tasked with informing residents and citizens through what started as daily press conferences. The Agency often used these conferences to present a mix of cherry-picked facts, speculations and quasi-science, but what was never presented to the public was their reasons behind their choice of strategy. One of the first internationally published critical articles was in the *New York Times*, where the writer described the Swedish strategy in terms of a biopolitical experiment where the decision-makers had chosen to expose the innocent citizens to a deadly and at the time unknown virus. When it was clear that the experiment had obviously failed and needlessly ended the lives of many people, the decision-makers, in particular the FHM, denied the causal connection of the strategy with its result and continued to practice the early cemented dogma. In science, the word experiment refers to the establishment of a procedure that is carried out in order to test a specific hypothesis. The FHM troika (including former chief epidemiologist Johan Giesecke; the then current chief epidemiologist Anders Tegnell; and the GD of the Agency Johan Carlson) appeared to have a belief that if one lets the virus spread it would be possible to achieve natural herd immunity. Their hypothesis seemed to be that it was possible for the population to achieve herd immunity by allowing the virus to spread in a "controlled" manner through the population. Giesecke was convinced from the beginning that the virus that was impossible to stop would infect almost everyone.[60] The trio held what could almost be described as an autocratic level of power and was not controlled by anyone. It is hard to fully understand how much influence this close-knit group had on the strategy, but it is clear that they were not very open to listening to those outside of their group. According to their vision, Sweden had the best, most efficient strategy for fighting off the SARS-CoV-2 virus. All critical questions from scientists and journalists concerning what appeared to be the goal of the Swedish strategy, achieving natural herd immunity, were constantly rebuffed. Ethicists, as well as the WHO, condemned such a goal as unethical, and probably it would qualify as a violation of human rights.

Nevertheless, investigative journalism and insider uncovering initiated from infection doctor Peet Tüll verified the suspicion.[61] Despite this, during the constitutional committee interrogation in April 2021 then PM Stefan Löfven continued to deny that the aim of the strategy was natural herd immunity.[62] It seems that he, unfortunately, did not fully understand the meaning of the term, as he consistently used it incorrectly in his answers (*folkimmunitet*/people's immunity instead of *flockimmunitet*/herd immunity).[63] What appeared to be an experiment to achieve natural herd immunity had failed on many crucial points. In scientific terms one could say that the experiment had shown the original hypothesis to be invalid. In Swedish virus politics, however, the decision-makers interpreted the empirical negative results of the experiment as verifying their hypothesis. Freelance journalist Johan Anderberg in November 2021 wrote an article where he praised at length the "noble experiment" where freedom had been saved, without mentioning with a word the avoidable thousands of lives lost and hundred thousands of long-term Covid sick.[64] Despite having found proof that there had been a natural herd immunity strategy, he still insisted that Sweden had chosen the correct pandemic management strategy.

What kind of an experiment is Sweden's pandemic response about? Who is captured in "the grammar of the crisis" and in what way? And – continuing along Michel Foucault's biopolitical thinking, applied by Lapo Lappin in his chapter – who is captured in the grammar of one's own construction of what the crisis is about? Conducting an experiment with a whole population requires a hypothesis, which can be verified or invalidated. However, beforehand this mechanism needs to be known, for example the new corona virus's mode of replicating. Answers to such a hypothesis can only be found through a process of international cooperation. The refusal of Sweden's public health experts to partake in the process of international scholarly knowledge production seemed to be a central characteristic of the Swedish strategy. This limited the knowledge that was available to inform the political decision-makers. The unwillingness to admit any failure reveals, in our opinion, one of the central reasons for their refusal to participate in international collaboration. What others can learn from this kind of experiment will be explored in the chapters of this book. Maybe it is possible that Sweden can still contribute with substantial insights to the global process of learning and to achieve one common "political grammar of the crisis"?[65]

More coherent studies of what happened in this experiment are still scarce. Among the first and most well-written studies we find US-Swedish historian Peter Baldwin's analysis of the responses to the first wave in 2020. Baldwin has meritoriously analyzed different countries and their pandemic management strategies, and he highlighted a "fatal contradiction" between two approaches in Sweden of aiming at natural herd immunity (before a vaccine was available) while at the same time reducing the spread so "that they never knew and decided what they were doing simultaneously".[66]

Andrew Ewing, American-Swedish scientist and member of The Royal Swedish Academy of Sciences, and writer Kelly Bjorklund published an extensive article in *Time Magazine* where relevant data, observations, and reflections are interwoven in an analytical way that supersedes the fragmented discussions that were being published in many well-respected scientific journals at the time. Their widespread *Time Magazine* article concluded that "the Swedish COVID-19 response is a disaster", a conclusion that is underpinned by a multiplicity of empirical data and logical reasoning. The article also included a clear imperative to other countries "to take care before adopting the 'Swedish way'" in order to avoid "tragic consequences for this pandemic or the next".[67]

Sweden is also included in the publications from the international research project *Evaluation of Science Advice in a Pandemic Emergency* (*ESCAPE*).[68] The project performs a comparative, international evaluation of the mechanisms of scientific advice during the pandemic emergency in 17 different countries. The Swedish part of the project, conducted by Nele Brusselaers, who is one of the authors of this book, offers a timeline and an analysis of the decision-making process, specifically regarding the interaction of science and politics. The project authors, including the editor of this book Sigurd Bergmann and several other authors featured in this book, state that Sweden, in fact, was very well equipped to prevent the pandemic of Covid-19 from causing serious damage to the health of its population, especially due to its long history of more than 280 years of collaboration between political bodies, public health and governmental authorities, and the scientific community that had yielded many successes in preventive medicine.[69] The country offers an impressively high level of trust in authorities and those in power, which was tested in 2020, when the death rates from Covid-19 climbed to ten times higher than those of Sweden's neighbouring country Norway.

The National Corona Commission, set in place by the Swedish Government in June of 2020, has issued several reports discussing the Swedish pandemic response. The Commission's final report underlines that the Swedish Government's abdication and reluctance to take action, and the decision to hand over the operative and decisive power to the FHM experts was one of the reasons that Sweden's strategy has had such tragic results. The leadership team of the FHM executed their power unilaterally, without working to collaborate with other relevant experts.[70] It was even verified by comparing Sweden, Germany, and the UK with regard to the interactions between national health governance, science, and the media how Sweden avoided plurality and excluded academia.[71]

Several books have been published in Swedish, and more are probably in production. In his book *Flocken* (*The Herd*) (Stockholm 2021) journalist Johan Anderberg offers a nationalist leaning defence of the FHM's decisions during the beginning of the pandemic, including several eye-opening interviews with the trio behind the strategy. Historian Henrik Charpentier Ljungqvist's book (*Corona: Ett historiskt perspektiv på vår tids pandemi*, Stockholm 2020), which discusses mortality rates, offers an uncertain source, with fragmented perspectives around the author's argument that Sweden's death tolls from the pandemic are nothing to be concerned with long term. Brusselaers and Edvinsson discuss in their chapters what counts as reliable or manipulative interpretation of statistic data. In contrast, Gina Gustavsson offers a solid exploration of the cultural dimension of Sweden's pandemic average.[72] Her book offers a unique and enlightening reflection on the

Swedish pandemic response. As political scientist and columnist, she dives deeper into the question of why there appears to be an asymmetric dissonance between Swedes' self-identity, including the way that they see their country, and the values and behaviours apparent during the current pandemic. Gustavsson opens our eyes to a hidden cultural dynamic and uncovers some of the central driving forces in the Swedish cultural soul. Understanding a pandemic demands an advanced transdisciplinary work where cultural, political, historical, and ethical analysis must go hand in hand with the perspectives of life sciences, social sciences, and law science. Gustavsson's book, and to some degree Per Wirtén's and Bengt Lindroth's books on Sweden's exceptionalism in the context of European and Nordic politics,[73] enrich our understanding of the Swedish pandemic experiment with substantial knowledge concerning the roots and practices of Swedish exceptionalism and its role in the handling of this pandemic emergency.

Gustavsson's thesis that patriotism explains the Swedish people's support for the deadly strategy is also empirically verified. While a study at the Pew Research Center from 2020 had stated that Swedes are less critical in Europe to their national response (where only 8% regarded it as "bad" and 25% as "somewhat bad"),[74] Gustavsson and Larsson Taghizadeh's study from February 2021[75] showed that inhabitants with a foreign background were more critical to the nation's pandemic response in general and more negative to the statement that lockdowns are dangerous. The study verifies a strong connection between patriotic proudness towards Swedish institutions and support for the Swedish strategy and the anti-lockdown narrative. Thereby it becomes clear that a strong desire for freedom and a liberal society may not be the key issue for Swedes. Rather it is patriotism – in the sense of institutional national pride, uncritical loyalty, and national chauvinism – that represents the deeper driving force for most of the citizens' massive support for what in fact threatened and took the lives of many.

Writer, filmmaker, and former virologist Lena Einhorn's work offers intriguing insights into Sweden's pandemic regime.[76] Her "journey in pandemic Sweden" titled *Between Hobby Epidemiologists and Expert Authorities* reveals the deeply personal struggle and amazement she felt while resisting the questionable exercise of power in the national pandemic emergency. Through records of written and oral statements Einhorn's book unveils the absolute power, and to some extent the emotional vulnerability in the leadership of civil servants who enchained themselves to a whole bunch of misjudgements that they had to defend autocratically against all critical reason. Memorably, the author quotes former PM Göran Persson's striking conclusion that "Tegnell [alone] has the political initiative in Sweden today". Einhorn's book traces, in diary form, the dysfunction of public media and politics and unfolds the driving forces behind the formation of the group of critical scholarly voices questioning the dubious pandemic management.

Journalist Amina Manzoor, whose articles indicate a loyalty to the Swedish strategy, covered the pandemic as medical reporter, despite not having a degree in any natural science topic, at the leading morning paper *Dagens Nyheter*, which she left after accusing the chief editor of having interfered with her ability to publish certain stories because of his critical attitude to the strategy. In her book she attempts to draw a line from the Spanish flu to the on-going pandemic, offering wide-ranging historical observations, thoughts about how scientists responded and how science was challenging for journalists, as well as a defence for her own position in so-called "polarised debates", such as the strive for natural herd immunity.[77]

Carl Johan Sonesson offers interesting information from his own experience as a political leader in one of Sweden's larger regions, *Skåne*. His book shares stories about uncertainty, irresponsibility, slowness, and confusion in decision-making between national and regional authorities. He shares how he had to struggle with the regional infection doctor's unwavering trust in Tegnell's decisions and rhetoric, and how she hindered and delayed the region's recommendation for its residents to use facemasks on public transport.[78]

One of the most significant scholarly contributions that was recently announced is the coming book *The Swedish Experiment* by French political scientist Yohann Aucante.[79] The author explores Sweden's unique response to the global pandemic (in 2020 and 2021) and studies also the strong wave of controversies that it has triggered. His book analyzes the "Swedish model" incorporating the country's value system, as well as its politics and administration in relation to the ideas of welfare, democracy, civil liberties, and respect for expertise. The author explains what others perceived as Swedish deviation, and emphasizes the justifications given by decision-makers. In his analysis of the controversies, Aucante emphasizes especially the impact on topical representations of a Swedish model (torn apart from the rest of the Nordic region), and the interplay with key themes of welfare/health reforms (elderly care, health care liberalization, unemployment insurance, among others). Moreover Aucante reflects on the comparative, and also implicitly normative, evaluations of national responses, while humbly avoiding personal judgement. His book offers "a thorough, insightful and topical reflection on a fascinating instance of policy exceptionalism" (Nicholas Aylott). Aucante discusses some of the themes that this book explores, and our hope is that both books can be seen as enriching and inspire further discussions about the Swedish way of pandemic management.

The *Science Forum Covid-19*, whose formation was discussed in Einhorn's book,[80] has throughout the majority of this pandemic educated the public through numerous YouTube programs and articles. The group developed a forum for scholarly exchange between scientists, and contributed to the public debate with critical articles. With 40 leading scholars, and nearly 800 supporting members, the Forum has communicated with an audience of many thousands of citizens, and in some of the most demanding periods even half a million of people. A rich archive of the Forum's widespread contributions is available online.[81]

Magnus Jerneck published a special issue of *The Swedish Journal of Political Science* with 34 scholars which critically investigated Sweden's pandemic management choices.[82] *Historisk Tidskrift* (the *Historical Journal*) published a debate between Rodney Edvinsson and Fredrik Charpentier Ljungqvist on how to interpret the statistical monitoring of mortality and deaths. Writer Lisa Bjurwald published an extensive report at *The Swedish Enterprise Media Monitor*, which included nine interviews about the media's role in the pandemic and thought-provokingly explored the media regarding their function either as "investigators of power or megaphones of power".[83] *The Journal of Law* early on published an article about the need to revise the country's constitutional law in order to be able to handle a pandemic.[84]

The Lancet has published several articles about Sweden and the pandemic that are rich in substance by authors. Carina King and a large group of scholars investigated Johan Giesecke's analysis in the early phase of the pandemic.[85] As a mentor for Carlson and Tegnell and paid advisor at the FHM we can regard him as one of the main architects of the Swedish strategy. King et al. point to the cynicism of the view "that slowing down the progression of COVID-19 is futile, as it implies that painfully acquired knowledge and efforts to develop or repurpose drugs and treatments will amount to nothing". In his response, Giesecke did not appear to actually respond to the critique, but rather insists that it is "doubtful if a strategy of removing lockdowns (whether regional or local) and re-implementing them will be accepted by citizens in the long run".[86] Was this the reason why Carlson and Tegnell never had trust in their own population with regard to tough restrictions?[87] Why was high trust from the general population answered in the opposite direction with low trust from the Agency? Why did they follow Giesecke's words that "our most important task is not to stop spread"?[88]

In December 2020, Mariam Claeson and Stefan Hanson published an analysis of what they described as the Swedish "enigma". They wrote a detailed description of the situation during the second wave when their observations showed that "too many people are dying unnecessarily in a country without timely concerted actions to interrupt the high transmission and reduce the burden of deaths". Their analysis points at the "decentralised and fragmented system of health and social services", as well as "failures in the governance and legal frameworks for health and social services" and accuses the Government of not engaging with "key stakeholders, including informed scientists, civil society, and behaviour change experts".[89] In a second article[90] they describe how Sweden, even after the third wave, chose to swim against the tide, continuing "on the same trajectory in the face of current trends, without timely action by agency and government leadership". They saw this as a method that "raises concerns about governance and accountability, and ultimately about fundamental ethics and values".

The national Corona Commission was established in June 2020 and published its first report in December the same year.[91] Only after strong pressure from the opposition and the Parliament, PM Löfven, who resigned from his position in November 2021, agreed to let the Commission present its final results (February 2022) before the next election in September 2022.[92] He tried to escape from his responsibility by suggesting it to present its findings first after the election. The Commission's first report, published in December 2020, investigated the pandemic with a focus on how it affected the country's elderly care. It stated clearly that it was the high level of contagion that was the central reason for the suffering and death of so many older citizens. In other words, the national Government and the FHM had erroneously blamed the municipalities as being responsible for the debacle in elderly care that could have been prevented. It is, therefore, clear that they must also be held accountable for this avoidable loss of lives. The Commission's first report also named the lack of protective equipment in the beginning of spring 2020 as playing a role in the debacle. It was also discovered that many doctors, who had in many cases never even examined their patients, still chose to prescribe palliative care including morphine instead of proper treatment for those with the virus (e.g. oxygen and hydration). This could potentially be seen as a kind of nationally structured euthanasia among the elderly.

The commission wrote: "We find it most likely that the single most important factor behind the major outbreaks and the high number of deaths in residential care is the overall spread of the virus in the society".[93] This again was a consequence of the FHM trio's belief in natural herd immunity. Influential German magazine *Der Spiegel* asked in an article, "Has Sweden sacrificed the elderly?" and they educated their readership about the meaning of the Swedish term *ättestupan*, that is, the edge where clans in premodern times pushed down the weak elderly to death in a ritualized form.[94]

On the 29th of October 2021 the Commission presented its second report.[95] The Commission sharply criticized the "slowness of response", which led to the inefficient limiting of the spread of the virus in the country. They also criticized the "inadequate" "pandemic preparedness" and legislation, as well as the unclear divisions of the country's different actors regarding who should bear responsibility for the different parts. The report discusses the large volume of cancelled and postponed care appointments due to the health system's overload, the "problematic lack of data", caused by the FHM's lack of testing and lack of statistical monitoring of the virus. The Commission questions the Government's decision to grant only one single authority a "leading role" for handling this pandemic. The commission noted that the Government could also have been more efficient and effective in their use of the infection law. The criticism also revealed that the Government's previous statement from May 2020 that "our preparedness is good"[96] was a lie. The commission concluded that in fact, Sweden was unprepared, and that health workers had been "left high and dry" due to the Work Environment Authority's (Arbetsmiljöverket) refusal to demand protective equipment in good time.

When many wish to forget about the pandemic, the health care workers, according to scholar Rebecca Selberg, will never be able to forget the overwhelming demands that appeared because of the pandemic. Having to care for a growing number of seriously ill and anxious patients caused health care workers to become exhausted and frustrated, as the public continued engaging in risk-filled behaviour which resulted in the continued spread of the virus.[97] Commission President, former Chief Parliamentary Ombudsman, Chief Justice and Chair of the Supreme Administration Court of Sweden (*Högsta Förvaltningsdomstolen*) Mats Melin described the pandemic management, during the press conference about the report, as "average".[98] This report did not discuss who should be held responsible. Critics have also responded that the renowned slowness on the one hand was in contradiction with the rapidity of applying the unethical method of natural herd immunization. Minister Hallengren rejected, much later (April 2022), in general the criticism of slowness, by stating "the Government has not been slow". "Not making decisions is not the same as being slow. This can also be about that one do not want to make a decision", she publicly declared.[99] Now it is evident that the Government obviously very deliberately had decided not to decide.

Also PM Löfven refused to accept the term "average".[100] Minister of Social Affairs Lena Hallengren has openly disagreed with the Commission's criticism and refused to take any responsibility.[101] Her party rewarded her directly by electing her onto its central board.[102] The Social Democratic Party postulates to learn from the pandemic (by not admitting any failure) and by "building the country safely" and developing the very best welfare state.[103] Former FHM General Director Johan Carlson stated – against science's better judgement – "no other countries know which measures are the most effective".[104] When columnists and commentators all around the globe shared the news about the shipwreck, they reported the "scathing criticism",[105] the "sharp judgement", and even "slaughter" of those responsible for the country's fatal pandemic management, contained in the report.[106]

The publication of the Commission's second report in October 2021, the 20th month of the pandemic, helped to bring the perceived public health nationalism and patriotic pride surrounding the Swedish pandemic strategy to an end. Only one of the leading newspapers in Malmö, Sweden's third largest city, continued its aggressive defence by not covering the Commission's criticism. Even the public television and radio stations, Sveriges Television (SVT) and Sveriges Radio (SR), which appeared to serve as megaphones of the Government and governmental agencies during the pandemic, seemed to become more careful in their reporting after this report. Only *Sydsvenska Dagbladet* in Malmö dared, during the slowly increasing fourth wave, to repeat the Government's mantra that "we have come pretty well out of this [pandemic]".[107] The entrance of the Omicron variant changed the situation and from December 2021 onwards the spread of the contagion in Sweden seemed to follow the same rapid increase seen in Denmark and Norway. In January 2022 the health care system reached its limits, as the size and speed of the spread of the virus exceeded all earlier waves. As the country heads into a second pandemic winter, the *BMJ* writer who monitored the first phase of the fourth wave is clear: "Sweden's situation remains precarious".[108]

On the 25th of February 2022 the Commission published its third and final report.[109] Despite its general support for recommendations given by the FHM, which were to be followed by the citizens voluntarily, the Commission expressed sharp criticism towards several aspects of the strategy. Interestingly, the report reveals an informative contrast between the "correct" economic crisis management with swift actions to save the Swedish economy on the one hand and on the other hand serious failures, delays, and nonactions regarding disease prevention and control. This contrast in response rate raises the question why economic interests in Sweden appear to have been given priority instead of acute matters such as the protection of life and health of residents and citizens. Regarding the prevention of disease, the report states that "the measures taken were too few and should have come sooner", and that "the Government should have assumed leadership of all aspects of crisis management from the outset". The Commission also believes that the Government should have taken a "clearer leadership of overall communication with the public" and that the FHM "should have communicated its advice and recommendations as clear rules of conduct". An important argument is presented in the report regarding the "precautionary principle" and its perceived absence of evidence in the FHM's belief in the FHM's belief in evidence; the Commission suggests that the precautionary principle should be seen as a compliment to the standard principles of crisis management.

The report strongly emphasizes, "the Government had too one-sided a dependence on assessments made by the Public Health Agency of Sweden". This one-sided dependence leads to the responsibility for those assessments resting on "a single individual, its Director-General", which the Commission found to be an unsatisfactory "arrangement for decision-making during a serious" societal crisis. The Commission ultimately found the concentration of responsibility to be "inappropriate, given the difficult balances that need to be struck between a wide range of societal outcomes".

The Commission also commented on the FHM's decision to ignore the opinions of other relevant actors when it stated that it "is of the [Commission's] opinion that the Agency should have secured input from an even wider range of specialists, including critical ones". Further, the Commission believed that the FHM "should not have dismissed the use of masks as a disease prevention and control measure". The responsibility for its "defensive view of the prospects of slowing the spread of the virus" resulting in "limited, late and not very vigorous measures, which failed to sharply reduce the transmission of the disease". These decisions, the Commission concluded, rest "with the Agency's then Director-General".

Although his contract was renewed just a month before, Johan Carlson resigned from his position directly after the Commission's second report in 2021 and can therefore hardly be held accountable. Former PM Stefan Löfven resigned, due to different reasons, in the autumn of 2021. Moreover, the Commission places emphasis on several systemic shortcomings, mainly the lack of cooperation between public officials and agencies responsible at the national, regional, and local levels. The report documents the Government's resistance to provide the Commission with all relevant documents and information for its investigation, which columnist Petter Wennblad at the national newspaper *Svenska Dagbladet* covered in a series of articles in January 2022. The Commission's report concludes, "the Governmental Offices documentation of their crisis management efforts must be substantially improved". Furthermore it states that conditions for international cooperation should be strengthened, and that there needs to be an increase in "truly cross-disciplinary research into the effects of the pandemic". The Commission discussed how "the overriding aim" of crisis communication "cannot be to allay concern". The Commission noted that even expressing such an aim "can mistakenly be understood to imply that the authorities are not averse to withholding information which might cause people to worry. Such an attitude is virtually the opposite of the transparency and honesty that should inform communication".

In two chapters on economic and social aspects, and in six additional expert reports, the Commission discusses its methods and the evidence for its conclusions. Even though the report was presented just one day after Russia started the war against Ukraine, it provoked almost two days of constructive public debates, with many authors focused on the Government's abdication of decision-making to the FHM.[110] The authors of this book agree with the Commission's opinion that their report should not be seen as the end of evaluation of the Swedish handling of the pandemic and discussions about the lessons that can be learned from the Swedish approach.

Minister of Social Affairs Hallengren and current FHM General-Director Karin Tegmark Wisell have completely refuted most of the criticism from the Commission and denied any responsibility. Hallengren asserted that Sweden's management strategy was "correct", and that the Government had never handed the "conductor's baton" over to the FHM.[111] She also renounced the criticism over the Government's slowness in responding to the spreading of the virus, referring to the statistics of excess mortality as proof for Sweden's success.[112] This is an argument that is commonly used as a way to redirect attention from the thousands of avoidable deaths in the country which scientifically does not provide any proof for its conclusions, as verified by many scientists.[113] After the Corona Commission's final report, Tegmark Wisell insisted on "the right to be careful" and refused to accept any criticism directed against the Agency of having responded weakly and slowly. In her response, she twisted the precautionary principle by re-interpreting it as a duty to act carefully rather than acting proactively in order to protect life and health and insisted that Sweden could not be compared with Norway.[114] In general she defended the strategy which the Agency claims had "a holistic perspective".[115] The Agency's definition of holistic perspective does not however seem to have a focus on individual citizens' lives and health; instead their definition is focused on societal well-being.

The art of and willingness to "learn from failure", discussed explicitly in Chapter 6, seems to be totally absent among the most influential decision-makers in charge of Sweden's pandemic experiment.

The Royal Swedish Academy of Sciences (*Kungliga Vetenskapsakademien*) established its own group of experts in September 2020 to discuss the Covid-19 pandemic.[116] On 30 November 2021 the Academy's Expert Group on Covid-19 presented its detailed report with 11 various thematic chapters.[117] The report discussing their "research syntheses and recommendations for the future" also included some severe criticism of some aspects of the Swedish strategy. The group concluded that the state did not apply the necessary precautions to protect the people, the Government's response was too slow when it was clear that the spread had reached Sweden, and the recommendations to the public were unclear. They also concluded that it appeared as though this was treated like an ordinary influenza epidemic, which led to the country being underprepared in many ways, including suffering a lack of protective equipment. Elderly care was especially poorly prepared which resulted in no possibility to protect the elderly once the spread of the contagion entered Swedish society.

The group identified a large range of needs and offered proposals for improvement. One of the proposals presented is for Sweden to establish an "independent expert unit with a high level of scientific expertise in relevant areas", as well as an ethics committee with scientific expertise in order "to support politicians and public authorities in achieving the difficult ethical balance necessary during a pandemic". The group places much of the blame for the Swedish pandemic management strategy on the FHM while still emphasizing that the Government bears the ultimate responsibility for crisis management. When asked about the report on the morning news show, *Nyhetsmorgon*, Minister of Social Affairs Lena Hallengren refused to comment on it, stating, "I have not fully read the report. There are many reports, and many expert groups, and I believe that the report is that group's opinion", showing no willingness to listen to or learn from the report's lessons.[118]

In the neighbouring country of Denmark, The Danish Parliament published a long parliamentary commission's evaluation that also analyzed Sweden's political pandemic handling, where they focused on the misleading claims that the country's legal structures did not allow a deeper involvement of the Government in the pandemic management (i.e. the independence of Government agencies, an explanation often expressed by the PM which stands in opposition to both experts in law[119] and the conclusions of the Danish commission).[120] The Swedish legislation is, however, special as it does not provide any possibility for the Government to announce a state of emergency in peacetime,[121] despite definitively giving the Parliament considerable powers to act in emergencies.[122] A Norwegian Commission similarly included relevant reflections on Swedish pandemic management in which they condemn Sweden for its lack of strong restrictions which resulted in high death tolls.[123]

Further highly relevant investigations have been published by Swedish governmental agencies such as the report from the Health and Social Care Inspectorate (IVO), which explored how it was possible for so many elderly citizens in care homes and those receiving in-home care to be actively excluded from receiving Covid-19-related health care, as well as why some were ordained to receive palliative care instead of being sent to a hospital.[124] The Christian Ecumenical Council raised concerns about this scandal, which they aptly described as "structural euthanasia".[125] Despite these findings, IVO did not choose to hand over the many cases to the legal system for investigation and the Government refused to accept any accountability and instead insisted that it was the municipalities who were responsible, as it is the municipalities who are in charge of elderly care.

Thousands of lives are estimated to have been lost due to the acceptance of a comparatively high level of infection in society,[126] the unwillingness to quickly establish effective measures, and the inability to provide safety equipment as quickly as possible, combined with the denial of the preventive impacts of facemasks by public health officials.[127] In Sweden about 50% of elderly care is provided by for-profit companies. Politicians on the left were quick to blame these companies for this scandal, despite the largest left-leaning party, the Social Democrats, not resisting the neo-liberal policies that caused the privatization of elderly care within the Swedish welfare system. Detailed studies show, however, that issues of deficient Covid-19 protection had taken place to about the same degree within both public and private elderly care.[128] Despite the fact that the eroded state of the elderly care system was well known and had been debated for years before the virus arrived, no analysis of the national and private institutions' resilience was carried out and no protective equipment was at hand once the virus arrived. The only decision taken by the Government in this situation was to prohibit visitors to the care homes when nearly 50% of the homes had already discovered cases of infection. This led to one of the most painful consequences of the pandemic, which is that too many citizens were left to die alone and without their loved ones close by.

While this book is focused mainly on exploring the pandemic history of Sweden, the comparison with neighbouring Norway has played a crucial role in many debates. There used to be a close and well-functioning relationship between the Nordic countries. This changed painfully in the beginning of the pandemic,[129] and became worse in November 2021, when the Swedish Minister for Nordic Affairs strongly criticized the Norwegian Government's decision to close its borders to protect its population.[130]

One of the most enlightening and rich sources that can help us understand Norway's pandemic management choices, which also discusses the relationship between Norway and Sweden, is found in Espen Rostrup Nakstad's book *Kode Rød – Kampen for det vakre* (*Code Red – Fighting for the Beautiful*).[131] The assisting director of the Norwegian Directorate of Health (*Helsedirektoratet*) was equipped by his Government with most of the operative power. In contrast to Tegnell and Carlson, he was skilled and experienced in crisis medicine and crisis management, and while the Swedish FHM was equipped with nearly absolute power, in Norway different units (including the larger hospitals) cooperated under Nakstad's leadership in close cooperation with PM Erna Solberg and Health Minister Bent Høie. In Sweden the different units (regions and municipalities) did not appear to have a similar level of cooperation with FHM and the national Government. While both the Norwegian Public Health Institute (FHI) and the Danish *Statens Serum Institut* (SSI) in the beginning wanted to follow the Swedish unique pandemic management strategy, like the Dutch and British Governments, who also trusted Tegnell and Giesecke's advice,[132] the Governments in Oslo and Copenhagen were quicker to realize the danger that the Swedish plan posed to their citizens, and overruled the public health agencies, which arguably saved thousands of lives.

In his book, Nakstad describes how in the pandemic's initial phase many countries in Europe acted hesitantly and slowly in comparison to Asian countries that acted rapidly implementing well-planned measures. The Swedish FHM, however, declared that Sweden has "a much better basic structure" than the Asian countries,[133] a hollow premise which was later disproven by the Corona Commission in

October 2021 which uncovered many substantial structural dysfunctions. Nakstad also dismantles the idea of being able to "flatten the curve" to prevent overloading the health care system. He shows that it is an idea that is out of touch with modern hospitals' economic reality and their lack of any supply buffers. Only maximal efforts to minimize the spread were acceptable.[134] Also Swedish leaders later ensured that this indeed was their intention, but their practice could not verify their words, not even in the fourth wave of the pandemic. Sweden is accused by Nakstad for obvious "cherry picking" of data and studies, and an unsatisfying use of science.[135] He recounts how Swedish leaders refused to accept the increasing criticism of their strategy as early as April 2020, which led to what Norwegian authorities regarded as an "ethical dilemma": how should they decide if they should criticize a neighbouring state in order to save human lives in that country?[136]

Nakstad's book revealed a healthy level of self-criticism in the Norwegian society.[137] One sad point in Norway's history, which he explains in detail, was that the FHI agreed to follow the Swedish way first but in June 2020 turned away from this vision. FHI leader Camilla Stoltenberg refused to comment on this. The Danish SSI envisioned a similar policy but thanks to the resolute decision-making PM Mette Fredriksen took advice from science and responded accordingly, efficiently and quickly. Thanks to a well-working interaction of science and politics, the Governments in Oslo, Helsinki, and Copenhagen saved the lives of many thousands of their citizens. In this book, we suggest to discuss if public health agencies at all should be entrusted with decision-making power or if they should content themselves with playing a prominent role as governmental advisors, alongside other scientist and academic institutions. No matter what role they will play in the future, they need to be equipped with excellent professional scientific resources, as Anders Vahlne's chapter concludes. Would changing this better serve the interaction of what Chapter 6 describes as "the triad of trust"? The issue of who should decide what on what grounds and how power sharing should work in a pandemic crisis seems to be a highly relevant topic for all democratic countries to discuss in the future, and the final research report from the *ESCAPE* project already offers many valuable insights on the topic.

As time goes by, the process of history writing becomes increasingly important. We hope that this book can contribute to the written history record with many relevant and constructive perspectives. At present, in February 2022, the defenders of the Swedish pandemic strategy are spreading several rather dubious narratives with the aim of painting Sweden as the country with the most successful pandemic strategy. The most common of the current narratives from the defenders of the Swedish strategy is that the excess mortality rate can tell us which strategy was the most successful. This statistic, as mentioned earlier, is often used to distract from the thousands of preventable deaths. It allows us to look at the number of deaths during a certain period of time, which allows us to see the deaths in a broader context. It does not, however, offer a reliable ground for drawing conclusions on what really has happened. Nevertheless, a couple of apologetic debaters recently postulated that Sweden's rate of excess mortality during selected periods compared to other countries proves that Covid-19 has not been a larger problem for Sweden than for the other countries, a conclusion that the statistics can not actually verify.

If one were to instead compare figures with Norway, it is possible to estimate the average number of lost years of life, or look at the significantly decreased life expectancy in Sweden that has been calculated in a reliable way. One can assume that between 10,000 and 12,000 lives were lost in Sweden due to the Swedish Government's inaction, and that many of these people died significantly earlier than they likely would have otherwise. In general, one can state that 10,000–12,000 lives have been lost due to the country's failed protection, and that these innocent men and women have lost a considerably high number of years of existence. A mathematical calculation from a study produced at Tromsø University shows that Sweden has in total lost 43,073 years of existence only in the period from March to November 2020 due to its pandemic management strategy.[138] Another study conducted by researchers in Oxford shows that life expectancy in Sweden has fallen drastically for the first time since World War II. While in previous years the average life expectancy had risen around 0.2 years per year, after the pandemic, it has fallen from 81.1 years to 80.3 years for men and from 84.5 years to 83.9 years for women, compared to Norway and Denmark who during the same time period continued to see a rise.[139]

Other narratives currently being spread about Sweden's successful strategy argue that it is impossible to verify the impact of lockdowns as a measure of infection prevention. Most of these narratives, purporting to show the success of the Swedish strategy, draw on cherry-picked data, which the proponents claim to have interpreted scientifically, although it is clear that it is their political ideologies that have influenced their results, rather than the actual data. It is not uncommon that these narratives converge with narratives from climate-sceptical, patriotic, or hyper-libertarian ideologies.[140] The Swedish Government has been one of the main sources of these theories, stating things such as the country has "come pretty well" out of this crisis (Lena Hallengren), and that "Swedish people have stayed together" taking united actions out of solidarity (PM Magdalena Andersson). Columnist Peter Wennblad strikingly states, that yes, we made it through the crisis together but "politics betrayed".[141]

Finally, we would like to mention two of the positive lessons that can be learned from the Swedish pandemic strategy. The first is the decision, which was made through a quick and efficient process by the National Health Insurance (*Försäkringskassan*) to allow anyone who was sick, or in a risk group, to stay home with most of their salary. It was a decision that likely helped to break many infection chains, potentially saving many lives. The second positive lesson is that the public's trust can be one of the most significant tools for the management of a pandemic. It is important that the Government does not misuse the public's trust, and that they strive to strengthen the trust through having a transparent decision-making process that can withstand public scrutiny. As we all know from our personal lives, broken trust does not repair itself quickly; rather it takes much time and energy from all parties to repair the relationship, and the same can be said about the public's trust towards their Government and governmental agencies. This should be even more important as the wounds of broken trust take enormous time and energy to heal. We are hopeful that these positive lessons from the Swedish strategy can be useful for others.

In the following chapter we would like to offer the reader a detailed commented timeline of important events and decisions. Authors will in their chapters refer to events that happened in Sweden's pandemic management history, and we think that it might be helpful to have a timeline at hand. More lessons learned from the Swedish strategy will appear throughout the rest of the following chapters. The next section offers short summaries of these.

The chapters

In the chapter following this introduction, we have included a detailed timeline of events. It includes information about the most crucial events, decisions, and judgements in the Swedish pandemic handling from December 2019 to February 2022. These are listed chronologically and are supplemented with comments in order to help the reader to achieve a better overview over the Swedish strategy's history.

Life scientist and virologist Anders Vahlne explores, in the third chapter, why FHM, Sweden's supposed expert authority for health, acted without any real expertise. For readers who are not familiar with the field of virology, the chapter starts with a short review on basic virology, with special reference to SARS-CoV-2, the virus that causes Covid-19. Vahlne also addresses how a SARS-CoV-2 infection is diagnosed in the laboratory and how the human body fights and rids itself of viral infections. His chapter also discusses the development of Covid-19 vaccines and SARS-CoV-2-specific anti-viral pharmaceutical therapies. The chapter ends with a recollection of the genesis of The Public Health Agency of Sweden (FHM) and how the previous Swedish infection control agency, The Swedish Institute for Infectious Disease Control, was replaced as recently as 2014, with an agency void of experts in virology.

In Chapter 4, social medicine scholar Martin Lindström, scrutinizes central aspects of the implementation of the Swedish strategy with a focus on evidence-based medicine criteria. His chapter reviews the events based on official statements, mass media reporting and literature with specific references to the situation during the spring (March–June) of 2020. Under the leadership of the FHM, Sweden officially abandoned testing and contact tracing in the end of the second week of March 2020 (with the exception of hospital patients and risk groups) and did not start to resume these WHO recommended actions until well into May 2020. Restrictions enhancing social distancing were looser than in other Nordic and European countries, and looser than recommended by the WHO. Indirect belief in natural herd immunity (not included in the official version of the strategy), belief in individual responsibility, and arguments against mouth protection also contradicted evidence-based medicine. The FHM put very high demands on evidence supporting protective measures but low demands on evidence supporting the implemented strategy.

In the fifth chapter theoretical physicist Emil J. Bergholtz critically explores the underlying assumptions of the Swedish Covid-19 response. The focus is on how simple back-of-the-envelope estimates using the knowledge available already well before the pandemic reached Sweden. Such elementary considerations should have alarmed any analytically minded observer. These calculations show that the Swedish goal of not overwhelming the health care system while allowing the infection spread at a controlled rate in order to achieve herd immunity in the population was unrealistic.

The impossibility of shielding risk groups while letting the disease run through society and the false dichotomy between freedom and saving the economy on the one hand, and decisive actions for infection control on the other are also discussed. The chapter documents the debate during the spring of 2020 followed by the blunt denial from the decision-makers of the chosen strategy. Finally, the present situation and future challenges posed by the pandemic are discussed. The author frames the potential for an escalating situation in which new and much more virulent and transmissive virus mutations develop as a version of the tragedy of the commons, and connects this all to the global challenge of climate change.

The sixth chapter explores how *learning from failure* represents a crucial skill for successful pandemic management, and how the lack of said skill can lead to devastating effects. Scholar of religion Sigurd Bergmann shares his anxious experiences of following the first weeks of the national response to the pandemic emergency. His chapter uses tools from cultural analysis to help us in our search for clues that can help us solve the mystery that the pandemic presented for Swedish society. Why did so many in the population follow their national leadership for a long time into the "pandemonium", the place where all demons gather, fuelling the fear of pain in individual and social bodies? Can this be related to the idea of shame within conformism? What role does high trust play when confidence is shaken? What does it mean for the conditions of restoring trust when responsible leaders, time and time again, deny having failed? Can one restore the legal system so that civil servants and politicians can be held accountable when their decisions violate the law? The chapter develops a hypothetical model of analyzing the pandemic interplay in the triad of science, politics, and trust, a model that might help comparisons of many countries' different responses in future research to be more comprehensive. Applying such a model to Sweden's experiment, the author concludes: Sweden is distinguished from others in a unique asymmetry of a) high trust in politics, b) very low trust from politics in science (in contrast to a traditionally high trust in science in other contexts), and c) an ambiguous high-and-low trust from politics (Government and Authorities) in the people. The chapter ends with an attempt to make us more aware of how individual and sociocultural processes such as accepting guilt and affirming shame play a substantial role in restoring trust in each other, as well as restoring the trust between politicians, scientists, and citizens.

Data and facts are powerful tools for decision-making yet can also easily be misrepresented and misinterpreted and depend highly on the quality of the data sources. Epidemiologist Nele Brusselaers problematizes in the seventh chapter why numbers are important but can be misleading. She begins from the crucial scientific discipline of epidemiology, investigating the distribution and determinants of health-related states and events, including but not limited to infectious diseases, in specific populations and settings. Using Covid-19 data from Sweden, this chapter discusses some common pitfalls in the interpretation of epidemiological data.

The eighth chapter also places a focus on the use of numbers, but from a different perspective. Considering the idea of political economics scholar in economic history, Rodney Edvinsson investigates the discrepancy between empirical evidence on immunity levels and statements from Swedish authorities. The author discusses evidence of infectious mortality, IFR, which was presented in the spring and summer of 2020, internationally and from Sweden. This evidence pointed to a very high IFR for high-income countries, around 1%, which would entail 50 000–100 000 deaths in Sweden. This evidence is contrasted with the assessments of representatives and certain employees of the FHM, which show how they downplayed the empirical evidence selectively to claim that Sweden, or at least Stockholm, would soon gain herd immunity. These claims implicated that Sweden would need to have a much greater spread of infection than the Western European countries and a much lower IFR. These extremely unrealistic assumptions legitimized the belief in natural herd immunity as a central part of Sweden's experiments (i.e. a strategy to allow the healthy part of the population to be infected at a rate that would not overburden health care, while isolating so-called risk groups). The reason why Sweden did not have higher mortality levels is that the original strategy had to de facto be abandoned when death rates started to rise.

Children at the front line of the pandemic are at the core of Chapter 9 written by cell biologist Johanna Höög. During spring 2020, schools all over the world closed and many countries went into a so-called lockdown. Sweden stood out as an exception. Schools for students in years 0–9 (ages 6–15) were not closed in the country a single day during the first wave of the Covid-19 pandemic. The FHM's decisions regarding testing made it nearly impossible to identify cases in children. Schools were instructed to try to make children keep at distance to each other and to encourage hand washing, and families were told to keep sick children home from school. Facemasks and other non-pharmaceutical interventions were not recommended. People worked under the impression, nurtured by the FHM, that children do not get sick in Covid-19 and that they do not contribute to the transmission of the disease. The author proposes that the FHM, with the help of others, built their policies like a "scientific house of cards", based on weak and sometimes non-existent evidence. The chapter explores situations that have been caused by these policies while reflecting specifically upon the strategy's consequences for children and their health. It investigates the origins of the momentous assumption presented by the FHM that children do not get sick and do not transmit the disease. It finally discusses the consequences of the strategy's consequences for the future of society as a whole.

Philosopher Lapo Lappin in Chapter 10 dives deeper into the ethical dimension of Sweden's strategy by emphasizing how utilitarianism has impacted the country's biopolitics. In the wake of the pandemic, *biopolitics* – the reflection on the ways in which politics relates to biology, introduced by Michel Foucault – has been declared dead, allegedly unable to grapple with twenty-first-century questions. Yet while biopolitical reflection has indisputably had shortcomings, it can prove illuminating when used to interpret a self-styled "liberal" pandemic strategy like that of Sweden. After showing that the notion of herd immunity was a core component of the Swedish strategy, the author argues that it is implicitly built on the ethical calculus of utilitarianism: sacrificing the lives and safety of weaker groups in society for the good of the whole. The chapter shows that this ethical perspective is permitted by a biopolitical conceptual apparatus that operates on the level of the "population", totalized as a homogenous whole (by way of concepts of *folkhälsa*, "society as a whole", "the economy", and *folkhemmet*). This conceptualization then allows for the systematic exclusion of certain groups, along the lines of the biopolitical "including exclusion" theorized by Roberto Esposito. The chapter shows how this mechanism is at work particularly in the exclusion of the elderly and risk-group parents of school children.

In Chapter 11 Kajsa Klein offers a differentiated analysis of the public discourse in pandemic Sweden. Drawing on research in media and communication studies, political philosophy, and in other fields, she explores the processes of crisis communication in the authorities and the sciences. Moreover the chapter investigates notably the strong voices, groups and opinions in the social media, and the perception and treatment of the critics of Sweden's way. The chapter examines Swedish Government misinformation and its impact on infection control and beyond. It looks at how three categories of actors upheld the legitimacy of the Public Health Agency (FHM): *collaborators* transmitting and promoting the FHM message, *supporters* love-bombing the FHM and heckling its critics, and, finally, the *science judges* who awarded the decision-makers and the loyalists and punished the critics. The author suggests that the public health patriotism and the mainstreaming of misinformation had the unfortunate unintended effect of reducing confidence in science.

Historian Jens Stilhoff Sörensen contextualizes in Chapter 12 Sweden's pandemic management in a wider frame where its tendency to act as a totalitarian democracy is unmasked. His chapter critically examines the Swedish state and society and explores characteristics that have been revealed through the pandemic crisis management. The chapter begins by problematizing Swedish democracy and discussing Sweden's crisis management first from a general perspective, then diving deeper into how it has worked during this pandemic. The chapter moves on to argue that we need to re-conceptualize the nature of the Swedish state and society through revisiting the concepts "state individualism" and "totalitarian democracy".

The final chapter takes us back into the long successful history of preventive medicine in Sweden that has come to an end during the pandemic due to the country's failed response. Epidemiologist Gunnar Steineck describes how for 280 years Sweden had been at the forefront of preventive medicine based on trusting cooperation between politicians, civil servants, and the research community. The means have been mandatory legislation, functioning national structures, and free preventive care. To put the sudden, drastic departure from this long tradition in context, this chapter briefly describes Sweden's history regarding preventive medicine, providing examples from throughout the history of success in different areas, such as infection prevention, maternal and child health care, cancer prevention, reducing childhood accidents, reducing traffic accidents, and preventing cardiovascular disease. The actions around the HIV pandemic constitute the last beneficial efforts. The approach to Covid-19 has meant a drastic end to this long tradition.

Do we dare to hope to learn from this end – and all the other chapters' lessons – for the sake of what is best for the lives and health of all forthcoming generations?

Notes

1 *WHO-convened Global Study of Origins of SARS-CoV-2: China Part, Joint WHO-China Study, 14 January–10 February 2021*, www.who.int/docs/default-source/coronaviruse/who-convened-global-study-of-origins-of-SARS-CoV-2-china-part-annexes.pdf?sfvrsn=3065bcd85 . Cf. Lytras, Spyros, Wei Xia, Joseph Hughes, Xiaowei Jiang, and David L. Robertson. "The Animal Origin of SARS-CoV-2", *Science* 373:6558 (27 August 2021): 968–970, www.science.org/doi/10.1126/science.abh0117 .

2 Roy, Arundhati. "The Pandemic Is a Portal", *Financial Times*, 3 April 2020.

3 Settele, Josef, Sandra Díaz, Eduardo Brondizio, and Peter Daszak. "COVID-19 Stimulus Measures Must Save Lives, Protect Livelihoods, and Safeguard Nature to Reduce the Risk of Future Pandemics", *Intergovernmental Science-Policy Platform on Biodiversity and Ecosystem Services (IPBES)*, Bonn, 27 April 2020, https://ipbes.net/Covid19stimulus .

4 Olsen, Björn. *Pandemi: Myterna, fakta, hoten*, new ed. 2020, Stockholm: Norstedts, 2010: 3. According to Olsen, 40–45, several reasons interact in accelerating the increase of zoonotic diseases leading to pandemics, such as population growth, the decline of bio-diversity and wild species, dominantly monocultural domestic animal stocks, global mobility, and urban density. Cf. Honigsbaum, Mark. *The Pandemic Century: One Hundred Years of Panic, Hysteria and Hubris*, new ed. New York: W.W. Norton & Company, 2020.

5 Stoellger talks about *Riss* and *Lebensweltwandel*. Stoellger, Philipp. "Eröffnung, Corona als Riss der Lebenswelt: Zur Orientierung über Naherwartungen, Enttäuschungsrisiken und Nebenwirkungen", in Held, Benjamin, Thomas Kirchhoff, Frederike van Oorschot, Philipp Stoellger, and Ines-Jacqueline Werkner (eds.). *Corona als Riss: Perspektiven für Kirche, Politik und Ökonomie*, Universitätsbibliothek Heidelberg, 2020: 149–184, https://books.ub.uni-heidelberg.de/heibooks .

6 www.nytimes.com/2021/10/12/health/when-will-covid-end.html .

7 Goethe, Johann Wolfgang. *Bedeutende Fördernis durch ein einziges geistreiches Wort,* 1823: 306; "Der Mensch kennt nur sich selbst, insofern er die Welt kennt, die er nur in sich und sich nur in ihr gewahr wird", in *Zur Naturwissenschaft überhaupt, besonders zur Morphologie: Erfahrung, Betrachtung, Folgerung, durch Lebensereignisse verbunden* (1817–24), München: Hanser (1989): 306–309. [The human being only knows herself as far as she knows the world, which she only becomes aware of in herself, and only in the world she becomes aware of herself.] Cf. Bergmann, Sigurd. *Weather, Religion and Climate Change*, London and New York: Routledge, 2020: 4–5.

8 On the Anthropocene cf. Deane-Drummond, C., S. Bergmann, and M. Vogt (eds.). *Religion in the Anthropocene*, Eugene: Wipf & Stock, 2017; Bergmann, S., K. Rigby,

and P. Scott (eds.). *Religion, Materialism and Ecology*, London: Routledge, forthcoming 2023.

9 Cf. Aaltola, Mika (ed.). *Understanding the Politics of Pandemic Emergencies in the Time of COVID-19: An Introduction to Global Politosomatics*, London: Routledge, 2022.

10 Ghebreyesus, Tedros Adhanom. "WHO Director-General's Opening Remarks at the Media Briefing on COVID-19 – 20 March 2020", *World Health Organization*, 20 March 2020, www.who.int/director-general/speeches/detail/who-director-general-s-opening-remarks-at-the-media-briefing-on-Covid-19–20-march-2020 .

11 The process *One world one health* gathered scientists in the first decade of our century in a dialogue about an international, interdisciplinary approach for combating threats to the health of life on Earth, with diseases among human, domestic animal, and wildlife populations at the core. Cf., www.oneworldonehealth.org/ .

12 One of the fruits of such acceleration is found in the opening of the WHO's *Hub for Pandemic and Epidemic Intelligence* in Berlin in September 2021, with "a mission is to provide the world with better data, analytics and decisions to detect and respond to health emergencies". www.who.int/news/item/01-09-2021-who-germany-open-hub-for-pandemic-and-epidemic-intelligence-in-berlin .

13 Krastev, Ivan. *Is It Tomorrow Yet? Paradoxes of the Pandemic*, London: Allen Lane, 2020: 2.

14 *Ibid*., 71.

15 The term *Totalereignis* aims at a historical event that affects and pervades all dimensions of social life such as war, revolution, or economic collapse. Cf. Bude, who analyzes the difference between generations who experienced such a total event, as for example the second World War and the following generations. Bude, Heinz. "Generationengerechtigkeit: Eine unbrauchbare Formel als Indiz eines verlorenen Zukunftsglaubens", *Lettre International/LI* 100 (2013): 21–22. Cf. Wils, Jean-Pierre. "Corona-Leere oder Corona-Lehre?" *Forschung & Lehre* 1 January 2021, www.forschung-und-lehre.de/zeitfragen/corona-leere-oder-corona-lehre-3299/ .

16 https://time.com/5899432/sweden-coronovirus-disaster/ .

17 "Act only according to that maxim whereby you can, at the same time, will that it should become a universal law." Kant, Immanuel. *Groundwork of the Metaphysic of Morals* (1785), transl. J.W. Ellington (3rd ed. 1993): 30.

18 www.spiegel.de/ausland/schweden-besuch-im-corona-wunderland-a-00000000-0002-0001-0000-000170816324 , www.tagesspiegel.de/wissen/intensivmediziner-schlagen-fuer-den-sommer-alarm-schwedens-leidensweg-aus-der-corona-pandemie/27197836.html , www.zdf.de/nachrichten/panorama/corona-schweden-inzidenz-sonderweg-100.html .

19 Goodman, Peter S. "Sweden Has Become the World's Cautionary Tale", *The New York Times*, 7 July 2020, www.nytimes.com/2020/07/07/business/sweden-economy-coronavirus.html . The term of "experiment" is also central in the detailed evaluation of Sweden's crisis management by scholars in political science, military science, and other disciplines: Aucante, Yohann. *The Swedish Experiment: The COVID-19 Response and Its Controversies*, Bristol: Bristol University Press, 29 June 2022. *Statsvetenskaplig tidskrift* (*The Swedish Journal of Political Science*) 123:5 (2021): "Tema: Coronapandemin – besluts fattande under svåra förhållanden", ed. by Magnus Jerneck, https://statsvetenskapligtidskrift.org/ .

20 www.sciencemag.org/news/2020/10/it-s-been-so-so-surreal-critics-sweden-s-lax-pandemic-policies-face-fierce-backlash .

21 www.thelancet.com/journals/lancet/article/PIIS0140-6736(20)31672-X/fulltext .

22 www.thelancet.com/pdfs/journals/lancet/PIIS0140-6736(20)32750-1.pdf .

23 www.zdf.de/gesellschaft/markus-lanz/presse-schweden-ungeschminkt-100.html .

24 www.dn.se/ledare/gina-gustavsson-regalskeppet-corona-har-kapsejsat-och-sjunkit/ .

25 www.tagesspiegel.de/politik/manchmal-fuehle-ich-mich-wie-ein-sandsack-anders-tegnell-was-treibt-den-chefepidemiologen-in-schweden-an/25890852.html .

26 The only lesson to learn from the national pandemic management is for FHM GD Carlson "to maintain the advanced levels" at his Agency and in the health care system, www.dn.se/sverige/fhms-johan-carlson-ovaccinerade-kan-inte-leva-som-vanligt/ . Science journalist Amina Manzoor had already earlier demanded to learn to live with the virus, https://fof.se/utdrag-pandemier . The Zero- or No-Covid method's option, which several countries practiced with great success and also mobilized a pan-European movement, was never really taken into account in Sweden, in spite of the undersigned ten scholars' demands and other voices, www.altinget.se/artikel/11-forskare-sverige-bor-ansluta-sig-till-ett-paneuropeiskt-nollcovid-upprop .
27 www.dn.se/sverige/hallengren-sverige-har-kommit-val-ut-ur-detta/ .
28 The term *bunkermentalitet* aims according to the authors at the FHM's unwillingness to revisit earlier adjudgements when new information from science appears, www.dn.se/debatt/lat-inte-prestige-hindra-en-omprovning-av-coronastrategin/ .
29 www.gu.se/som-institutet/resultat-och-publikationer/som-undersokningen-om-coronaviruset file:///Users/sib/Downloads/Den%20svenska%20coronastrategin.pdf , https://novus.se/nyheter/2021/01/fortroendet-kring-corona-for-myndigheter-och-regeringen-rasar/ .
30 Krastev. *Is It Tomorrow Yet?* 6.
31 Bergmann, Sigurd. "Memoria Passionis Subversiva: The Moral Power of Remembrance in the Pandemic – in a Swedish Lens", in Erbele-Küster, Dorothea, and Volker Küster (eds.). *Between Pandemonium and Pandemethics: Responses to Covid-19 in Theology and Religions*, Leipzig: EVA, 2022, 101–121. Cf., www.dagensarena.se/essa/om-doendets-konst/ [On the Art of Dying/Ars Moriendi].
32 Cf. the *New York Times'* careful visualization of *Those We've Lost,* www.nytimes.com/interactive/2020/obituaries/people-died-coronavirus-obituaries.html , and their *Wall of Grief,* www.nytimes.com/2021/02/21/insider/covid-500k-front-page.html , and the German *Tagesspiegel*'s interactive long list of photos, names, and short bios, https://interaktiv.tagesspiegel.de/lab/den-toten-der-coronapandemie . German president Frank-Walter Steinmeier initiated a campaign, *Aktion #lichtfenster,* where he encouraged citizens to light a candle in the window every Friday in January 2021, www.ekd.de/aktion-lichtfenster-62441.htm .
33 This number is an estimate and the number of diseases is increasing all the time due to new infections. Even many children are affected. Ca. 10% of Covid patients seem to be affected, www.uu.se/nyheter/artikel/?id=16740&typ=artikel . The challenge for the health care system in the long run is obvious, although one, sadly enough, that seldom includes long-Covid patients in reliable calculations. Cf. www.langtidscovid.se/om-lngtidscovid .
34 https://tt.omni.se/manga-svenskar-utan-luktsinne-koar-for-hjalp/a/rEmB4a .
35 www.nature.com/articles/d41586-022-00414-x .
36 www.dn.se/sverige/kungen-om-pandemin-vi-har-misslyckats/ .
37 A UN officer in Geneva sent me a mail where she expressed her anger about the GB Declaration and ensured that she and all other inhabitants of the US county of Great Barrington, where she was born, are angry about the biofascist declaration. No one born or living here, she ensures me, would even imagine to sign such an inhumane text.
38 https://kvartal.se/artiklar/den-svenske-Covidrebellen-i-usa/ . Still in November 2021 Kulldorf incurably attacks Anthony Fauci and the US management, propagates the GBD's unethical method of striving for (natural) herd immunity, claiming the uselessness of lockdowns and shares lies about "Zero Covid deaths among children and a Covid risk to teachers lower than the average of other professions" in Sweden, where 25% of all teachers were infected and almost 16 children have died (several times more than in other Nordic countries). It seems unbelievable how a serious journal like *Newsweek* can publish such dangerous disinformation. Freedom of opinion does not necessarily imply the freedom to offend the families of innocent children, www.newsweek.com/

how-fauci-fooled-america-opinion-1643839 , www.dn.se/debatt/vara-siffror-om-dodsfall-i-covid-bland-barn-ar-de-officiella/ .

39 https://bylinetimes.com/2020/10/09/climate-science-denial-network-behind-great-barrington-declaration/ .

40 Ludvigsson's and others' impact on Swedish School Minister Anna Ekström was fatal and led to an incredible amount of infection, suffering, and also painful death for school children and teachers. Still the Government ensures internationally how proud they are to have kept schools open as much as possible. Ca. 35% of all children (according to FHM officer Karin Tegsell Wikmark, in the press conference 16 September 2021) and 25% of all teachers in elementary schools (according to the Teachers Union) have been infected, https://skolvarlden.se/artiklar/ny-studie-var-fjarde-grundskolla rare-smittad-av-covid-19 . Ordinary recommendations from the FHM have not been followed in schools and the responsible Agency for the Work and Environment did not protect neither disciples nor teachers, www.lararen.se/nyheter/coronaviruset/ny-undersokning-stor-covid-oro-i-lararkaren . Ludvigsson is influential also in the Swedish Paediatric Society that initially resisted vaccinating children, but changed their mind in September, and the FHM decided to vaccinate children 12 years and older – the last country in Europe to do so, https://lakartidningen.se/aktuellt/nyheter/2021/09/barnlakarforeningen-oppnar-for-vaccination-fran-12-ar/ .

41 www.science.org/content/article/critics-slam-letter-prestigious-journal-downplayed-Covid-19-risks-swedish .

42 https://twitter.com/agneswold/status/1254422187165077505 , www.expressen.se/nyheter/agnes-wold-forsvarar-tegnell-efter-uttalandet-om-invandrare-i-aktuellt/ . Benjamin Kallischer Welander has in detail analyzed the danger when voices such as Wold and Frans are given a platform in the public media as alleged experts, www.gp.se/deb att/farligt-att-ge-plats-%C3%A5t-frans-och-wold-ist%C3%A4llet-f%C3%B6r-riktiga-coronaexperter-1.38261880 .

43 https://volante.se/bocker/alla-tvattar-handerna/ .

44 www.ergo.nu/bok/20210216-emma-frans-tv%C3%A5r-sina-h%C3%A4nder .

45 www.dn.se/sverige/tom-britton-har-skrivit-hundratals-mejl-till-anders-tegnell-ibland-har-han-fatt-svar/ . Cf. Emil J. Bergholtz's and Rodney Edvinsson's chapters on Britton's calculations .

46 www.dn.se/debatt/varfor-racker-inte-saklighet-nar-forskare-debatterar/ , www.dn.se/debatt/vi-bor-radda-de-unga-om-varden-inte-kan-klara-alla/ . On the overarching bio political context of Sweden's pandemic management, see Lapo Lappin's chapter.

47 www.aftonbladet.se/nyheter/a/6jmxp3/det-avslojar-den-nedlatande-synen-pa-aldre .

48 www.johnsnowmemo.com/ .

49 This offers a similar pattern as in climate sceptics, and it somehow reminds of the arguments from the GBD, even if FHM leaders have denied to apply the GBD method. The GBD drivers' activities are financed through the same sources from the Koch brothers who heavily support climate and corona scepticism.

50 *Sveriges Radio*, 17 December 2020.

51 https://sverigesradio.se/artikel/lofven-uppger-att-strategin-vaxte-fram-trots-webbpub licering-av-densamma . Cf. Jerneck, Magnus. "Inledning: Konsten att bemästra en pandemi", *Statsvetenskaplig tidskrift* (*The Swedish Journal of Political Science*) 123:5 (2021): 7–30, 11.

52 www.di.se/debatt/sverigebilden-i-tyskland-ar-for-evigt-forandrad/ . On the loss of reputation and the change of Sweden's image in the Nordic countries, see www.dn.se/sverige/hanteringen-av-pandemin-slar-mot-sverigebilden/ . Nevertheless, without any humbleness or confession about Sweden's high infection process, conservative parliamentarian Hans Wallmark attacks Norway for having closed borders (to protect their citizens) at the Nordic Council in November 2021, www.nrk.no/norge/ny-rapport_-noreg-burde-ikkje-ha-stengt-grensene-mot-dei-andre-nordiske-landa-1.15716396 .

53 www.abccommercial.com/contentsales/program/swedish-model, www.arte.tv/en/videos/101800-000-A/covid-sweden-suffers/ , www.arte.tv/en/videos/096952-004-A/geopolitics-of-covid-19/ , www.arte.tv/de/videos/102406-000-A/schweden-corona-zufluchtsland-fuer-junge-menschen/ , www.arte.tv/de/videos/098383-000-A/corona-wie-ergeht-es-schweden-ohne-lockdown/ , www.ardmediathek.de/video/weltbilder/freiheit-statt-lockdown-schwedens-weg-in-der-corona-krise/ndr-fernsehen/Y3JpZDovL25kci5kZS84NTVlZmI3OS1jZmYxLTQwNGUtYjg0ZC02YzllZmI2NzBmMGI/ , www.ardmediathek.de/video/europamagazin/schweden-ist-der-corona-sonderweg-ein-irrweg/das-erste/Y3JpZDovL2Rhc2Vyc3RlLmRlL2V1cm9wYW1hZ2F6aW4vYzg1ZmUxY2QtNjcxMC00ZWYzLThjMjItN2QwODgzZDdjMWQw/ , www.ardmediathek.de/video/weltspiegel/schweden-schulbeginn-ohne-einschraenkungen/das-erste/Y3JpZDovL2Rhc2Vyc3RlLmRlL3dlbHRzcGllZ2VsL2RhM2FjMzIxLTk2NzYtNDU4YS04Y2FmLTBkMzMwYmViNGU2ZA/ , www.ardmediathek.de/video/weltspiegel/schweden-corona-sonderweg-auf-kosten-von-senioren/das-erste/Y3JpZDovL2Rhc2Vyc3RlLmRlL3dlbHRzcGllZ2VsLzIzZTAyNDdkLTkyY2EtNDViYi1hY2YxLThmNDlhYmJjMzIzOQ/ , www.zdf.de/nachrichten/panorama/corona-schweden-inzidenz-sonderweg-100.html , www.zdf.de/gesellschaft/markus-lanz/presse-schweden-ungeschminkt-100.html . Prominent film director Maj Wechselman produced a thought-provoking movie, *The Swedish Way*, where she draws on the historical story of a captain arriving at Stockholm in 1710, escaping from his quarantine and starting the spread at a pub. The critical points about collective irresponsibility between then and now become obvious, www.youtube.com/watch?v=kBPUQNQzalg . French-Swedish film director Olivier Guerpillon contributes to five great European filmmakers' collective documentary *Isolation*, 2021, with a subtle piece about alienation in between trust and distrust with regard to the national response, https://bio.nu/isolation/ . Viktor Nordenskiöld presented in February 2022 his documentary *Bakom den svenska modellen* (*Behind the Swedish Model*), where he intimately follows Tegnell and Hallengren, trying to figure out the depth of decision-making and how they responded to criticism, praise, and frustration, https://program.goteborgfilmfestival.se/en/program/behind-the-swedish-model .

54 https://journals.plos.org/plosone/article?id=10.1371/journal.pone.0249732 .

55 www.svd.se/sverige-har-inte-fatt-till-en-stark-signal-mot-smittan, www.svd.se/vi-kan-genast-ta-till-oss-norges-framgangsfaktorer .

56 www.svd.se/a/GGoPVJ/vi-kan-genast-ta-till-oss-norges-framgangsfaktorer .

57 www.dn.se/debatt/overdodlighet-ett-svagt-matt-pa-pandemins-effekter/ .

58 www.sydsvenskan.se/2021-10-29/carlson-om-kritiken-for-tidigt-att-saga .

59 The utilitarian view has been contributed to the Swedish debates by influential philosopher Torbjörn Tännsjö and paediatrician Johnny Ludvigsson, who both valued the lives of younger humans higher than of elderly. Cf. also Lapo Lappin's chapter in this book, www.dn.se/debatt/vi-bor-radda-de-unga-om-varden-inte-kan-klara-alla/ , www.dn.se/debatt/varfor-racker-inte-saklighet-nar-forskare-debatterar/ . Debaters did not offer much noteworthy support, but in ordinary life contexts one could often encounter the more crude answer to what to say about Sweden's high death tolls among the elderly: They would have died anyway. Tännsjö and FHM GD Tegmark Wisell seem to rank people's health higher than the individual citizen's health, by arguing for the need to consider what they without any clarification circumscribe as "wholeness", www.dn.se/debatt/lat-inte-covid-19-pandemin-kullkasta-folkhalsoarbetet/ , https://sverigesradio.se/artikel/tegmark-wisell-sverige-valde-en-delvis-annan-strategi . Hereby they violate a legal principle in international law where a state can never rank collective health over individual health according to the European Convention on Human Rights' article 2.

60 www.svd.se/a/Xg1z1x/giesecke-de-flesta-kommer-att-smittas .

61 www.svd.se/a/mBB4Ev/fhm-s-tidiga-strategi-var-flockimmunitet?metering=offerklarna .

62 www.gp.se/nyheter/sverige/stefan-l%C3%B6fven-i-ku-flockimmunitet-ingen-strategi-1.45623983 .
63 www.expressen.se/nyheter/lofven-pressas-i-ku-svarar-om-strategin/ .
64 www.sydsvenskan.se/2021-11-01/katastrofen-som-aldrig-kom .
65 www.journals.uchicago.edu/doi/pdf/10.1086/711432 .
66 Baldwin, Peter. *Fighting the First Wave: Why the Coronavirus Was Tackled so Differently across the Globe*, Cambridge: Cambridge University Press, 2021. Cf., www.cambridge.org/se/academic/subjects/politics-international-relations/comparative-politics/fighting-first-wave-why-coronavirus-was-tackled-so-differently-across-globe?format=HB .
67 https://time.com/5899432/sweden-coronovirus-disaster/ .
68 https://escapeCovid19.org/ . Brusselaers, Nele, David Steadson, Kelly Bjorklund, Sofia Breland, Jens Stilhoff Sörensen, Andrew Ewing, Sigurd Bergmann, and Gunnar Steineck. "Evaluation of Science Advice During the COVID-19 Pandemic in Sweden", *Humanities and Social Sciences Communications* 9, Article number: 91 (2022), www.nature.com/articles/s41599-022-01097-5 . The extensive report has gained intense international attention, though scarcely in Sweden. It was not even commented by Minister Hallengren in a specific parliamentarian interrogation on it, www.latimes.com/business/story/2022-03-31/sweden-covid-policy-was-a-disaster , https://abcnews.go.com/Health/scathing-evaluation-swedens-covid-response-reveals-failures-control/story?id=83644832 , https://newsy-today.com/now-there-are-proofs-corriere-it/ , www.zeit.de/2022/16/corona-politik-schweden-analyse , www.abcnyheter.no/nyheter/verden/2022/04/12/195838566/sverige-slaktes-i-ny-skremmende-rapport, https://plus.tagesspiegel.de/politik/vernichtendes-urteil-uber-schwedens-corona-politik-ein-moralisch-ethisch-und-wissenschaftlich-fragwurdiger-laissez-faire-ansatz- , www.spiegel.de/wissenschaft/medizin/coronavirus-kritischer-bericht-zum-schwedischen-sonderweg-in-der-coronapandemie-a-8c814d12–948a-42ca-acbf-228f9992e29d,455451.html , www.riksdagen.se/sv/dokument-lagar/dokument/skriftlig-fraga/rapport-om-den-svenska-pandemihanteringen_H9111372 .
69 See especially Gunnar Steineck's chapter in this book.
70 Nevertheless the Government, itself remaining passive, was continuously provided with detailed information. Maja Fjaestad – Minister Hallengren's close assistant and centrally involved in the Ministry's decisions – tells about her daily lunch meetings with GD Johan Carlson, www.svd.se/regeringen-hade-okanda-moten-med-fhm-kritiker , www.svd.se/grubblar-mycket-pa-om-sverige-gjorde-ratt .
71 Hanson, Claudia, Susanne Luedtke, Neil Spicer, Jens Stilhoff Sörensen, Susannah Mayhew, and Sandra Mounier-Jack. "National Health Governance, Science and the Media: Drivers of COVID-19 Responses in Germany, Sweden and the UK in 2020", *BMJ Global Health* (2021), https://gh.bmj.com/content/bmjgh/6/12/e006691.full.pdf .
72 Gustavsson, Gina. *Du stolta, du fria: Om svenskarna, Sverigebilden och folkhälsopatriotismen*, Stockholm: Kaunitz-Olsson, 2021.
73 Wirtén, Per. *Mitt hemland: Ett utanförskapsområde*, Stockholm: Bonniers, 2021; Lindroth, Bengt. *Vi som inte var med i kriget: Om Sverige, Norden, Europa & Coronan*, Stockholm: Carlssons, 2021.
74 www.svt.se/nyheter/utrikes/matning-kanslan-av-splittring-vaxer-under-pandemin , www.pewresearch.org/topic/coronavirus-disease-Covid-19/ . For a short time Sweden was approached as a model for combining the population's trust and some measures, even in the WHO, that at that time received large extra financial support from the Swedish Government. In the acceleration of the second wave, however, these voices were silenced when it became obvious how this strategy harvested all too many lives in its disaster, www.weforum.org/agenda/2020/04/29-april-who-briefing-trust-sweden/ .
75 www.di.se/debatt/patriotism-forklarar-stodet-for-svenska-coronastrategin/?fbclid=IwAR2bsgrSpZFdtGsf69dMLa-oZYBMPd4FxAMNQ32B5x5bB1Vg-8P-oreDW2U .
76 Einhorn, Lena. *Bland hobbyepidemiologer och expertmyndigheter: En resa i pandemins Sverige*, Stockholm: Norstedts, 2022.

77 Manzoor, Amina. *Pandemier! Från spanska sjukan till covid-19*, Stockholm: fri tanke, 2021. Cf. Lapo Lappin's chapter.

78 Sonesson, Carl Johan. *Skånes kamp mot coronan: En personlig berättelse*, Malmö: Samizdat, 2022.

79 Aucante, Yohann. *The Swedish Experiment: The COVID-19 Response and Its Controversies*, Bristol: Bristol University Press, 29 June 2022.

80 https://vetcov19.se/en/ .

81 https://vetcov19.se/en/media/artiklarna/, https://vetcov19.se/en/media-in-english/, www.youtube.com/channel/UCarSBJ6PFC8_6oFJ9pwvqvQ .

82 *Statsvetenskaplig tidskrift* (*The Swedish Journal of Political Science*) 123:5 (2021), https://statsvetenskapligtidskrift.org/ .

83 https://naringslivets-medieinstitut.se/wp-content/uploads/2021/05/Coronarapporten_2.pdf . Cf., https://naringslivets-medieinstitut.se/tag/lisa-bjurwald/ .

84 https://svjt.se/svjt/2020/1080 . Cf., www.dn.se/debatt/svensk-krisberedskap-har-inte-fungerat-som-den-borde/ .

85 www.ncbi.nlm.nih.gov/pmc/articles/PMC7836894/ .

86 www.ncbi.nlm.nih.gov/pmc/articles/PMC7832477/ .

87 Comparing with Germany, the Government all the time through all waves had clear majorities in the population, between 60 and 80% of citizens understanding and accepting restrictions, with groups of 10–20% asking for tougher ones. In December 2020 one could find 35% who accepted the restrictions as "completely right" and 49% demanded "tougher responses", www.zdf.de/nachrichten/politik/politbarometer-haertere-massnahmen-100.html .

88 www.ncbi.nlm.nih.gov/pmc/articles/PMC7200128/ .

89 www.thelancet.com/pdfs/journals/lancet/PIIS0140-6736(20)32750-1.pdf .

90 www.thelancet.com/journals/lancet/article/PIIS0140-6736(21)00885-0/fulltext .

91 https://coronakommissionen.com/publikationer/delbetankande-1/ .

92 www.dn.se/nyheter/sverige/lofven-coronakommission-tillsatts-innan-sommaren/ .

93 https://coronakommissionen.com/wp-content/uploads/2020/12/summary.pdf .

94 www.spiegel.de/ausland/corona-in-schwedens-pflegeheimen-der-eingeladene-tod-a-00000000-0002-0001–0000–000173444539 .

95 https://coronakommissionen.com/publikationer/delbetankande-2/ .

96 https://sverigesradio.se/artikel/regeringen-beskrev-beredskap-som-god-trots-brister .

97 www.sydsvenskan.se/2022-02-13/skracken-i-patientens-ogon-vad-hander-med-mig .

98 www.svt.se/nyheter/inrikes/mats-melin-stallt-utom-allt-tvivel-att-regionerna-var-ansvariga-for-testning .

99 www.svd.se/a/dn9epX/hallengren-regeringen-var-inte-senfardig .

100 www.svt.se/nyheter/snabbkollen/lofven-s-haveri-ar-att-ta-i .

101 www.svd.se/hallengren-jag-haller-inte-med-om-kritiken .

102 www.socialdemokraterna.se/kongress/kongresshandlingar/valberedningens-forslag .

103 www.socialdemokraterna.se/kongress/live-fran-kongresshallen/2021-10-22-omraded–vi-bygger-landet-tryggt-forts .

104 www.svd.se/carlson-om-kritiken-for-tidigt-att-saga .

105 www.aftonbladet.se/nyheter/a/V95jX3/svidande-kritik-sverige-var-senfardiga-i-sin-pandemihantering . Even the Commission's first report was characterized as "etching criticism" in December 2020, www.altinget.se/artikel/svidande-kritik-av-regeringens-stodaatgarder-under-pandemin .

106 www.vg.no/nyheter/utenriks/i/k6dm9v/svenske-myndigheter-faar-slakt-fra-coronakommisjon . Even after the Commission's first report, Norwegian media used the term of "slaughter", in surprise over Tegnell's compact unwillingness "to offer any self-criticism", www.nrk.no/urix/tegnell-tek-ikkje-sjolvkritikk-etter-slakt-av-korona handteringa-1.15291376 .

107 www.dn.se/sverige/hallengren-sverige-har-kommit-val-ut-ur-detta/ .

108 Paterlini, Marta. "What Now for Sweden and Covid-19?" *BMJ* 375:3081 (2021), www.bmj.com/content/375/bmj.n3081 .
109 https://coronakommissionen.com/publikationer/slutbetankande-sou-2022-10/ . Quotes from the report's Summary in English, https://coronakommissionen.com/wp-content/uploads/2022/02/summary_20220225.pdf .
110 www.dn.se/sverige/coronakommissionen-regeringen-borde-lyssnat-mindre-pa-folkhalsomyndigheten/ .
111 https://tt.omni.se/hallengren-om-kritiken-det-var-ratt-vagval/a/Or2w11 .
112 https://sverigesradio.se/avsnitt/1499446 .
113 www.hep.lu.se/staff/akesson/overdodlighet.pdf , www.altinget.se/artikel/relativisera-inte-synen-paa-manniskoliv, www.dn.se/debatt/overdodlighet-ett-svagt-matt-pa-pandemins-effekter/ .
114 https://tt.omni.se/fhm-s-generaldirektor-ratt-vara-forsiktiga/a/V92Kzp .
115 https://sverigesradio.se/artikel/tegmark-wisell-forsvarar-coronastrategin-avgorande-att-vi-tittat-pa-helheten .
116 www.kva.se/sv/pressrum/pressmeddelanden/vetenskapsakademien-bildar-expertgrupp-om-Covid-19 .
117 https://s3.eu-de.cloud-object-storage.appdomain.cloud/kva-image-pdf/2021/11/covidrapport_slutrapport_sammanfattning_211130_eng.pdf .
118 *TV 4*, 1 December 2021, www.tv4.se/klipp/va/13732043/lena-hallengren-s-vi-hade-trottnat-om-vi-infort-vaccinbevis-tidigare .
119 https://democracy.jcie.or.jp/wp-content/uploads/2020/08/Challenges-to-rule-of-law-democracy-and-human-rights-after-the-outbreak-of-COVID-19-from-a-Swedish-perspective.pdf .
120 www.ft.dk/da/aktuelt/nyheder/2021/01/udredning-om-covid_19 . In their extensive well-written analysis of Sweden's management in the Danish report's supplements (Bilag 4, pages 505–534), Carl Dahlström and Johannes Lindvall point at the specific Swedish system of power sharing between the Government and the Agencies, where nevertheless the Government is responsible for controlling the Agency and where "informal contacts" are an often used important instrument for communication. A journalist's request to take part of the (open accessible) mail correspondence between the Governmental Office and the FHM however was answered negatively in October 2020 as there had not been any such correspondence at all in the first wave. Nevertheless, daily lunches with FHM GD Carlson and governmental officers took place, as became public (cf. earlier). Obviously PM Löfven equipped the FHM with absolute power from the beginning and relied, as he often repeated, totally on "his" Agency. "It would have directly been a breach of duty in not to listening to the FHM," he answered in the Parliament's interrogation, without mentioning that he refused to listen to any other voices at all, www.dn.se/sverige/lofven-i-ku-beslut-om-strategi-saknar-betydelse/ . FHM GD Carlson put it this way: "It is we who are clearly holding the conductor's baton" (*taktpinnen*), www.dn.se/nyheter/sverige/sa-gick-det-till-nar-regeringen-gav-taktpinnen-till-expertmyndigheten/ .
121 Hydén, Håkan. "Corona – en rättspolitisk utmaning!" *Statsvetenskaplig tidskrift* (*The Swedish Journal of Political Science*) 123:5 (2021): 315–342, 338.
122 Baldwin. *Fighting the First Wave*, 61.
123 www.aftonbladet.se/nyheter/a/VqJ7pW/norges-och-sveriges-strategier-jamforda–sverige-doms-ut .
124 www.sydsvenskan.se/2021-01-02/lakaren-tog-betalt-for-att-porta-patienter-fran-sjukhusvard, www.sydsvenskan.se/2021-02-18/efter-hemliga-coronabesluten-lakaren-tas-omedelbart-ur-tjanst , www.sydsvenskan.se/2021-10-31/efter-sydsvenskans-avslojande-vardpersonal-misstanks-for-bedrageri . Even if this practice obviously represents a crime, nothing is brought into indictment. Merely the region complains and demands a financial compensation due to fraud. No patients or institutions report to the police. The health of human beings seems to have a dubious value in the region's health care.

125 www.dn.se/debatt/hur-nara-dodshjalp-har-coronavarden-av-aldre-varit/ . Doctor Johnny Ludvigsson (cf. earlier), however, opposes and claims the "individual's right to a worthy death", www.dn.se/debatt/skilj-pa-prioriteringar-palliativ-vard-och-eutanasi/ . Archbishop Antje Jackelén replicates stating that the way of treating a society's elderly offers a measure for trust and safety of all, www.dn.se/debatt/svenskar-daliga-pa-att-respektera-manniskor-over-70-ar/ . In a replica to columnist Hanne Kjöller's insinuations about elderly who want to die, www.dn.se/ledare/hanne-kjoller-var for-ryggar-vi-for-begreppet-vara-kvinnor-men-inte-for-vara-aldre/ , she reminds us about sociological data offering evidence about Sweden's ageism among the worst five countries in the world, www.dn.se/ledare/sveriges-kristna-rad-nekad-behandling-vacker-fragor-om-varderingar/ . Did *Der Spiegel*'s title "The Invited Death" (see earlier) summarize aptly what happened? Did Sweden sacrifice its elderly?

126 One can verify the fact that Sweden could have saved ca. 10,000–12,000 lives with another strategy in different ways, by mathematical modelling; by investigating the real effects of lockdowns, facemasks, and other NPIs; or by calculating the consequences of their absence in Sweden. The most reliable and simple way although is to compare Norway and Sweden as these countries offer a highly similar structure of demography. Confounding factors are slim. Medicine professors Dag S. Thelle and Gunnar Steineck have already shown how such an analysis provides us with a reliable facet for the first wave, www.svd.se/sverige-har-inte-fatt-till-en-stark-signal-mot-smittan , www.svd.se/vi-kan-genast-ta-till-oss-norges-framgangsfaktorer . The OWiD figures (in Chapter 2) indicate the surprisingly high difference in number of cases and death tolls. The Danish, Norwegian, and Swedish commissions have in their reports compared and analyzed the different outcomes of different measures. The number of 10,000 lost lives that could have been saved if Sweden simply would have responded in the same way as neighbouring countries therefore offers an epidemiologically reliable figure.

127 On the history of and reasons for officially denying the use of facemasks in Sweden see Einhorn. *Bland hobbyepidemiologer och expertmyndigheter*, 38–39. It was obvious that Tegnell simply had not understood the process of infection, refused to change his view, and therefore even declared facemasks as risk. Cf. www.svd.se/a/GG4K99/kan-nya-fakta-overtyga-fhm-om-munskydd , and www.expressen.se/debatt/nej-anders-tegnell-munskydd-hjalper-inte-bara-pa-marginalen/ .

128 www.dn.se/sverige/fakta-i-fragan-var-privata-aldreboenden-samre-an-kommunala-pa-att-skydda-de-aldre/ .

129 www.coronatimes.net/Covid-19-nordic-trust-collective-denial-sweden-norway/ . For a comparison of some epidemiological factors in the Nordic countries see https://journals.sagepub.com/doi/full/10.1177/1403494820980264 .

130 www.nrk.no/norge/ny-rapport_-noreg-burde-ikkje-ha-stengt-grensene-mot-dei-andre-nordiske-landa-1.15716396 .

131 Nakstad, Espen Rostrup. *Kode Rød: Kampen For Det Vakre*, Oslo: Gyldendal, 2021.

132 www.theguardian.com/commentisfree/2021/jan/03/swedish-model-failed-Covid-19 , https://medium.com/@barbara_c/how-the-mitigation-strategy-tempted-northern-europe-and-convinced-only-sweden-f6fb9197d49a .

133 Nakstad. *Kode Rød*, 69.

134 *Ibid.*, 99.

135 www.dagbladet.no/kultur/anklager-sverige–skummelt/74380162 . Tegnell responds in a strangely twisting way to the Norwegian criticism of Sweden's pandemic management, also from PM Solberg by postulating that "we are actually doing the same thing as Norway" but without locking down anything, www.dn.se/nyheter/sverige/norska-kritiken-jag-tror-sverige-gor-helt-fel/ .

136 Nakstad. *Kode Rød*, 206–207.

137 www.nrk.no/anmeldelser/anmeldelse_-_kode-rod.-kampen-for-det-vakre_-av-espen-rostrup-nakstad-1.15687297 , www.vg.no/rampelys/bok/i/qWmL7E/tam-og-feberfri-bokanmeldelse-espen-rostrup-nakstad-kode-roed , www.dagbladet.no/kultur/selvskryt-fra-nakstad/74378878 .

138 www.dagbladet.no/nyheter/sverige-har-tapt-43-073-levear/73165171 .

139 Aburto, José Manuel et al. "Quantifying Impacts of the COVID-19 Pandemic Through Life-Expectancy Losses: A Population-Level Study of 29 Countries", *International Journal of Epidemiology* (26 September 2021), https://academic.oup.com/ije/advance-article/doi/10.1093/ije/dyab207/6375510?searchresult=1 . Cf., www.svd.se/dramatisk-minskning-av-livslangden-i-sverige . Further studies of a large number of different countries' decreased life expectancy, www.nature.com/articles/s41598-021-83040-3 , www.bmj.com/content/375/bmj-2021-066768 , www.ncbi.nlm.nih.gov/pmc/articles/PMC8743065/ .

140 Cf. on the three economists' alleged "meta-analysis" pretending that lockdowns have no impacts at all, by scholars located in a dubious neo-liberal thinktank supported by the climate-sceptical Koch brothers, www.sciencemediacentre.org/expert-reaction-to-a-preprint-looking-at-the-impact-of-lockdowns-as-posted-on-the-john-hopkins-krieger-school-of-arts-and-sciences-website/ and www.tagesspiegel.de/wissen/was-ist-dran-an-der-us-studie-lockdowns-sollen-fast-keine-corona-todesfaelle-verhindert-haben/28031754.html . In spite of heavy criticism from a wide number of international experts, economist Lars Jonung postulates that this shows how Sweden did right, www.dn.se/vetenskap/forskare-nedstangningarna-raddade-nastan-inga-liv-alls/ .

141 www.dn.se/sverige/hallengren-sverige-har-kommit-val-ut-ur-detta/ , "Men en sak som är uppenbar är att svenska folket har kunnat hålla ihop när det verkligen gäller" (PM Magdalena Andersson) [One thing that is obvious is that the Swedish people have been able to hold together in a pinch], www.dn.se/sverige/statsministern-dags-att-oppna-upp-sverige/ , www.svd.se/tva-ar-som-visat-samhallets-styrka .

2

A TIMELINE OF EVENTS

December 2019 to February 2022

Sigurd Bergmann

This chapter presents an annotated timeline of the most crucial events, decisions and statements in the Swedish handling of the pandemic from December 2019 to February 2022. The events are listed chronologically in order to help the reader to get a better overview.[1]

The following images show the infection and death curves for both Norway and Sweden, since they are compatible on many parameters. When you look at the curve, I encourage you to imagine what might have happened if "the Norwegians [had] run Sweden's public health system," as Peter Baldwin suggests in his foreword.

Please note: the system of testing in Sweden was not fully scaled up until the summer of 2020, so the testing data for February–June period is unreliable. Despite the Corona Commission's sharp criticism of FHM's deficient statistics, the Agency stopped testing of fully vaccinated and children on the 1st of November 2021,[2] thereby making it difficult to monitor the fourth wave. As of February 2022 all testing has been discontinued, with the exception of people in select risk groups, people in health care and those in elderly care. This means that reliable monitoring of the virus is no longer possible.

In order to allow the reader to grasp the extent of the coronavirus spread in Sweden, I have also included the data for Norway in Figure 2.1. As Sweden and Norway are quite similar in many epidemiologically significant parameters and counter factors are relatively insignificant, one can get both a mathematically and epidemiologically reliable comparative image of what could have happened in Sweden if it would have simply applied the same pandemic response as its neighbour. Tegnell consistently refused to engage in such a comparison, using the quasi-argument that Norway (and sometimes Finland) is the deviant, not Sweden. He stated that it is too soon to do any sort of evaluation of who handled things best, despite the fact that one could do such a comparative evaluation week by week.[3]

DOI: 10.4324/9781003289364-3

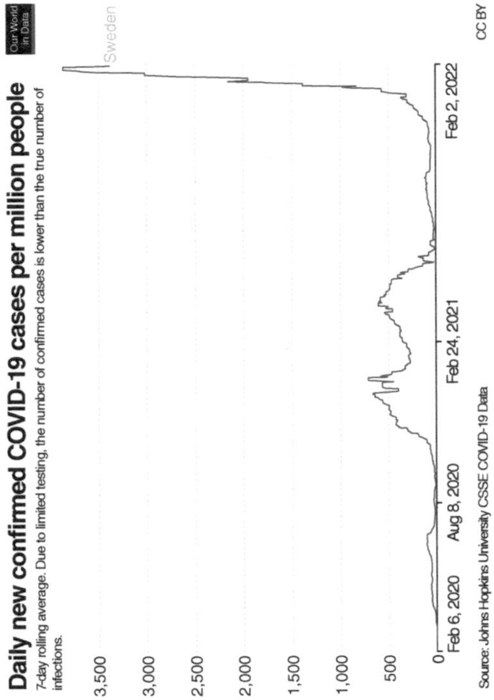
Daily new confirmed COVID-19 cases per million people
7-day rolling average. Due to limited testing, the number of confirmed cases is lower than the true number of infections.
Our World in Data
3,500
3,000
2,500
2,000
1,500
1,000
500
0
Sweden
Feb 6, 2020
Aug 8, 2020
Feb 24, 2021
Feb 2, 2022
Source: Johns Hopkins University CSSE COVID-19 Data
CC BY

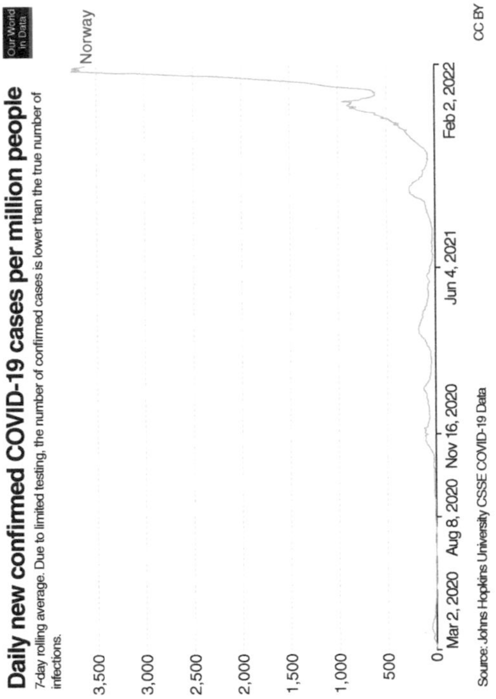
Daily new confirmed COVID-19 cases per million people
7-day rolling average. Due to limited testing, the number of confirmed cases is lower than the true number of infections.
Our World in Data
3,500
3,000
2,500
2,000
1,500
1,000
500
0
Norway
Mar 2, 2020
Aug 8, 2020
Nov 16, 2020
Jun 4, 2021
Feb 2, 2022
Source: Johns Hopkins University CSSE COVID-19 Data
CC BY

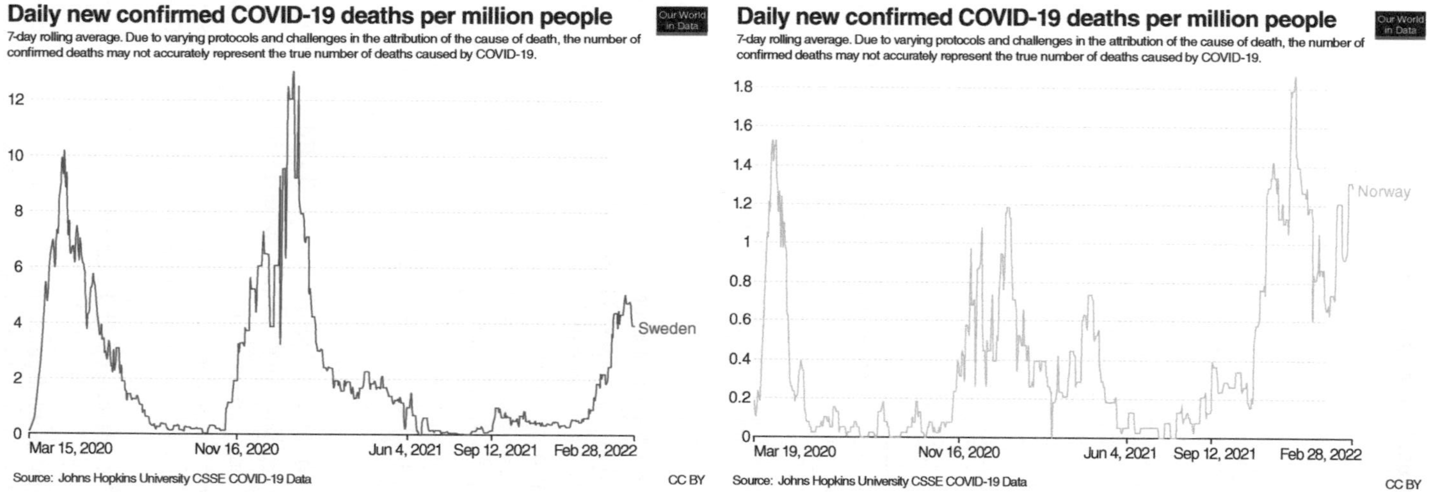

FIGURE 2.1 a) Daily new confirmed Covid-19 cases, b) Daily new confirmed Covid-19 deaths, c) Number of Covid-19 patients in hospital per million people, Sweden, Norway, February 2020–February 2022

Source: Hannah Ritchie, Edouard Mathieu, Lucas Rodés-Guirao, Cameron Appel, Charlie Giattino, Esteban Ortiz-Ospina, Joe Hasell, Bobbie Macdonald, Diana Beltekian and Max Roser (2020) – "Coronavirus Pandemic (COVID-19)". Published online at OurWorldInData.org. Retrieved from: https://ourworldindata.org/coronavirus [Online Resource].

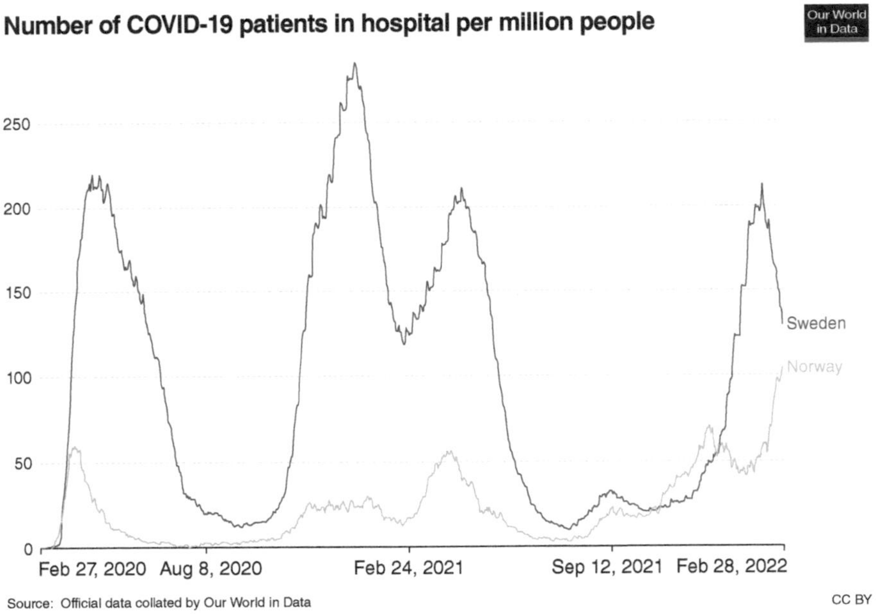

FIGURE 2.1 (Continued)

Recently the apologists for the strategy have proposed that Sweden has been more successful than other countries. Hereby they have cherry-picked which countries are in this comparison, which skews the data, ignoring the fact that Sweden has, in actuality, been overwhelmingly worse than others in many measures.[4] It is certainly not easy to compare different countries during the pandemic. However, there is no valid reason to refuse comparisons at all. It appears the reason for denying any comparison between Sweden and Norway is to deny one's own incompetence and to avoid shame. Will the state some day in the future do justice to this experiment's many victims?

19 December 2019, the Public Health Agency (FHM) published three documents about pandemic preparedness[5] which were to be seen as a "support for preparing for an influenza pandemic for government agencies, regional infection doctors, contingency managers, contingency coordinators, as well as operational and planning managers within the regions' and municipalities' health care systems."

31 December 2019, Sweden received the first report about a new virus outbreak in Hubei, China.

16 January 2020, FHM published an update stating that a new coronavirus was found in China. In an interview, chief epidemiologist Anders Tegnell said that he

did not believe that the virus outbreak in Hubei, China was similar to the SARS outbreak in 2003: "It is fully possible to break this infection spread," he declared.[6]

29 January, FHM published an update stating that they were following the situation with the virus.[7] They mentioned that they are in a close working relationship with the WHO, and that they will hold all the relevant workers informed. They also wrote that they would decide which measures are relevant. Tegnell held an interview with *Aftonbladet* where he denied the effectiveness of facemasks, and that the clinical picture they have of the virus is that it is very similar to influenza, and that it spreads like a normal influenza virus according to the calculations they have done.[8]

31 January, Sweden's first case.

1 February, the Government classified the virus as "generally dangerous infection" and "socially dangerous infection." Hereby also arbitrary measures became possible according to the infection law (even if one in the following history never applied any such legal sanctions).

5 February, FHM issued a statement: "In Sweden, most of the measures within infection prevention are taken without force. Experience shows that a well-informed and motivated person understands and follows the recommendations and that giving the individual personal responsibility is better than forced measures" as well as that they believed that the "risk for spreading within Sweden is still very low."[9]

23 February, Tegnell said that FHM had "no plans to test those who are travelling to Sweden from Italy, because that just is too complicated." And that FHM's "stance is that the risk for a large spread within Sweden is still low." He claimed that the spread in Italy was random chance, and that they did not have any information saying that the typical ski resort cities had had many infections.[10]

26 February, the second case in Sweden was confirmed, in a man who just returned from Northern Italy. One week later 62 new cases. Another 620 new cases a week after that. While many countries responded as quickly as possible, Sweden chose to remain passive. No lockdowns were executed, schools remained open, no borders were closed, visitors were not banned from the nursing homes, and no asymptomatic travellers were tested. Its measures were so mild that only Belarus, Iceland and Andorra had more mild responses. The tardiness in this "creeping crisis" could be explained by "psychological repression" and "cognitive delays";[11] nevertheless the procrastination was fatal. It might also have depended on the trio of FHM leaders' (verified) initial analysis that one could not stop the virus from spreading and therefore one should let it spread through the population at a reasonable pace in order to achieve natural herd immunity, an analysis that appeared to be applied during the entire first wave.

This was the same day that the first press conference, arranged by the FHM, was transmitted live on Swedish National Television and Radio. These would soon become an important part of the day for many Swedes, as from the 6th of March, daily press conferences were held until 17 May 2021, with a summer break 1st of

July to 17th of August, after which they became weekly. The daily press conferences kept the public well informed about the statistics about the spread of the virus, as well as FHM's views surrounding the situation. However, the FHM never communicated their strategy or the basis for their strategy during the press conferences. No underlying reasons for the strategy were communicated and GD Carlson called all criticism against Tegnell "indecent" (*ovärdigt*).[12] This came the same day as a report from *Dagens Nyheter* where they claimed that a hospital in Stockholm was already starting to become overwhelmed with patients (not all of them were Covid patients).

Asymptomatic infected travellers returning to the Stockholm region from skiing vacations in Northern Italy and Austria were not quarantined, but instead encouraged by the FHM to go to work and school.[13] Tegnell denied continuously until 2021 that travellers from the Alps imported the virus in February although this is well documented by the FHM's own sequencing analysis.[14] Italy reported "sustained community spread" in the country by 28 February, and many countries issued quarantine for returning travellers. The first returnees from skiing vacations came home to western Sweden the 16th of February.

7 March, the Swedish final selection event for the Eurovision Song Contest 2020, *Melodifestivalen*, took place in the Friends Arena in Stockholm, live with an audience of 27 000 spectators, after two ticketed rehearsals which also had live audiences. Denmark on the other hand, who held its final selection event on the same day, did so without a live audience. Also the international final Eurovision Song Contest 2020, planned for 12–16 May in Rotterdam, was cancelled.

10 March, FHM issued public advice to avoid visits to those in the hospital or elderly care homes.

11 March, first Covid-19 related death in Sweden. WHO declared a pandemic. Gatherings of more than 500 were banned.

12–13 March, Sweden's FHM strongly pressured the Finnish Public Health authorities and Finnish Government to not close their schools or lock down their society. They encouraged the Finnish authorities to follow the Swedish strategy. This information first became public in January 2021.[15]

13–19 March, FHM advice was to: avoid international travel, maintain distance, stay at home if feeling sick, work from home if possible, wash hands, implement distance learning at higher institutions.

13 March, the Government eliminated regular unpaid sick days in the national health insurance system. This was an efficient way of minimising social contacts as it allowed citizens to stay at home with their salary.

19 March, travel to Sweden was banned from countries outside the EU and Norway. Swedish citizens were allowed to enter without any restrictions. (While neighbouring countries under several periods closed their borders, Sweden only closed the border to Norway for a limited period, 25 January–1 March 2021, because of the appearance of a new virus mutation. Otherwise, Sweden kept its borders open.)

22 March, Prime Minister Stefan Löfven gave his first short speech about the virus to the nation where he talked about the threat to "life, health and jobs," predicted many deaths (without any expression of compassion) and declared the goal to keep the spread at a level that did not overload the health care system.[16]

23 March, more than 2000 scientists at Swedish universities signed a petition to the Government criticising the FHM's way of responding to the corona outbreak. Social minister Lena Hallengren expressed her appreciation and complete trust in the "expert agency," that is, the FHM.[17] The call for action was neither taken into account nor shared by media.

26 March, FHM's GD Carlson decided to stop registering every case, and instead left it up to doctors at a microbiological laboratory or doctors who decide about hospital care or elderly care.[18] This caused such a dramatic decrease in testing that it became impossible to follow the spread statistically. Scholars in law science have criticised this decision as an illegal violation of the infection control law without any mandate.[19] In his second instruction (28 April) Carlson made it optional for the legally responsible infection doctors in every region to register or let it be.[20] 24 September he instructed that henceforth only verified cases but no suspected cases should be registered.[21] The system of testing and tracing was in this way reduced to a minimum in the whole country. The only reason one can see for such a fatal and illegal decision was not to spend money on what the trio anyway regarded as useless, but to let the spread reasonably blow through the population.[22]

27 March, gatherings of more than 50 were banned.

30 March, visitors to the elderly care homes were banned.

1 April, the ECDC recommended timely and accurate testing, and on 8 April facemask use in the public to prevent asymptomatic transmission.

The same day as the report from ECDC recommending more testing, the FHM issued consolidated official "advice" to the public and businesses and organisations (HSLF-FS 2020:12): "The Public Health Agency's regulations and public advice regarding everyone's responsibility to prevent the infection of Covid-19 etc."[23] It contained advice for the public such as "avoid crowding in public spaces," "those over 70 should limit their social contacts," and "wash your hands"; as well as advice for businesses such as "provide hand sanitizer, and place markers on the floor indicating distance." Unfortunately while theoretically the advice in this document was obligatory, it lacked monitoring or enforcement mechanisms.

4 April, Tegnell claimed "herd immunity is the only way to stop the spread in any reasonable way. Measures can only reduce it for shorter periods."[24]

7 April, according to a quickly formulated proposition, the Government passed a specific mandate that was to be in place from 18 April–30 June 2020 that would allow them to issue harder infection control measures. These measures were never used. The mandate also gave the expert authorities at FHM a large influence over the strategic decisions to combat the virus. In fact, all power of pandemic management, characterised by a combination of "recommendations and free will," was hereby handed over to the FHM.[25]

April–September 2020, three times in the spring, summer and early autumn (without legal mandate), the FHM's GD Carlson issued the instruction to change the law's duty to register infected persons. The procedures of testing and tracing were hereby suspended as efficient tools. Instead of increasing its testing ability, access was often complicated with long waiting times. The number of infections was underreported and Sweden quickly lost control of the spread of the disease. Also, contact tracing was limited, although mandatory by the law. In most places the regional infection control physicians left contact tracing to the infected individual without follow-up. Quarantine was not recommended, not even for household contacts (until 1 October 2020, and only for adults). By ignoring testing, reporting, contact tracing and quarantine, Covid-19 was left to spread unnoticed at first.

14 April, 22 scientists working in different fields at Swedish universities published an opinion article in Sweden's largest newspaper, criticising the FHM's failure and demanding that the politicians take action to stop the spread.[26]

16 April, Tegnell expected that herd immunity would be achieved in Stockholm in May 2020.[27] Stockholm's population immunity showed in May only 10% of immunity rate after infection, and 2–5% in other regions.[28] Herd immunity was, according to Baldwin, "the get-out-of-jail card the Swedish authorities were counting on since they did not consider their citizens willing to tolerate extensive lockdown."[29] The WHO banned it as "unethical" in October 2020.[30] Tegnell, Carlson and Löfven have constantly denied having used the method of natural herd immunisation in spite of a large number of irrefutable verifications (cf. on the details in Emil J. Bergholtz's chapter).

24 April, the data now showed that the first wave peaked on this day, with a rolling seven days' average of 107.43 deaths.

1 May, Tegnell denied that the virus was imported by travellers returning home from Italy and pointed to other winter vacation destinations.[31] Experts in Norway and Sweden pointed out the slow introduction of strong and efficient measures early on as a decisive point of difference. These differences caused Sweden to begin with a higher number of people infected than its neighbours and the consequences became obvious. On 28th May, the former chief epidemiologist, Annika Linde, noted that the country had no actual strategy at all for preventing spread in the elder care.[32]

6 May, Tegnell announced the FHM's refusal to help The Swedish Civil Contingencies Agency (MSB) develop a corona warning app.[33] Although the MSB had invested 15 million crowns, the FHM rapidly scrapped the whole project.[34] Sweden is still one of only three European countries that does not have a corona detection app, and has no plans to put one in place.[35]

8 May, former chief epidemiologist and then FHM advisor Johan Giesecke postulated that the other Nordic countries will achieve the same high death tolls as Sweden within one year,[36] and that all the world inhabitants will be infected, of which 98% will not feel anything.[37]

7 June, leader of the Christian Democratic Party (KD) Ebba Busch accused the Government of allowing a comprehensive spread "*med berått mod*" (with deliberate

intention), when thousands of Swedes landed in February at Stockholm airport from areas with high spread, and then allowed them to walk freely into the society. PM Löfven said he preferred to wait before comparing deaths in different countries.[38]

(13 January 2021 Busch angrily and publicly revealed that PM Löfven had explicitly shared his intention to open for a larger spread of the infection "due to obvious advantages" with the other party leaders at his regular Corona meetings. Löfven denied this immediately; the other leaders stayed silent and only one politician from the Liberal Party dared to confirm Busch's statement.)[39]

8 June, *Vetenskapsforum Covid-19* (Science Forum Covid-19)[40] was founded by several of the 22 critical scientists and others, with 40 high-ranked scientists in the lead, circa 800 supporting members and a broad range of public activities educating the populace with video and social media channels, discussions, seminaries, press conferencing and debate articles. The Forum's mission is

> to save lives and prevent all forms of suffering in the Covid-19 pandemic. We aim to provide an unbiased assessment of the on-going scientific discussion to find the best path to handle the pandemic through scientifically informed and ethical decisions. The overall goal is to minimize the impact of Covid-19.

Many thousands of citizens, domestic and international media and scientists are following the Forum continuously.

17 June, Foreign minister Ann Linde defended the Swedish strategy in a remarkable interview with *Deutsche Welle* (DW), where she praised "the best strategy," admitting no failure in spite of the high death tolls, instead blaming the results on private elderly care homes, and proudly highlighting the population's high trust of the authorities.[41]

24 June, Tegnell described his feelings from the beginning of the pandemic during a popular radio talk show. He said he felt "as if the whole world has gone crazy"[42] in the springtime, when other countries had started to take measures to stop the spread of the virus.

(Staying "controlled and unaffected by press and stress," is by the way one of Tegnell's character traits – in the views of others close to him as one of his important individual skills to enable him for the demanding mandate. He did not regard caring for sick people in need of "fluff and compassion" as merited during his practice as clinical doctor, he told the journalist.)[43]

June–August, the FHM constantly indicated "low infection spread" during the summer although Sweden's rate was circa four times higher than neighbouring Nordic countries and Germany, and Norwegian epidemiologist Frode Forland characterised this as an "underlying spread" and accused Sweden of not taking any precautionary action.[44] Tegnell declared in summer that he did not believe in any second wave, and still in October he withheld that the on-going process was not a second wave but only an "increasing spread."[45]

30 June, the Government established the national Corona Commission with Mats Melin, Chief Justice and Chair of the Supreme Administration Court, as chair. (Löfven intended to establish such a commission later, avoiding the forthcoming election campaign in 2022, but opposition leader Ulf Kristersson and the other parties forced him to start this process of evaluation before the summer).[46]

1 July, travel recommendations eased, and restrictions for restaurants and cafés were removed.

21 July, 25 doctors and scientists in the Science Forum Covid-19 published an article in *USA Today* titled "Sweden Hoped Herd Immunity Would Curb COVID-19. Don't Do What We Did. It's Not Working."[47]

23 July, the FHM injunction (HSLF-FS 2015:4) about contact tracing, "Guidance for contact tracing of Covid," was replaced. This was the first of several changes to this injunction.

12 August, journalist Emanuel Karlsten published his investigative analysis of the FHM mail correspondence, verifying a desire to reach herd immunity was at the core of Sweden's pandemic strategy.[48] This was in addition confirmed in a mail published by former chief of the Health Agency's unit for infection protection, Peet Tüll, on 5 November.[49]

21 August, PM Löfven stated that he believed that his Government had done everything right and that Sweden's strategy was correct.[50] He refused to accept the criticism of the Government's handing over all the decisions surrounding crisis management to the FHM and said that he felt safe trusting the FHM.[51]

26 August, the Agency's three scenarios for the autumn failed totally with fatal underestimates when the second wave accelerated from October onwards.[52]

31 August, the FHM recommended for the first time that children with symptoms be tested for Covid-19.

23 September, Giesecke advised Ireland against pinning hopes on imminent advent of vaccine and to let coronavirus spread through the under-60 population. In his view his country's "soft lockdown" worked because the country trusted its people.[53]

24 September, Tegnell downplayed the risks for the already increasing wave as a "small increase," and misjudged the relative increase, missing again all possibilities to respond quickly and instantly. Instead he praised his own method as "sustainable" and successful due to citizens' "obedience" (which was falsified according to the MSB Agency's statistical surveys of behavioural change).[54] Twenty-six critical scientists had already accused the Agency by 17 August for not responding adequately to the risk of increasing spread when schools opened again.[55]

24 September–October, although the spread was increasing the Government in its decisions moved back and forth several times without any consistency with regard to the contagion,[56] by changing its decisions about the number of people allowed to gather (conforming to criticisms from cultural workers led by comedian Jonas Gardell). First, restrictions were maintained until 8 October but then the Government lifted these and allowed a maximum of 50 persons at restaurants and a maximum of 500 persons gathering in sports and cultural

events. Bars and nightclubs opened up and the spread increased worryingly by the end of October due to the opening and the Government's misleading crisis communication. As a response to the increase, PM Löfven declared first the end of larger gatherings but surprised Sweden then again by allowing max 300 persons at sport and cultural events. As expected the spread increased even more.

25 September, The Royal Swedish Academy of Sciences established its own expert commission (including former chief epidemiologist Annika Linde).[57]

1 October, the restrictions on visiting elderly care homes were lifted.

6 October, Tegnell rejected that the technology to measure virus levels in sewage plants, used by engineering scientists, could be used to help predict increasing spread.[58]

13 October, local/regional restrictions were allowed.

3 November, a max of eight persons were allowed at a restaurant table.

6 November, former Norwegian PM and former WHO head Gro Harlem Brundtland strongly criticised Tegnell and the FHM for their relaxed line, stating she was surprised that so many have followed them. She held the political leaders in Sweden responsible for the country's death tolls that were 10–20 times higher than the other Nordic countries.[59] Brundtland characterised the situation in Sweden as "unbelievable," and questioned why Tegnell could hold so much power in a country with a Parliament and a Government.[60]

15 November, former chief epidemiologist Annika Linde criticised Tegnell, who wrongly believed the country would have herd immunity to protect it from a second wave of Covid-19.[61] Linde had obviously changed her mind.

16 November, PM Löfven unexpectedly shared at a press conference some new restrictions that the Government had decided on, rather than the FHM. These restrictions included only allowing eight people to be in a group together at public events, and bars and restaurants were now required to stop selling alcohol after 10pm. Otherwise, as before, individual responsibility was urged as the best instrument for preventing the spread.[62] Otherwise, individual responsibility was urged again (as the best instrument in the "Wohlfühlstaat" (feel-well-state)).[63] By this constant praise and advising of individual responsibility two things were achieved; at first one could continue along the traditional path of so-called state individualism, that is the safe guaranteeing of maximum individual rights of freedom, and at second to ascribe most of the responsibility's success or failure to the individual while the national state and its lack of mandatory restrictions could go free.

Another surprise in November was that the so far not very much investigative but rather power-supporting media and journalists wakened up when the worst of the raging second wave harvested its victims. Obviously a majority of them, and more and more inhabitants, from now on understood that their total trust had been betrayed.[64] Supporting polls fell down from 82% (for FHM, 62% for the Government, May 2020) to 50.60% (58% FHM, 36% Government, January 2021), even if this loss of trust did not impact on the leaders' practice.[65]

22 November, PM Löfven held his second speech to the nation (of only two short speeches in the 20 pandemic months), where he encouraged every individual to take responsibility. "It depends on you and me."[66] In spite of recommendations to avoid shopping centres Löfven himself and also his Minister of justice Morgan Johansson visited these for Christmas gifts in December, rejecting any lapse.[67] Swedish Broadcasting later offered him a scene in a Christmas show where Löfven could perform as devoted to his wife, who ensured that her husband had followed coronavirus recommendations.[68] In spite of recommendations to avoid unnecessary travel Minister of Finance and Löfven's successor as PM Magdalena Andersson enjoyed winter vacation in a skiing resort.[69] MSB GD Dan Eliasson though was replaced after a vacation trip to the Canarias to visit his daughter.[70] While GD Carlson never had been questioned in his office at all until he resigned, Eliasson's replacement might be regarded as a fall guy.

24 November, the Health and Social Care Inspectorate (IVO) presented its report on the many cases of palliative instead of adequate Covid care, and on the state of the elderly cares. It stated that no regions had taken their full responsibility to offer safe and appropriate health care. Twenty percent of the patients who were doomed to palliative care/death had not received a doctor's individual visit and diagnosis. Health care laws for care in the final phase of life were violated. The report offered a horrible picture of avoidable suffering but the IVO did not take any action in handing over the cases to the legal authorities.[71]

24 November, alcohol was forbidden after 10pm in restaurants, and bars were told to close at 10.30pm.

1 December, PM Löfven denied all responsibility for the crisis in elderly care and the many deaths and passed this issue over to the regions and municipalities. Regarding the question of accountability, he referred to the forthcoming Corona Commission's report and declared that he did not want to repent of anything.[72]

15 December, the Corona Commission presented the first part of their report.[73] It states that the state failed to protect the elderly, that it should have taken actions to prepare the elderly cares. The Commission found that the regions and municipalities were partially responsible, but that the Government bore the utmost responsibility. The Commission emphasised that it undoubtedly was the high level of spread in society that caused many of the deaths.

17 December, the second wave's peak of deaths, rolling seven days' average reached 77.

On the same day, in the Royal family's traditional Christmas broadcast program, King Carl XVI Gustaf criticised distinctly that "the country has failed in its response to Covid-19."[74] The statement was very widely shared internationally, though without any reaction from the Government or Agency.

23 December, FHM began to recommend facemasks in health care institutions and elderly care homes.

24 December, a max of four persons were allowed at a restaurant table.

7 January 2021, the FHM recommended facemasks in rush hours on public transport when a seat could not be reserved. Public obedience was low, and not

controlled, and FHM GD Carlson himself was caught several times travelling without a facemask.[75] No one bothered about this, but many followed his example and left it at that.

Early January, vaccination started with the oldest persons, and continued its programme based on generation. (By 28 February 2022, it included 74.69% of the whole population.) From August 2021 younger people from 16 years of age were also included. Only Astra Zeneca from 25 March was given to persons 65 years or order (a praxis that by many is regarded as unethical and a violation of the law about equal health care); this was terminated 27 July. From mid-October 2021 children from 12 years age were also vaccinated (as the last country in Europe).

8 January, the Government passed an extension of the pandemic law valid from 10 January to 31 September (prolonged later to 31 January 2022). This gave them more extensive mandates to decide restrictions (for example regarding the number of persons gathering or opening hours). Some of the earlier recommended "norms" were now turned into "regulations."[76]

20 January 2021, the third wave's peak of deaths, rolling seven days' average reached 130.54. No new restrictions were decided for the third wave, and the Government insisted that Sweden was going to follow the same path as before. Tegnell, Hallengren and Löfven blamed individuals for not taking enough responsibility despite Löfven himself not following the restrictions during his Christmas shopping.[77]

9 February, *Sveriges Radio* (National Swedish Radio) reported about how they infiltrated a "hidden Facebook group" where critical scientists and citizens were portrayed as enemies of national security, and where methods (otherwise usual in the sphere of psychological defence) were practised by the Radio's science section leader Ulrika Björkstén in a way that raised serious issues about the media's public task and its alleged national and ideological independence. A large number of condemnations on serious media followed. Several complaints were issued. A wave of hate and threat was triggered by Björkstén's unobjective attack as a consequence. FHM GD Carlson took the chance and told the public about threats against his staff members, whereupon also critical scientists reported about all hate that they had been exposed to by public health nationalists. A large number of serious writers and journalists responded with critical questions about the FHM's disastrous crisis communication, the Swedish Radio's dubious involvement in preparing for a new national Agency of Psychological Defence, and damaging the freedom of opinion. Others were nevertheless panegyrising the national state and condemning its critics. According to the most acknowledged media experts the level of a decent public self-critical discourse in Sweden's pandemic management had reached its "*lågvattenmärke*" (low watermark) in this scandal.[78] Former TV4 chair and distinguished writer Jan Scherman uncovered the embarrassing role of FHM's leading press officer Christer Janson's role in manipulating and treating critical voices in the public debate.[79]

14 February, citizens were recommended not to travel unnecessarily; vacation trips to the skiing resorts were however unbanned. Public transport companies

were allowed to use only 50% of available seats on a bus or train. Region Stockholm experienced an increase of 25% of new cases three weeks later.

18 February 2021, Tegnell still denied the significance of pre- and asymptomatic spread although the FHM already noticed this as a threat in June 2020.[80]

25 February, the Parliament decided to recommend all members use facemasks in the chamber and the foyer, when one could not keep at distance. The recommendation was lifted 14 June.

11 March 2021, on the King's initiative the Royal family arranged a memorial liturgy at Drottningholm castle for the remembrance of the corona victims the last year, transmitted by Swedish Television. PM Löfven ignored this anniversary but promised on the same day to build Europe's best welfare state on his Facebook account.

25 March to 26 April, the Parliament's constitutional committee (*Konstitutionsutskottet*/KU) executed an official interrogation and presented its final evaluation of the Government's pandemic management on 3 June.[81]

27 March, PM Löfven banned public gatherings with more than 50 people, predicted more sick, bankruptcies, loss of jobs and lives, and urged everyone to take personal responsibility.[82]

20 April, Tegnell again denied the significance of asymptomatic spread and infectiousness.[83]

21 April, the National Board of Health and Welfare declared a state of emergency (in the on-going wave of infections) as serious; intensive care Covid patients had to be moved between different places due to an overloaded capacity.[84]

25 May, Lisa Bjurwald published a rich report on Swedish media as "investigators or megaphones of power."[85]

1 July, several of the restrictions in place were lifted. It was no longer mandatory to wear facemasks on public transport, and the limit for the number of people allowed at public gatherings was lifted.

From August, a fourth wave slowly accelerated, which mostly hit younger citizens and children. Patients in intense care were mostly unvaccinated. The delta variant was dominant and infected a larger amount of persons more rapidly. The FHM refused to vaccinate children and the Government refused to decide about a corona certificate allowing only the vaccinated to attend gatherings.

22 August, PM Löfven announced his resignation in November 2021, which was not due to his pandemic management.

23 August, the FHM presented three scenarios for the period 20 August–20 November 2021.[86]

19 September, the fourth wave's first peak of deaths, rolling seven days' average reached 10.1. Deaths among elderly occurred again, even among the vaccinated, as the spread had entered care homes again.

26 September, Löfven defended the Swedish corona strategy and repeated in an interview on CNN that he had done nothing wrong and that Sweden's pandemic management by no means could be regarded as a failure.[87]

28 September, the FHM decided to offer everyone over 80 years of age, and persons in elderly care (but not health workers), a third dose of vaccine.

29 September, most restrictions lifted (such as limits for gathering, and recommendations to work from home), the non-vaccinated were recommended to be careful and avoid meeting the elderly (without any control measures). The Government prepared for a vaccination certificate in case this might be needed. (Although many voices demanded to use such a tool, it was not practised in September–November, and Sweden "mixed" the vaccinated and unvaccinated without any control measures.)

30 September–13 December, The Swedish National Association for People with Intellectual Disability and The Swedish National Down Syndrome Association sent a first letter in September and a second in November to the FHM with a request to booster vaccinate these persons with much higher risks for severe disease and death; they had been vaccinated early with priority and evidence suggested they were lacking vaccine protection from 2021 September.[88] None of these letters was responded to by the Agency. Critical questions about the Agency's "contempt for the weak" were raised in the national debate 16 November.[89] Minister Hallengren announced 23 November that people with disabilities would receive booster vaccines in the near future. Conducting regional vaccination though was slow, and in Region Skåne (S. Sweden) it first started 13 December. No plan for booster vaccinating health workers at the institutions for individuals with disabilities was presented. The FHM's slowness thereby allowed four months to elapse where the country's disabled citizens had a lack of vaccine protection.

9 October, King Carl XVI Gustaf stated that the country's opening had gone "a bit too quick," and that it would have been better to move "slower but safer."[90]

12 October, the Government suggested prolonging the temporary pandemic law until 31 January 2022, and proposed changing it, so that it could no longer shut down and place limits on attendees at public gatherings.

21 October, the FHM presented new scenarios where they predicted a continued spread and stated that the Agency's present recommendations were sufficient for avoiding an increasing spread the next three months (until January).[91] Two weeks later this conclusion was also falsified by slowly but constantly increasing infections in the fourth wave. The rate of positively tested in Stockholm increased, for example, to 7.7.

27 October, the FHM decided to offer everyone over the age of 65 a third dose of vaccine. The regions prepared to start this vaccination in late November.

From October 2021 onwards the Royal family continued its series of visits to every single of the country's 21 regions in order to learn about the citizens' and local social bodies' experiences in the pandemic. No other national or regional institutions had so far shown such an interest for the people's experiences from below.

29 October, the national Corona Commission presented its second report which contained caustic criticism of the country's "shipwreck,"[92] resulting in an

intense debate in many media and fora. PM Löfven, Social minister Hallengren and GD Carlson rejected the points and refused to accept any criticism.

1 November, the testing and tracing of vaccinated persons was abandoned by the FHM. Reporting to the ECDC became unreliable this way, and OWiD has marked their statistics with a warning for the unreliability of Swedish statistics on new cases.[93]

1 November, FHM GD Johan Carlson retired and Karin Tegmark Wisell, former 2nd chief epidemiologist at the Agency, took office, after a secret selecting procedure.

3 November, Tegnell refused to offer a third vaccine dose to health care workers,[94] although the increase in breakthrough infections and the decrease of immunity levels after four to six months had been verified. His explanation sounded confused and power-crazed as Sweden had stored all too many vaccines so that the country could start immediately to protect the exhausted health workers. Many other countries were therefore offering such a dose in autumn 2021, and Israel had "boostered itself out" of worries of infections as half of their population had been vaccinated a third time and a demand for three doses for citizens to get access to cafés, gatherings, etc.[95] Sweden threw it away that health workers demanded to use for their third dose, but Tegnell played this down as "one always must expect some loss of vaccine in a program."[96]

4 November, WHO Head for Europe Hans Kluge criticised Sweden for lifted restrictions and demanded explicitly the use of facemasks in the whole society. Europe was again, with 49 (including the Vatican City State) countries reporting increasing infections, the centre of the world's pandemic, and the WHO expected half a million deaths in Europe until February 2022.[97] Many doctors and nurses were angry about the FHM recommendation to send children with symptoms to day-care, although the country suffered from a RS-epidemic and hospital resources were overloaded. The Agency responded that "they have landed in thinking this is a way forward."[98]

6 November, FHM GD Tegmark Wisell responded to the Corona Commission that the Agency "could not have done anything in another way" and that their emphasis was, in contrast to other countries, on several other aspects of "public health" rather than entirely on Covid-19.[99]

10 November, while Germany, Denmark, Norway and others were fighting worrying exponential growth of infections in the fourth wave, the number of cases in Sweden was increasing slowly. The FHM decided about booster vaccinations already after five months for all over 65 but still rejected them to risk groups[100] and health workers. According to Tegnell, Sweden should also prepare, even as he continued the slack passive style, though "we actually have not learnt much from earlier times about if it really helps to do things in advance."[101]

11 November, GD Tegmark Wisell postulated that the infection law did not allow testing of vaccinated persons, an interpretation that was refuted by several lawyers who accused her of violating the law.[102]

12 November, Tegnell alleged (again) that one could not compare Sweden to other countries due to the high number of immigrants and the urban density,[103] a statement that one rather must regard as fake, as national statistics in, for example, Norway and Sweden provide a different empirical view.[104] Although conscious about the fourth wave's threat he did not rely on the people's willingness to accept any restrictions (an assertion without any evidence as to other countries' polls, for example in Germany, which indicated 49% of the people demanded even tougher restrictions than those already practised).[105] A scenario worked out by Region Stockholm's epidemiologists predicted a number of 5 400 loss of lives in the fourth wave 2021/22.[106]

15 November, after GD Carlson and Minister Hallengren's rejection of the Commission's criticism, it was no surprise that Tegnell also refused to accept it, by stating that their conclusions were based on false grounds. As explanation, he argued with the tautology that Sweden's high death tolls therefore depended on a much stronger spread than other countries.[107]

16 November, a detailed study from Uppsala University, Norway's Public Health Agency and Sydney University[108] analysed the impact of public health interventions in the Nordic countries during the first year of SARS-CoV-2 transmission and evolution. It showed a clear substantial net export of the spread from Sweden to other countries due to the inefficient Swedish strategy. Among the Nordic countries, which all experienced a substantial virus import from Sweden, Finland received the majority of Sweden's virus export despite strict travel restrictions. A formal question on this in the Parliament was never answered by Minister Hallengren.[109]

25 November, the FHM allowed the regions to also give a booster dose of the Covid-19 vaccines to health care workers in specific situations. After strong criticism from politicians and union representatives Tegnell defended the decision to wait on the vaccination still for some time.[110]

26 November, the FHM recommended all travellers arriving by flight from South Africa, Lesotho, Botswana, Zimbabwe, Mozambique, Namibia and Eswatini to get tested after arrival.

30 November, The Royal Swedish Academy of Sciences' Expert Group on Covid-19 presented its detailed report with 11 various thematic chapters, including severe criticism of the Swedish strategy. The report offered many important lessons to learn from the failures and successes of the Swedish strategy.

30 November, the FHM recommended all travellers arriving by flight from any country except the other Nordic countries to test after arrival, but as Sweden had not established any information strategy a majority of travellers were not aware and did not get tested.[111] The first two omicron cases in Sweden were verified 29–30 November; 16 cases were discovered 9 December. 7.79% in all analysed sequences in Sweden were omicron by 13 December (OWiD). The emergence of the omicron variant would not lead to any major changes in Sweden's Covid response, according to Tegnell, who insisted that their strategy "has worked in the past."[112]

1 December, the FHM decided that a *Covid certificate* (verifying double vaccination, but not a former infection) must be used at gatherings indoors (cultural events) with more than 100 persons. Such gatherings could also take place without a certificate but they would be required to apply specific rules for social distancing. Restaurants, bars and training studios remained open without such a certificate. The Christian Ecumenical Council criticised this restriction due to an alleged conflict between the right of religious freedom and the need to ask believers to identify at the entrance, while Jewish and Muslim organisations did not see any problem at all and prioritised the regulation's positive effect on health protection. Christian churches could however decide locally if they wanted to follow the certificate regulation or the alternative one, whereby many were confused on the criteria how to decide. Many restaurants wanted to use the certificate but were confused by the FHM's unclear crisis communication.[113] The Swedish Work Environment Authority decided that national agencies (such as elderly care homes, universities, hospitals, etc.) could not demand Covid certificates from its employees or visitors. Unvaccinated health workers could in this way continue to take care of patients without any specific demand.

2 December, *Dagens Nyheter* reported on a super-spreader event which occurred two weeks prior, a Christmas dinner for 400 employees at a clinic of Sahlgrenska University Hospital in Gothenburg which had Tegnell as the guest speaker, where 20 persons got infected.[114]

2 December, Region Skåne re-established the demand of facemasks for employees, patients and visitors in the health care system.

7 December, in spite of different critical voices to vaccinate children from 5 year's age[115] the FHM refused to partake in any discussion or action.[116] Children between 12 and 15 years of age could be vaccinated from 2021 October. As many municipalities in November and December reported a steadily increasing number of infections at schools all over the country, it became obvious that schools were central drivers of the on-going infection, an observation constantly denied by the FHM. A reason against vaccination of children below 12 years of age is that they are very seldom seriously diseased, a point that has to be differentiated since more children would suffer seriously if the spread of the contagion was higher. More would suffer from the well-known children's long-Covid. As the Swedish decision makers in the Agency and Government proudly declared, also in the fourth wave, keeping schools open at any price was the right way. One must ask if the intention was rather to increase (unethically and illegally) natural herd immunity than to provide the best care for the children and their families. While Sweden was the last country in Europe to start vaccination of older children it remained among the very few who did not vaccinate children from 5 years of age. Cynical voices were pretending that Sweden's fourth wave was taking a less worrying course, owing to the children's high immunity level in combination with the many other formerly infected citizens. However, we do know about a relatively short-lived endurance of immunity after an infection, and we do know about re-infections with both the delta and the omicron variants.

7 December, FHM recommended its population a) to keep a distance from others, b) to avoid crowding in public transport and to use facemask if crowding could not be avoided (the decision was individual and not controlled), c) to avoid crowding in restaurants, d) to avoid crowding in working places, where employers should require vaccination and "to some degree" a work-from-home office "if possible." Many were not using facemasks on public transport and the FHM commented, "it is unrealistic to expect that all accept their recommendations the first day."[117]

9 December, the number of Covid hospitalisations increased quickly, and the number of available ICU beds decreased to 20%.

10 December, Health Workers Union (*Vårdförbundet*) criticised the regions for an all too slow rate of getting booster vaccinations to health workers. FHM put the blame on the regions, and the regions blamed the FHM for slow and diffuse planning and communication.[118]

10 December, the Swedish Council on Medical Ethics (Smer) arranged a webinar on "Priority setting in healthcare in pandemics and other situations of mass casualties" in honour of its award winner, Torbjörn Tännsjö, a long influential, utilitarian ethicist.[119] Tännsjö argued strongly for totally deleting the notion of human dignity from ethics, and supported his disciple Lars Sandman and the Swedish Health Agency's decision to practise triage in emergencies created by the pandemic according to the controversial QALY-method, that is, to apply the criteria of biological age (how that could be determined for a seriously ill patient) in deciding who will receive survival care and who will not.[120] Sandman refused to reflect on the method's legal implications (probably in conflict with the Constitution that, against the philosopher's vision, very well emphasises the equal value of every human's dignity), and at this point in the pandemic no one knew in fact how doctors in demanding ICU situations had applied the national instructions or followed their own sound reasoning and conscience. No statistics were available either, but anecdotes from the floor indicated that the philosopher's instruction did not become manifest.[121]

12 December, Tegnell denied again that there was any reason to change anything in the Agency's recommendations despite the omicron variant.[122]

12 December, the FHM recommended children with symptoms to return to their *Kindergarten* after a short time at home and could not see any risk for increased spread. This decision was strongly criticised by the Teachers' Association (*Lärarförbundet*).[123]

14 December, the number of new cases increased 30% compared to the last week. On average 2 733 persons had tested positive every day the last seven days. According to the FHM the number of infections had reached the highest level since May.[124] The FHM could not answer virologist and writer Lena Einhorn's question (in the ordinary press conference 16 December) concerning how many percentages of the omicron variant had been observed in the country in the last two weeks.

15 December, the FHM expanded its previous decision and recommended that from 16 December all travellers get tested as soon as possible after arrival.

16 December, all travellers from Europe and the Nordic countries must provide a Covid vaccination certificate upon arrival. Minister Hallengren and GD Tegmark Wisell declared that they "may present" new restrictions the next week.[125]

16 December, a group of merited lawyers and doctors criticised the FHM's lack of references and value-loaded formulations about "humanist worldview" and "holistic public health perspective" in a reasoning that was not compatible with legal demands for a national Agency's decision-making.[126]

16 December, only a minority of people were following the recommendations from the FHM concerning facemasks on public transport. Tegnell reminded the media about his and the Agency's doubts about the impact of facemasks, insisting that he preferred that people avoid crowds. He did not encourage the use of facemasks but referred to some selected studies on limited efficiency (which he misinterpreted, avoiding mentioning the overwhelmingly many positive studies).[127]

17 December, the number of new cases and the rate of hospitalisation were rising constantly and rapidly. Several hospitals were switching to crisis mode and ICU hospitalisations were increasing.

18 December, columnist Anna Dahlberg in *Expressen* referred to Tegnell's numerous failures, accused him not considering the people but defending his own anti-facemask decision, and discussed the Agency's responsibility for the testing chaos in the fourth wave.[128]

21 December, new recommendations from the FHM were to be applied from 23 December. Among these recommendations were: work from home when possible; avoid crowds; only seat guests at restaurants and bars; at gatherings a max. of 500 guests were allowed without required vaccine certificates, and distance demanded between groups; at gatherings with more than 500 people vaccine certificates were needed and a max. of 8 persons per group were allowed. From 24 December, mandatory seat booking for certain trains and busses was required. From 28 December, a max. of 50 visitors indoors at private gatherings was allowed; a mandatory negative PCR-test was necessary for all foreign travellers to Sweden older than 12 years without residence (Swedish citizens are recommended to test); it is recommended that children from 5 years and up with specific respiratory problems be vaccinated.

23 December, the Government announced its instructions for the FHM to arrange a national vaccination week in March 2022, without any information on what this might imply.

27 December, FHM warned about reliance on antigen tests.[129] After Christmas vacation the testing system collapsed in several regions, owing to the high spread of Covid-19 and other respiratory diseases. The test positivity rate rose to 19–26% in many regions at the end of the year and in Stockholm every third tested person was infected.

28 December, circa 60% of all new cases in Stockholm were infected with omicron, but FHM refused to publish its results on the proportion of the variant in positive tests.[130]

2 January 2022, Tegnell declared that no specific recommendations were needed for schools opening after Christmas vacation (other countries in Europe were

practising weekly antigen testing, facemasks, small groups and ventilation). The teacher associations questioned if it at all was possible to apply FHM recommendations to stay at distance in schools.[131] They were afraid of infections in every class after vacation, (i.e., after 10 January).

The number of new cases, the proportion of the highly infectious omicron (circa 30% late December), and the numbers of hospitalisation were increasing rapidly in an accelerating fourth wave. In some regions there was a doubling of numbers in a week, and several hospitals were switching to crisis mode. Skiing regions experienced a rapidly increasing spread, but no tourists were encouraged to cancel their vacation in the skiing resorts.[132]

5 January, Social minister Hallengren decided to enact the (non-mandatory) use of vaccine certificates from 12 December at restaurants and bars, private and cultural gatherings, shopping malls, and long-distance public transport. (No facemasks, no vaccination of 5–12-year-old children, and no law for mandatory vaccination of health workers were planned.) Records of daily reported new cases were set at 17 320 (4 January) and 23 877 (5 January).

9 January, many experts had begun to question the FHM's scenarios from 21st of December, where the worst indicated number, 13 376 cases, was to be on 12 January, a number which was already passed on the 29th of December. The Agency predicted a decline of infections in mid-January due to herd immunity, a development that seemed totally unrealistic considering the steep increase of new cases. In spite of all critics the Agency withheld that the contagion is "still within the frames of our scenarios,"[133] a statement which later would be proven false. A large number of hospitals need to switch to crisis mode because of the rapidly increasing admissions.

10 January, the Government stated a worsened situation in the increasing spread and 40% more hospital admissions the previous week and announced new restrictions. PM Andersson demanded an "exertion of force" by all. From 12 January:

- If possible work at home.
- Gatherings of more than 20 persons were for only seated groups of max. eight persons (except religious meetings where one could also stand); for more than 50 persons a vaccination certificate was needed.
- Restaurants were required to close at 11pm, max. 8 persons in a group.
- Avoid private parties, etc.
- Higher education should take place at distance but not always.

Although the Government and the Agency underlined the seriousness of the situation the restrictions seemed to be rather weak than (allegedly) strong. No facemasks were recommended; no vaccination of children 5–11 years, no specific restrictions for schools and day-care centres, no plan for increasing the number of vaccinations (73%), no obligation for health care workers to be vaccinated were imposed, and there was no strategy for protecting vulnerable groups. The leaders stated a central objective was the protection of the threatened health care system, not the protection of individual suffering, sickness and death. Liberal right-wing party leader Nyamko Sabuni criticised the restrictions in general and argued for withdrawal of the pandemic law and removal of power from the Government to the Parliament, and the young conservative politician's student groups refused to follow the restrictions.[134]

11 January, the number of new cases exploded and climbed to records that far exceeded the FHM's worst scenario (18 661 new cases by 11 January instead of the predicted 13 300). In Region Skåne (southern Sweden) for example, the number of new cases rose to 55% compared to the foregoing week. GD Tegmark Wisell emphasised that their scenarios never intended to offer a prognosis. The number of hospitalised patients climbed from 723 (1 January) to 1 241 (11 (January). The demand for a negative test for all travellers at entry was lifted again.

12 January, the political debate in the Parliament opened up; the recent restrictions were criticised as unmotivated, and the prolongation of the pandemic law was questioned. The PM and two of the party leaders were infected at the session.

13 January, the FHM presented two new scenarios with 69 000 infected daily at its worst. In contradiction to what was known in science the Agency assumed 100% immunity of all infected earlier. Tegnell warned against a "dramatic infection increase" but indicated some hours later he would examine whether the pandemic could be downgraded as no longer "dangerous for the society" after the omicron wave.[135] Apparently, he and his Agency were (again) banking on natural herd immunity (a method that international experts strongly advised against),[136] as he repeated that it "for a long time has not been our intention to stop the contagion."[137]

14 January, Minister Hallengren was called to the Parliament's social committee to explain why the Governmental Office refused to hand over documents to the Corona Commission.

18 January, the spread increased with new case records, doubling the year's second week. The test positivity rate in the Stockholm region was 58.5% (18 January 2022). Testing worked unsatisfyingly in many regions; schools and day-care had to shut down due to outbreaks, many workers in the society's critical infrastructure were infected or quarantined. The spread also reached elderly care homes. Even if omicron led to less serious sickness, its rapid increase overwhelmed the hospitals' capacity where both vaccinated and unvaccinated were cared for. Death tolls were rising in analogy, even if ICU patients remained few.

20 January, due to the loss of employees in many sectors of public life: quarantine regulations were reduced by the FHM from seven to five days. School classes were not any longer sent home if anyone was infected. Although the FHM did not recommend facemasks, some infection doctors in the regions decided to do so. Also, the national rescue forces instructed their workers to use them.

19–21 January, the populist right party (The Sweden Democrats/SD) brought a charge against Minister Hallengren to the Parliament's Constitutional Committee (KU) for withholding documents surrounding the pandemic strategy from the Corona Commission. Hallengren had declared that protocols from the Crisis

Group's 149 meetings did not exist, but a civil servant showed these to a columnist, and the Governmental Office finally allowed the Commission to take part of these. Heated debates in the media were rising. 28 January, the right-wing opposition party (*Moderaterna*) also brought a charge against PM Andersson to the KU for "darkening for the Commission."

20 January, FHM shortened the time for family quarantine to five days, and prioritised PCR-testing.

22 January, several thousand citizens demonstrated, including groups of right-wing extremists, in Stockholm and Gothenburg against vaccine certificates.

25 January, Swedish health care had carried out 169 000 fewer surgical operations in the pandemic with tens of thousands of patients queuing. Circa 280 000 new cases (of Sweden's total circa 1 992 990) had been reported the previous week (whereby many private antigen tests were not included).

26 January, in a press conference Hallengren and Tegmark Wisell stated there was an "extreme spread" at present and for the next two weeks, and due to the limited testing one could only estimate that circa half a million persons were being infected every week. The restrictions were prolonged for two weeks, and lifting most of them was announced for 9 February.

27 January, despite many countries within the EU and the US already vaccinating children, the FHM declared their decision not to vaccinate children from 5–11 years of age. Teachers told about chaotic situations in schools and their constant anxiety. Many families experienced infections and felt like they were getting left in the lurch. According to critical voices the hospitalisation of children increased worryingly in the omicron wave, including increasing secondary diseases of diabetes and MIS-C, a fact disregarded by the Agency.

28–31 January, the fourth wave's peak of new cases, rolling seven days' average reached 40.27 (probably much higher due to unsatisfying testing).

3 February, PM Andersson announced the lift of most of the restrictions, including travel restrictions, from the 9th of February, and FHM asks the Government to downgrade SARS-CoV-2 as a disease no longer "dangerous for the society." It was still recommended for unvaccinated individuals to abstain from large gatherings, and stay home when they have symptoms.

6 February, GD Tegmark Wisell announced the decision to terminate testing starting 9th February, with the exception of symptomatic health workers and patients, due to the "non-defendable economic cost."[138] Experts in the Science Forum Covid-19 and others objected.[139]

9 February, the Government suggested the Parliament downgrade SARS-CoV-2 as an infection no longer dangerous for the society from 1 April, which was the same date that the pandemic law was set to expire.

9 February, most restrictions were lifted, a decision that gained some outrage from doctors, and people in risk groups, although the number of patients in hospital care climbed up to 2 220 (cf. peaks of 2 252 in the first wave, 2 998 in the 2nd, and 2 164 in the 3rd wave), although circa ten times as many children (0–9 years) were admitted to hospital care, including ICUs, as in earlier waves, and although

children younger than 5–12 years were not vaccinated, 25.4% of the whole population was unvaccinated. Experts and representatives for people in medical risk groups objected.

10 February, FHM official Sara Byfors explained the Agency's recent decision to limit testing to those in health care and elderly care as well as a small set of those in risk groups. According to Byfors, testing did not add anything in relation to its costs; it was most likely that every person with symptoms was infected, and one "has to live with not knowing" about the wave's peak of infections. Because of the existing immunity after infection and vaccination the Agency did "not believe that it will get much worse."[140] The FHM's "belief" in immunity though should be seen in correlation to omicron's significant ability to cause re-infections, where in Sweden it became common for more and more to be re-infected.[141]

14 February, the FHM recommended a fourth vaccination dose for people above 80 and people in elderly care.

17 February, due to the very high level of infections one could notice in the recent weeks: a) a constant rise of death tolls, b) a sharply rising number of children admitted to hospital care[142] and c) an ever-increasing number of hospitalisations. The FHM and associated doctors pointed at the fact that many are admitted with and not because of Covid-19 (supposedly also true for many deaths), pretending cynically that these figures were not worrying. But as far as no differentiated statistics were offered and general testing had been closed down, the public discourse on the suffering in the fourth wave's extremely high spread was covered by a smoke screen. The situation is similar to that of Denmark, where all restrictions were lifted 1 February and the number of infections, hospitalisations and death tolls have constantly risen. While experts in the USA and Germany sharply criticise this strategy, those in power in Denmark refer to the mostly mild disease processes.[143] Neither in Sweden nor in Denmark was the risk of many expectable long-Covid cases discussed in the context of the wave's decidedly large spread. No strategic plans for the pandemic future were discussed, by those in power or in public debates.

17 February, the fourth wave's peak of deaths, rolling seven days' average reached 52.5.

20 February, the willingness to be vaccinated subsided considerably in all regions due to the FHM's lift of restrictions.[144]

21 February, the FHM presented two scenarios for the spring, where they anticipated either no new variant after omicron, or a new infectious variant causing a new wave.[145]

25 February, the National Corona Commission presented its final report (cf. Chapter 1). In stark contrast to Minister Hallengren and GD Tegmark Wisell's beforehand public asseverations that all pandemic management has been suitable and successful,[146] the report expressed sharp criticism of several aspects of the pandemic management strategy, including the Government's handing over of power to the FHM. Hallengren and Tegmark Wisell denied accepting any criticism.

25 February, in contrast to the Commission's praise of health workers, a survey with chief doctors responsible for Sweden's Intense Care Units revealed severe

consequences with tough prioritisations and worryingly decreased quality of health care when the country's ICUs were forced to escalate. Health workers reported about long-term chronic exhaustion, which caused a large number to resign.[147]

In March the FHM announced that Tegnell would soon work as a vaccine expert at the WHO. Tegnell left his position as chief epidemiologist the 14th March and was, after an internal staffing, replaced by FHM officer Anders Lindblom. After a short time the FHM announced surprisingly that Lindblom would retire 30 June.[148] Later in April the FHM declared that they had not come to an agreement with the WHO, and that Tegnell instead would work with international issues at the Agency.[149] He was sure that the WHO "not at all regards Sweden or him as controversial" and looks "even more" forward to his new mission, that is, to assist other countries in establishing Government public health agencies.[150] I beg to differ, wondering if his merits at the FHM really qualify for strengthening other countries' public health.

The fourth wave slowly waned in spring (although one could not follow it clearly due to FHM's ceased testing), but in late April the dominant omicron BA.2 variant caused a new rise of infections.[151] No children from 5 years of age were vaccinated, a fourth booster vaccination was offered only to people from 65 years of age (not to risk groups, except those with serious immunodeficiency), and deaths were falling from 52.5 in February to 24.8 in April (according to OWiD). The number of vaccinated citizens stagnated after February, and only 75.06% of the whole population was fully vaccinated (14 April 2022).

I hope that this commented timeline can offer some understanding of the dramatic history that took place in the country during the pandemic. Sweden was of course not alone in navigating more or less badly in the stormy ocean of SARS-CoV-2, and not everything that Sweden did was wrong.

Understanding the threat and the preparedness of individuals to change their behaviour was impressive to experience in the country in early spring 2020. Initially, the emergence of creative solidarity practised in neighbourhoods also awakened hope. Many state-independent associations and organisations for example practised harder restrictions than what was recommended: first, gatherings were restricted to a maximum of 500 and somewhat later restrictions of a maximum of 50 were recommended. The promising start, however, turned quickly into an attitude that now our good welfare state will "fix it all" for us. Tegnell was quasi-religiously adored as some kind of saviour, and all traditional faith communities kept silent with regard to the idolatry.[152] It was sad to follow the quickly increasing conformist and patriotic attitudes, rhetoric and practices, where critics of the state were ridiculed, silenced, threatened and excluded. The former high-trust society turned into what Gina Gustavsson analyses as blind patriotism, and as history goes on the leaders' misuse of this high trust turned into withdrawal of trust, sadness, retirement and loneliness. Processes of shame and the violent aggression to avoid shame by admitting failures have done much harm to the country, a theme that I will explore in one of the following chapters.

Notes

1 As main sources for this timeline I have used:

- The overview in the Swedish ESCAPE report (Figures 2ab, op. cit.).
- Johan Ekman. "Hur blev vi pandemins försökskaniner?" [How did we become experiment rabbits?], *Aftonbladet*, 9 July 2021, https://special.aftonbladet.se/coronastrategin .
- https://coronadokumenten.miraheze.org/wiki/Huvudsida .
- Marina Ghersetti and Tomas Odén, *Coronapandemin våren 2020: En undersökning av nyheter och opinion*, https://rib.msb.se/Filer/pdf/29525.pdf .

  Coronapandemin: Den andra vågen, Swedish Radio's investigation of the second wave in two parts, 13 and 14 April 2021, https://sverigesradio.se/avsnitt/1706454 , https://sverigesradio.se/avsnitt/1706750 ,

  https://emanuelkarlsten.se/tegnell-mejlen-sa-fick-flockimmuniteten-faste-hos-folkhalsomyndigheten/ .
- https://tegnellcitat.se/ .
- https://floderochtekoppar.blogspot.com/2021/09/pod-med-alla-fyra-delar-av-sveriges.html?m=1 , Four podcasts on Sweden's pandemic management by a well-informed scholar in technical physics (earlier active in developing systems for the National Disease Institute), who describes and discusses the rationality, reasoning and communicating of the strategy by those in power. Explored in detail are themes such as delayed responding; ignoring international and scientific knowledge; heroisation of Tegnell; blind conformism; fatal misjudgement in many contexts; lack of transparency; ambivalent handling of evidence, facts and science; contradictory judgements, failed prognoses and unrealistic calculations; individual prestige of never changing one's view; passive government; history revisionism; construing and communicating false images of reality; herd immunity; absence of accountability and more. In 2.23 hours the author explores and depicts the central characteristics of the FHM's underlying pathology.

2 http://web.archive.org/web/20211026075646/www.folkhalsomyndigheten.se/smittskydd-beredskap/utbrott/aktuella-utbrott/covid-19/skydda-dig-och-andra/det-har-galler-fran-den-1-november/ .

3 www.svt.se/nyheter/inrikes/tegnell-kommer-agna-manga-ar-for-att-se-vad-de-ratta-atgarderna-var .

4 Anderberg postulated that in November 2021, 50 countries had bigger death tolls than Sweden and that excess mortality rates placed Sweden in position 21 of 31 countries in Europe (a continent that in fact includes 44 countries). Hereby he sadly verified the famous saying that you can prove everything you want with statistics. He insinuated that media tendentiously ignored his figures in order to maintain their image of Sweden as the bad guy, www.sydsvenskan.se/2021-11-01/katastrofen-som-aldrig-kom . The freelance journalist's decided opinion was that Sweden never experienced any "catastrophe" and that all talk about average, failure and disaster lacked any empirical evidence. Rodney Edvinsson analyses in his chapter how insufficient (and often also unethical) the use of (cherry-picked) excess mortality statistics is, and the 10 000 who have died due to the Swedish strategy will not have any comfort or justice if they are compared by Anderberg with deaths in another period of time. What Anderberg ignored is that with regard to excess mortality, Sweden was among the worst 23% in the world when comparing all countries. Additionally, in the fourth wave during the autumn of 2021 more lives were lost (although on a different scale due to the number of vaccinated inhabitants) than in other comparable countries, as the decision makers did not learn anything from failures and continued their inefficient method of avoiding testing, tracing and measures as much as possible. Social Democrat columnist Anders Lindberg drew on Anderberg's misleading interpretation and argued for excluding the country's pandemic management from the forthcoming election campaign, as one could not have done anything otherwise

anyway. Humans die, that's it, www.aftonbladet.se/ledare/a/1OW4lG/anders-tegnell-blir-inte-hogerns-trumfkort-2022 .

5 www.folkhalsomyndigheten.se/publicerat-material/publikationsarkiv/p/pandemiberedskap-hur-vi-forbereder-oss-ett-kunskapsunderlag/; https://www.folkhalsomyndigheten.se/contentassets/b6cce03c4d0e4e7ca3c9841bd96e6b3a/pandemiberedskap-hur-vi-forbereder-oss-19074-1.pdf; https://www.folkhalsomyndigheten.se/contentassets/2f2a536f14e54a83b983594b4b71c3d4/pandemiberedskap-kommunicera-19074-2.pdf; https://www.folkhalsomyndigheten.se/contentassets/1c7ea06c959541c0bfac32ed4f92f73c/pandemiberedskap-tillgang-anvandning-lakemedel-19074-3.pdf

6 https://sverigesradio.se/sida/artikel.aspx?programid=1650&artikel=7385928 .

7 https://www.folkhalsomyndigheten.se/nyheter-och-press/nyhetsarkiv/2020/januari/folkhalsomyndigheten-foljer-utvecklingen-kring-det-nya-viruset-i-kina/; Aftonbladet: https://www.aftonbladet.se/nyheter/a/XgBO3B/det-har-vet-vi-om-coronaviruset

8 www.aftonbladet.se/nyheter/a/WbBgwL/kinesiska-viruset-har-spridits-till-flera-lander–aven-via-manniskor .

9 www.folkhalsomyndigheten.se/nyheter-och-press/nyhetsarkiv/2020/februari/information-om-karantan/ .

10 https://tt.omni.se/anders-tegnell-slump-att-italien-drabbats/a/9vQWqr .

11 Ekengren, Magnus, Alina Engström, and Mark Rhinard. "Coronapandemin – en smygande kris vintern 2020", *Statsvetenskaplig tidskrift* (*The Swedish Journal of Political Science*) 123:5 (2021): 33–66.

12 https://lakartidningen.se/aktuellt/nyheter/2020/03/johan-carlson-kritiken-mot-tegnell-ar-narmast-ovardig/ .

13 www.krisinformation.se/en/news/2020/february/information-for-travellers-concerning-the-new-coronavirus .

14 https://bulletin.nu/historierevisionism-om-coronahanteringen .

15 www.hbl.fi/artikel/sitra-beslutsfattandet-har-fungerat-relativt-bra-under-coronakrisen-aven-om-starten-var-improvise/ .

16 www.regeringen.se/tal/2020/03/statsministerns-tal-till-nationen-den-22-mars-2020/ .

17 www.dn.se/nyheter/sverige/forskare-i-upprop-till-regeringen/ .

18 www.folkhalsomyndigheten.se/contentassets/4e0a7e97fe654fa2b9d28ace831c185f/hslf-fs-2020-10.pdf .

19 www.altinget.se/artikel/experter-sveriges-smittskyddslag-har-inte-efterfoljts .

20 www.folkhalsomyndigheten.se/contentassets/4e78ed361f164d29a9128481d1384477/hslf-fs-2020-23.pdf .

21 www.folkhalsomyndigheten.se/contentassets/6250183ea135423f8ed6f20c86ef2d04/hslf-fs-45-2020.pdf .

22 The Swedish Press Agency *TT* reported 15 March that "the time for stopping the virus has gone, and epidemiologists begin to understand that this virus is here for to stay. It will not fade away before a majority of all Swedes have been infected." Leader of the Christian Democratic Party (KD) Ebba Busch accused the Government in June 2020 for having opened up for a comprehensive spread "*med berått mod*" (with deliberate intention) and 13 January 2021 she angrily revealed to the public how PM Löfven had shared his intention to open for a larger spread of the infection "due to obvious advantages" with the other party leaders at his regular meetings. Löfven denied this immediately, the other leaders stayed silent and only one politician from the Liberal Party dared to confirm Busch's statement, www.svd.se/kontroversiell-strategi-som-kan-radda-liv , www.svt.se/nyheter/inrikes/bush-regeringe-tillat-smittan-att-spridas , www.youtube.com/watch?v=iJWqmGi_yjI .

23 www.folkhalsomyndigheten.se/contentassets/0ac7c7d33c124428baa198728f813151/hslf-fs-2020-12u.pdf .

24 https://svenska.yle.fi/artikel/2020/04/04/nej-sveriges-strategi-ar-inte-flockimmunitet-men-flockimmunitet-ar-enda-sattet (TV interview with reporter Marianne Sundholm, Finland's Broadcast *Yle* in Sweden).

25 www.altinget.se/artikel/fhm-onskade-och-fick-avgorande-inflytande-over-regeringens-beslut .
26 www.dn.se/debatt/folkhalsomyndigheten-har-misslyckats-nu-maste-politikerna-gripa-in/ . Cf. on how this and all further reflections were not heard at all in the following year, www.dn.se/debatt/vi-var-22-oroade-forskare-som-ville-na-de-politiskt-ansvariga/ .
27 https://twitter.com/ar_Covid/status/1374291554127466501 .
28 www.folkhalsomyndigheten.se/nyheter-och-press/nyhetsarkiv/2020/juni/forsta-resultaten-om-antikroppar-efter-genomgangen-Covid-19-hos-blodgivare/ .
29 Baldwin, Peter. *Fighting the First Wave: Why the Coronavirus Was Tackled so Differently across the Globe*, Cambridge: Cambridge University Press, 2021: 150.
30 https://news.un.org/en/story/2020/10/1075232 .
31 www.dn.se/nyheter/sverige/tegnell-italienresenarer-var-inte-den-stora-introduktionen-i-sverige/ .
32 www.svt.se/nyheter/inrikes/annika-linde .
33 www.svt.se/nyheter/inrikes/anders-tegnell-vi-har-for-stor-smittspridning-for-att-anvanda-corona-app .
34 www.expressen.se/nyheter/msb-utvecklade-app-for-15-miljoner-blev-stoppade/ .
35 https://ec.europa.eu/info/live-work-travel-eu/coronavirus-response/travel-during-coronavirus-pandemic/how-tracing-and-warning-apps-can-help-during-pandemic_sv .
36 www.dn.se/nyheter/sverige/giesecke-om-ett-ar-ar-ovriga-norden-i-kapp-sveriges-dodstal/ .
37 https://twitter.com/ar_Covid/status/1376956277612503044 .
38 www.svt.se/nyheter/inrikes/bush-regeringe-tillat-smittan-att-spridas .
39 www.svd.se/kontroversiell-strategi-som-kan-radda-liv , www.svt.se/nyheter/inrikes/bush-regeringe-tillat-smittan-att-spridas , www.youtube.com/watch?v=iJWqmGi_yjI .
40 https://vetcov19.se/en/ .
41 www.dw.com/en/swedens-fm-linde-we-managed-to-flatten-the-curve/av-53846751 .
42 www.svt.se/nyheter/snabbkollen/tegnell-som-om-varlden-blev-galen-1 .
43 Anderberg, Johan. *Flocken*, Stockholm: Bonniers, 2021: 35. Giesecke, who enthroned Tegnell, "his boy," at the FHM position appreciated most about Tegnell that he was totally "unpolitical," that is, "not affected at all by what others regarded as opportune" (36, 38). As mentor Giesecke also assisted Tegnell in finalising his PhD on heart surgery. With regard to epidemiology Tegnell had only passed a distance education where he used the double time (four years) in which to take his exam.
44 www.dn.se/sverige/fhm-raknar-med-lag-smittspridning-i-sommar/ , www.expressen.se/nyheter/coronaviruset/norge-ni-har-inga-atgarder-mot-det/ .
45 www.dn.se/sverige/tegnell-okade-smittspridningen-ar-inte-en-andra-vag/ .
46 www.regeringen.se/pressmeddelanden/2020/06/mats-melin-leder-coronakommissionen/ , www.dn.se/nyheter/sverige/lofven-coronakommission-tillsatts-innan-sommaren/ .
47 https://eu.usatoday.com/story/opinion/2020/07/21/coronavirus-swedish-herd-immunity-drove-up-death-toll-column/5472100002/ .
48 https://emanuelkarlsten.se/tegnell-mejlen-sa-fick-flockimmuniteten-faste-hos-folkhalsomyndigheten/ .
49 www.svd.se/fhms-tidiga-strategi-var-flockimmunitet .
50 www.dn.se/varlden/bolsonaro-till-attack-mot-coronautredning-har-gjort-ratt-fran-forsta-stund/ .
51 www.dn.se/nyheter/sverige/lofven-coronakrisen-har-skapat-stora-revor-i-valfarden/ .
52 www.folkhalsomyndigheten.se/publicerat-material/publikationsarkiv/s/scenarier–tre-smittspridningsscenarier-inom-regeringsuppdraget-plan-infor-eventuella-nya-utbrott-av-Covid-19/ , www.svt.se/nyheter/inrikes/svt-granskar-hosten-blev-varre-an-folkhalsomyndighetens-varsta-scenario-1 .
53 www.irishtimes.com/news/health/let-coronavirus-spread-through-under-60-population-d%C3%A1il-committee-told-1.4361858 .
54 https://sverigesradio.se/avsnitt/1706454 .

55 www.dn.se/debatt/coronaoron-infor-hostens-skolstart-ar-befogad/ .
56 https://sverigesradio.se/avsnitt/1706750 .
57 www.kva.se/sv/pressrum/pressmeddelanden/vetenskapsakademien-bildar-expert grupp-om-Covid-19 .
58 www.svd.se/tegnell-om-kths-avloppsstudie-vad-tillfor-det-har .
59 www.expressen.se/nyheter/coronaviruset/brundtlands-kritik-mot-sveriges-strategi/ .
60 www.vg.no/forbruker/helse/i/jBvGk9/maa-bare-si-fra .
61 www.mirror.co.uk/news/world-news/sweden-wrong-herd-immunity-says-23014969 .
62 www.dw.com/de/meinung-corona-im-wohlf%C3%BChlstaat-schweden/a-59342931 .
63 *Ibid.*
64 www.dn.se/ledare/det-svenska-pandemifiaskot-slar-mot-sjukskoterskor-och-gamla/ , www.dn.se/ledare/ansvaret-for-coronakrisen-ar-ingen-kurragommalek/ , www.svd.se/coronalaget–i-den-andra-vagen, www.gp.se/ledare/sveriges-coronastrategi-beh%C3%B6 ver-synas-i-s%C3%B6mmarna-1.37573165, https://kvartal.se/artiklar/i-det-ansvarslosa-sverige/ , www.expressen.se/ledare/anna-dahlberg/tegnell-haller-inte-mattet-sa-dags-att-inse-det-nu/ .
65 www.kantarsifo.se/sites/default/files/reports/documents/allmanhetens_tillit_tankar_och_beteende_under_coronakrisen_8_maj_2020_kantarsifo.pdf , www.msb.se/site assets/dokument/aktuellt/pagaende-handelser-och-insats/coronaviruset–Covid-19/resultat-fran-kantar-sifos-undersokningar/januari-2021/1544449-msb_rapport-coro naundersokning_210205.pdf .
66 www.regeringen.se/tal/2020/11/statsminister-stefan-lofvens-tal-till-nationen-den-22-november-2020/ .
67 www.expressen.se/nyheter/stefan-lofven-om-vad-han-kopte-vid-kritiserade-julklapps besoket/ .
68 www.svt.se/nyheter/inrikes/ulla-lofven-om-omtalade-julklappen-du-foljde-de-regler-som-galler .
69 https://sverigesradio.se/artikel/7637325 .
70 www.aftonbladet.se/nyheter/kolumnister/a/lE4Lv7/eliasson-fick-sparken–pa-ett-snyggt-satt .
71 www.ivo.se/publicerat-material/nyheter/2020/ingen-region-har-tagit-fullt-ansvar-for-individuell-vard/ .
72 www.dn.se/sverige/lofven-regionerna-bar-ansvaret/ .
73 https://coronakommissionen.com/ .
74 www.theguardian.com/world/2020/dec/17/king-sweden-failed-Covid-strategy-rare-royal-rebuke-lockdown-hospitals-cases .
75 https://sverigesradio.se/artikel/johan-carlson-anvande-inte-munskydd-under-rusning stid .
76 Hydén, Håkan. "Corona – en rättspolitisk utmaning!" *Statsvetenskaplig tidskrift* (*The Swedish Journal of Political Science*) 123:5 (2021): 315–342, 329.
77 www.aftonbladet.se/nyheter/a/OQOmk1/tegnell-om-tredje-vagen–tror-pa-vandn ing-i-maj , www.svt.se/nyheter/inrikes/stefan-lofven-varnar-for-en-tredje-vag-viktigt-hur-man-beter-sig , www.dn.se/sverige/tegnell-oroande-att-sjunkande-tendensen-avs tannat/ .
78 https://sverigesradio.se/avsnitt/dold-facebookgrupp-oroar-experter-Covid-19-pan demin-och-informationspaverkan-vetenskapsradion-pa-djupet , https://kvartal.se/artiklar/nar-fri-asiktsbildning-blev-ett-hot/ , www.opulens.se/opinion/media-och-nat kultur/sveriges-radio-leker-med-elden/ , www.dagensmedia.se/opinion/debatt/jan-sch erman-myndighetsmegafonen-tog-over-i-pandemirapporteringen/ , www.dagensme dia.se/medier/dagspress/fhm-om-spridandet-av-vetenskapsradions-granskning-vi-har-ett-ansvar-att-mota-informationspaverkan/ , www.dagensmedia.se/medier/dagspress/kritikerna-som-ifragasatte-svenska-strategin-medierna-blev-megafon-at-fhm/ , www.dn.se/insandare/chockerande-att-kritiker-mot-coronastrategin-utmalas-som-folk fiender/ , www.hd.se/2021-02-09/kritisera-garna-coronastrategin-men-gor-det-oppet ,

www.sydsvenskan.se/2021-02-11/det-borjar-i-kritik-det-slutar-i-krav-pa-folkmord stribunaler-och-inlasning-av-dem-som-inte-ger-vika .
79 www.dagensmedia.se/opinion/debatt/jan-scherman-myndighetsmegafonen-tog-over-i-pandemirapporteringen/ , www.dagensmedia.se/medier/digitalt/fhm-forsvarar-sig-har-ar-mejlvaxlingen-mellan-presschefen-och-jan-scherman/ .
80 www.expressen.se/nyheter/coronaviruset/fhm-kande-till-symtomfri-smitta-agerade-6-manader-senare-nar-kurvan-okade/ .
81 www.riksdagen.se/sv/aktuellt/2021/jun/3/kus-granskning-av-regeringen-ar-klar/ .
82 https://svenska.yle.fi/artikel/2020/03/27/sverige-forbjuder-sammankomster-pa-fler-an-50-personer-stefan-lofven-vi-kan-inte .
83 https://twitter.com/ar_Covid/status/1384490744153575424 .
84 https://twitter.com/ar_Covid/status/1384972253239054336 .
85 https://naringslivets-medieinstitut.se/rapport-nyhetsmediernas-coronarapportering/ .
86 https://www.folkhalsomyndigheten.se/contentassets/0f5da1a87e8b4da0a6225aaaf86f 61f0/scenarier-for-fortsatt-spridning-delrapport-5.pdf
87 https://edition.cnn.com/videos/tv/2021/09/26/exp-gps-0926-lofven-swedish-Covid-experiment.cnn , www.dn.se/varlden/lofven-forsvarade-svenska-coronastrate gin-i-cnn/ , upon this also denying that Sweden was different from other nations and even had used facemasks, which it definitively had not (!).
88 www.fub.se/nyheter/prioritera-vaccin-till-vuxna-med-downs-syndrom/ , www.fub.se/wp-content/uploads/2021/09/skrivelse-FHM-4-nov-2021-om-pafyllnadsdos-vaccin.pdf .
89 www.altinget.se/artikel/varfor-vagrar-folkhalsomyndigheten-ge-boostersprutа-till-uppenbara-riskgrupper .
90 www.tv4.se/artikel/4VjvMdBk2PDSyxqG146CKp/kungen-om-ateroeppnandet-av-sverige-gick-lite-snabbt .
91 www.folkhalsomyndigheten.se/contentassets/9ff003627b8a4a1a881f34844f0fcc0a/scenarier-fortsatta-spridning-delrapport-6.pdf .
92 https://coronakommissionen.com/2021/10/21/sverige-under-pandemin-corona kommissionens-andra-delbetankande/ .
93 www.dn.se/debatt/testa-aven-fullvaccinerade-med-luftvagsinfektion/ , www.dn.se/debatt/vi-far-inte-gora-om-samma-misstag-en-gang-till/ .
94 https://lakartidningen.se/aktuellt/nyheter/2021/11/tegnell-svarar-pa-kritiken-darfor-drojer-tredje-dos-till-vardpersonal/ .
95 www.tagesspiegel.de/politik/kaum-noch-corona-infektionen-israel-boostert-sich-zum-impfvorbild/27758526.html .
96 https://sverigesradio.se/artikel/tusentals-vaccindoser-slangs-trots-att-vardpersonal-vill-anvanda-dem .
97 www.svd.se/whos-varning-till-sverige-fel-tid-att-oppna .
98 www.sydsvenskan.se/2021-11-04/varden-rasar-mot-fhms-forskolerad .
99 https://sverigesradio.se/artikel/tegmark-wisell-sverige-valde-en-delvis-annan-strategi .
100 Although disabled and, for example, persons with Down syndrome had been vaccinated early in the process they were even after seven months refused a booster vaccine, without any explanation from the FHM. Socialstyrelsen, the Agency responsible for all health care and these groups, kept silent and did not intervene to protect its doctors, health workers and risk groups, in continuity with the Agency's former passivity in 20 pandemic months, https://hejaolika.se/artikel/vaccinerade-med-downs-syndrom-loper-mangdubbel-risk-for-covid-19/ .
101 www.dn.se/sverige/tegnell-utvecklingen-i-europa-ar-en-varningsklocka/ .
102 www.altinget.se/artikel/experter-alla-med-misstankt-smitta-ska-testas .
103 www.ft.com/content/0c07de5f-e852-4c23-823b-5f8f7d18ebef .
104 The number of immigrants in Norway (14%) and Sweden (17%) could not verify anything of what Tegnell alleged by repeating his controversial and disproved view from December 2020, www.aftonbladet.se/nyheter/a/gW3E1A/tegnell-om-uttalandet-det-var-olyckligt,

but the difference in dwelling density among immigrants in Sweden (30%) and in Norway (16%) might eventually have some impact. Even if dwelling density matters with regard to virus transmission, the Swedish strategy not to minimise the spread most possibly appears as even more unbelievable, as the Agency has full access to the numbers of dwelling density from the national statistics, https://nordicwelfare.org/integration-norden/fakta-och-forskning/ , www.scb.se/hitta-statistik/artiklar/2021/sverige-har-flest-trangbodda-i-norden/ , https://journals.plos.org/plosone/article?id=10.1371/journal.pone.0242398 .

105 *ZDF Politbarometer*, 12 November 2021, www.zdf.de/nachrichten/politik/politbarometer-corona-massnahmen-klima-102.html .

106 www.dn.se/sthlm/nytt-varstascenario-5-400-fler-doda-i-covid-19-till-sommaren/ .

107 www.dn.se/vetenskap/tegnell-kritisk-mot-coronakommissionens-satt-att-rakna/ .

108 www.eurosurveillance.org/content/10.2807/1560-7917.ES.2021.26.44.2001996#html_fulltext .

109 www.riksdagen.se/sv/dokument-lagar/dokument/skriftlig-fraga/sveriges-export-av-covidsmitta_H911377 .

110 https://lakartidningen.se/aktuellt/nyheter/2021/11/tegnell-svarar-pa-kritiken-darfor-drojer-tredje-dos-till-vardpersonal/ .

111 https://sverigesradio.se/artikel/manga-kanner-inte-till-nya-testrekommendationer .

112 https://afp.omni.se/omicron-won-t-change-swedish-covid-strategy-epidemiologist/a/8Qx8yx .

113 www.dn.se/ekonomi/restauranger-vill-infora-vaccinpass-efter-hundratals-avbokningar-till-julborden/ .

114 www.dn.se/sverige/coronautbrott-efter-personalfest-pa-sahlgrenska-universitetssjukhuset/ .

115 www.dn.se/debatt/testa-alla-sjuka-skolbarn-och-erbjud-vaccin-fran-5-ar/ , www.dn.se/debatt/vaccinera-barn-fran-fem-ar-och-anvand-munskydd/ .

116 www.dn.se/vetenskap/nu-slar-smittan-mot-barnen-viruset-beter-sig-annorlunda/ .

117 www.dn.se/sverige/fhm-orealistiskt-att-rad-om-munskydd-efterlevs-direkt/ .

118 www.svt.se/nyheter/inrikes/vardforbundet-vaccinering-av-vardpersonal-gar-for-langsamt .

119 https://smer.se/calendar/award-winner-seminar-2021-priority-settings-in-health care-in-pandemics-and-other-situations-of-mass-casualties/ .

120 Cf. Bergmann, Sigurd. "Navigating Ethics in a Pandemic – Contempt for the Weak Versus Love of Neighbor in a Swedish Lens", *Dialog*, 7 November 2021, https://onlinelibrary.wiley.com/doi/full/10.1111/dial.12697 .

121 ICU doctors report clearly about the situations of overload resulting in triage/prioritisation (to death), www.dn.se/nyheter/sverige/overlakare-logn-att-patienter-inte-prioriterats-bort/ , www.sydsvenskan.se/2021-01-01/sent-en-natt-var-det-ett-faktum–sjukhuset-hade-inga-intensivvardsplatser-kvar .

122 www.dn.se/sverige/tecken-pa-att-omikron-ar-mer-luftburet-an-tidigare-varianter/ .

123 www.svt.se/nyheter/inrikes/trots-hardare-rekommendationer-ska-snoriga-barn-anda-till-forskolan .

124 www.svd.se/smittan-okar–hogsta-nivan-sedan-i-maj .

125 www.svt.se/nyheter/inrikes/nya-restriktioner-kan-inforas-nasta-vecka .

126 www.altinget.se/vard/artikel/experter-med-vilket-mandat-folkhalsomyndigheten .

127 www.dn.se/sverige/tegnell-svart-att-andra-attityden-till-munskydd/ .

128 www.expressen.se/ledare/anna-dahlberg/hur-forklarar-tegnell-misstagen-under-hosten/ .

129 www.dn.se/sverige/apoteken-snabbtester-for-covid-19-saljer-slut-direkt/ .

130 www.gp.se/debatt/folkh%C3%A4lsomyndigheten-m%C3%A5ste-l%C3%A4gga-alla-fakta-om-omikron-p%C3%A5-bordet-1.62359726 .

131 www.svd.se/oerhort-svart-att-halla-avstand-i-skolan .

132 https://sverigesradio.se/artikel/rekordsnabb-smittspridning-ak-inte-pa-skidresa-om-du-ar-sjuk .

133 www.dn.se/sverige/fhm-mojligt-att-vi-ser-en-storre-okning-framover/ .
134 www.svd.se/l-vill-stoppa-nya-coronarestriktionerna , www.svd.se/vi-kommer-inte-att-folja-restriktionerna .
135 www.svd.se/folkhalsomyndigheten-haller-presstraff-d48q , www.expressen.se/nyheter/coronaviruset/tegnell-da-borde-vi-se–over-hur-corona-klassas/ .
136 www.zeit.de/gesundheit/2022-01/corona-lage-karl-lauterbach-christian-drosten-rki , https://fortune.com/2022/01/05/experts-omicron-herd-immunity-not-long-terrible-cost/ .
137 www.dn.se/sverige/tegnell-covidpass-ar-ingenting-att-luta-sig-mot-just-nu/ .
138 www.svt.se/nyheter/inrikes/tegmark-wisell-testningen-ar-inte-ekonomiskt-forsvar bar .
139 https://vetcov19.se/wp-content/uploads/2022/02/Skrivelse-till-regeringen-8-febru ari-2022-fran-Vetcov19.pdf .
140 www.dn.se/sverige/fhm-det-ar-inte-relevant-att-testa-alla/ .
141 www.svt.se/nyheter/inrikes/fler-aterinfekteras-i-covid-19 .
142 www.dn.se/vetenskap/allt-fler-barn-far-sjukhusvard-pa-grund-av-covid-19/ .
143 https://twitter.com/DrEricDing/status/1493465973952757760 , www.tagesspiegel.de/wissen/todeszahlen-fast-wieder-auf-rekordniveau-der-daenische-weg-als-war nung-fuer-deutschland/28073686.html , www.dr.dk/nyheder/udland/danske-coro natal-vaekker-frygt-og-mistro-i-udlandet-nu-blander-ssi-sig-i-debatterne .
144 https://sverigesradio.se/artikel/nar-restriktionerna-forsvann-vill-farre-vaccinera-sig .
145 www.folkhalsomyndigheten.se/nyheter-och-press/nyhetsarkiv/2022/februari/nya-scenarier-pekar-pa-minskad-spridning-av-covid-19/ .
146 www.svd.se/hallengren-vi-har-hanterat-pandemin-rimligt, www.dn.se/sverige/karin-tegmark-wisell-restriktionerna-lyckades/ .
147 www.dn.se/sverige/chefer-for-intensivvarden-vi-blev-kallhamrade/ , www.dn.se/sverige/tack-och-lov-har-de-flesta-i-sverige-inte-sett-det-vi-sett/ .
148 www.folkhalsomyndigheten.se/nyheter-och-press/nyhetsarkiv/2022/mars/anders-tegnell-till-internationellt-vaccinuppdrag-for-who/ , www.svd.se/a/v5Knw5/tegnell-utsedd-till-who-jobb-som-inte-finns, www.svd.se/a/y4MMze/tegnells-toppjobb-ett-miss forstand, www.svd.se/a/wOjJg5/tegnells-eftertradare-slutar-i-sommar .
149 www.svd.se/a/v57PBB/who-sager-nej-till-anders-tegnell .
150 www.dn.se/sverige/anders-tegnell-det-kanns-bra-att-det-har-klarnat/ .
151 www.svd.se/a/28xz6l/folkhalsomyndighetens-scenario-nu-okar-smittan-igen .
152 See more in: Bergmann, Sigurd. "Memoria Passionis Subversiva: The Moral Power of Remembrance in the Pandemic – in a Swedish Lens" (forthcoming) in Erbele-Küster, Dorothea, and Volker Küster (eds.). *Between Pandemonium and Pandemethics: Responses to Covid-19 in Theology and Religions*, Leipzig: EVA, 2022: 101–121.

3

ON THE VIROLOGY OF SARS-COV-2 AND AN EXPERT AUTHORITY WITHOUT REAL EXPERTS

Was there a deliberate disinformation from the Public Health Agency of Sweden on the SARS-CoV-2 infection's spread in the population?

Anders Vahlne

"Flabbergasted"

> The new corona virus SARS-CoV-2 does not infect children to any extent and children do not spread the infection.[1]

When I heard this statement by an official from the Swedish Public Health Agency (*Folkhälsomyndigheten*, FHM) at a press conference, I could not believe my ears. This was early 2020, and it didn't stop there. On live transmitted public press conferences one could hear:

> If you do not have any symptoms or don't feel sick, you can go to your work or school, because then you cannot infect other people.[2]
>
> Facemasks have no effect on the spread of this virus, but if you keep a distance of five to six feet from other people you are safe.[3]

I thought: don't they read the scientific literature? At this time only just over 200 scientific articles on this new corona virus, and its pandemic, had been published. I had read them all. So should the odd 500 officials of the FHM. Then, how could this Swedish expert agency on communicable diseases deny that children could spread the virus, deny that there could be pre- and asymptomatic transmission of the infection and also deny that the virus was airborne? Why did they even infer that the use of facemasks could have the opposite effect, that is, increase the spread of the virus?

Some of the experts in virology and infectious diseases in Sweden had already been publicly critical in the latter part of February 2020 to the agency's lack of

DOI: 10.4324/9781003289364-4

concern and its refusal to take actions against the new pandemic, such as quarantining of people arriving from places where the virus was spreading, and this included thousands of Swedish families returning from skiing in the Alps of northern Italy after school holidays late in February. FHM did not even recommend normal infection control measures like testing, tracing and isolation. Were they just not up to date with the expanding literature, or were they just indifferent, or did they actively intend to let the virus spread in the population? Did they aim for herd immunity? This was unacceptable with a virus that we knew had a very significant morbidity and mortality, and about which we knew little or nothing about its long-term effects. This was before we had learnt how to optimally treat the patients, before antiviral drugs or even vaccines had been developed? Having spent half a century doing science on how viruses cause disease, on virus laboratory diagnostics, on antiviral treatment, and on virus vaccines and other measures of disease prevention, I was flabbergasted.

The virology of SARS-CoV-2

How genes in our cells are expressed

To understand the shortcomings of the FHM and why I was not only concerned but also deeply worried, I need to briefly educate those readers who are not familiar with the field of virology. Don't worry, I will make it simple. First a few words on molecular biology, here in particular how genetic information, harboured in the DNA of the chromosomes, is expressed in cells. DNA (deoxyribonucleic acid) molecules are long chains of smaller molecules we call deoxynucleotides. The genetic alphabet has four letters (i.e., the different deoxynucleotides), which are designated A, T, C and G. Three of these letters in a row code for one of 20 different amino acids, the elements that make up proteins. Proteins are long folded chains (strings) composed of amino acids. The combination of three nucleotide letters is called a codon. Since there are 64 possibilities to make a combination of the three nucleotides ($4 \times 4 \times 4$) and there are only 20 different amino acids, there is more than one combination of A, T, C and G to code for many of the one and same amino acid. This is how the DNA in the chromosomes determines which proteins a cell can make. Since all cells in the body contain the same chromosomes, and thus the same genetic information, not all information they carry can be expressed in every type of cell. A neuronal cell will express different parts of the chromosomes compared to a muscle cell. How the genetic information in a cell is expressed is tightly controlled. The tools, which make all other type of molecules in a cell, are called enzymes and in general they are all proteins.

The DNA in a cell is composed of two complementary deoxynucleotide chains or strands. The deoxynucleotide A in one strain base pairs with T in the other, and C with G. So, where there is an A in one strand there is a T in the complementary strand and vice versa and where there is a C there will be a G. This is how genetic information can be inherited.

To make a protein, the cell reads the DNA by making a copy of the gene, coding for the protein in question, in one of the strands of the DNA. The copy called messenger ribonucleic acid (mRNA) is a chain of letters in RNA called nucleotides. The sugar moiety of the nucleotides in RNA has a hydroxyl (−OH) group on one of its carbon molecules where DNA has only a hydrogen (−H), hence DNA lacks an oxygen (it is deoxy−). The mRNA will be complementary to the DNA strand read. A difference between DNA and RNA in the cell is that RNA consists of a single strand as opposed to DNA, which has two complementary strands. Another difference is that RNA is short-lived in the cell, in contrast to DNA. T in DNA is called U in RNA. So, where there is an A in the DNA, the complementary nucleotide will be a U in the mRNA. The reading of the gene (DNA) to make an mRNA is called *transcription*. The mRNA is transported out from the nucleus to the cytosol and binds to an organelle called a ribosome. There the ribosome reads the mRNA and makes a strain of amino acids, which will fold and make a protein. The order of the amino acids is thus determined by the order of nucleotides in the mRNA. This process in the ribosomes is called *translation*.

What is a virus?

Viruses are small particles consisting of genetic material (DNA or RNA) encapsulated in a protein shell (called the nucleocapsid) and for some viruses the nucleocapsid can also be enclosed in a lipid membrane envelope. The virus does not contain any organelles and cannot multiply by itself. They need to get into (infect) a living cell, which in turn will produce new viruses under the instruction of the cell and virus's genetic material.

SARS-CoV-2

The virus causing Covid-19 is called SARS-CoV-2 from **S**evere **A**cute **R**espiratory **S**yndrome **Co**rona **V**irus 2. It is an enveloped virus, that is, its nucleocapsid is enclosed in a lipid membrane or envelope. Its genetic material is in the form of single-stranded RNA. To get into a cell, the virus envelope must bind closely to the cell's surface. This is accomplished by the binding of a virus protein, called the spike protein, extruding from the viral envelope to a protein on the cell. When the viral envelope gets in close contact with the cellular plasma membrane, the envelope fuses with the plasma membrane, a little bit like two soap bubbles merging into one bigger soap bubble when they adhere to one another. In the case of SARS-CoV-2 this cell protein (virus receptor) is angiotensin converting enzyme 2 (ACE-2).[4] This protein (ACE-2) is abundant on cells in the upper respiratory tract but also in the lungs, blood vessels, in the heart and in the intestine.[5] For the SARS-CoV-2 envelope to fuse with the plasma membrane besides the receptor ACE-2, there also must be a coreceptor present on the cell surface, TMPRSS2, cutting the virus's spike protein after it has attached to ACE-2, to allow for the envelope-cell membrane fusion to begin.[6]

How viruses cause disease (viral pathogenesis) and how the body fights a virus infection

Why do we get sick when we are infected with a virus? The course of events in the body that leads to a viral disease (viral pathogenesis) is different for all viruses. It depends on which cells in the body are infected. The infectious dose is in most cases (but not all) of crucial importance. In animal experiments one often refers to infectious dose 50% (ID_{50}) and lethal dose 50% (LD_{50}), the dose of virus necessary to infect 50% of the animals and to kill 50% of the animals, respectively. Obviously, this is very hard, if not impossible, to determine in human virus infections, but nonetheless the infectious dose should be of importance also in human disease, and so also for SARS-CoV-2.

Once we have had an infection, for most viruses, we get immune to a new infection with the same virus. This is because we develop and maintain virus-specific antibodies and T-cells against the virus. This is called *adaptive immunity*. The antibodies can bind to the virus and hinder it from attaching to cells: these are called neutralising antibodies, or they can bind to infected cells expressing virus proteins or parts thereof on their surfaces and kill the infected cell through what we call *complement activation*, or by in turn binding natural killer (NK) T-cells, which kill the infected cells. Antibodies are at first produced by white blood cells called B-lymphocytes. The B-lymphocytes are matured to plasmablasts, which in turn mature into highly antibody-producing plasma cells. Some B-lymphocytes mature into long-lived memory B-cells. These latter cells can be activated and mature into plasma cells if the individual encounters the same pathogen again. Some virus-specific T-cells help antibody-producing cells to develop and multiply (T-helper cells); others can directly specifically kill virus-infected cells. However, it takes about two weeks to develop this antiviral adaptive immunity. In most instances we recover from a virus infection within a week. This is because we are born with a non-specific immunity to viruses and other infectious agents. We call this our innate immunity. It consists of antiviral proteins we call interferons, the NK cells mentioned earlier and the inflammatory response. SARS-CoV-2 is extremely sensitive to interferons. To avoid this, a big part of the SARS-CoV-2 genome is there for the virus to get a stealth property (i.e., go under the radar), to prevent the innate immunity from being induced.[7]

The inflammatory response is the cause for most of the symptoms we get when infected with viruses, and mostly the inflammatory response is what makes us sick. Sometimes our inflammatory response overreacts, and we get severe disease and may even die. An example is the severe disease adults can get from an otherwise mostly benign viral childhood disease like mumps or chickenpox.

In the case of SARS-CoV-2 we do not yet fully know what causes the disease (called Covid-19 from **co**rona **vi**rus **d**isease 20**19**) and all the symptoms we get when infected by the virus. The disease is multifactorial. One factor is that the infection can make infected cells melt together with neighbouring cells to form syncytia (these are also known as "Giant Cells").[8] We also know that there can be an overreaction of the inflammatory response in the lungs. The infection of the cells in the lung induces them to produce small proteins called cytokines that signal to the body to recruit inflammatory cells like monocytes to the lungs where they will mature into macrophages, which will digest infected cells.[9] The injury to the lung alveoli caused by this inflammatory response, as well as the syncytia formation already mentioned, will result in extracellular fluid leaking into the alveoli. The inflammatory damage to the lungs will in turn cause inflammatory cells to produce more cytokines, with more monocytes recruited, leading to a viscous cycle of inflammatory-cell lung tissue destruction and more inflammatory response. This leads to what we call *acute respiratory distress syndrome.*[10] In severe disease there will thus be an overproduction of cytokines, called a *cytokine storm*, that can affect many other vital functions in the body. Viruses leaked out into the blood stream (viremia) can infect the cells making up the inner lining of the blood vessels, thus damaging the vessels. Another effect of the viremia is the formation of small blood clots, a *disseminated intravascular coagulation* (DIC).[11] Therefore, anticoagulant treatment of Covid-19 patients was introduced in the spring of 2020. DIC is seen in many serious infectious diseases like bacterial septicaemia.[12] The Covid-19-induced DIC, however, has a different pathogenesis than that seen in septicaemia.[13] SARS-CoV-2 virus can also pass the blood-brain barrier and cause brain damage.[14] These injuries to different organs in the body caused by the virus and the inflammatory response are what also causes the long-term effects of the infection (i.e., long-Covid).[15] In short, you do not want to get infected with this virus, not even with the new variant Omicron.

We do not know why some people get a relatively mild infection or even asymptomatic infection, whereas others get severe disease and even die. Apart from known risk factors, my personal belief is that the infectious dose initially inhaled deeply into the lungs is responsible for the severity of the lung infection in Covid-19. The more virus, the higher risk for a detrimental local inflammatory response. Another reason for damage to the alveoli is that the spike protein of SARS-CoV-2 induces fusion of their cells (pneumocytes) as mentioned previously. Also, this should be dose-dependent infectious. It is obvious that the major route of infection leading to severe disease is by inhaling aerosols containing the virus.[16] The smaller the virus-containing aerosol particles are, the deeper into the lungs they can reach. We have known for a long time that the transmission of other corona viruses like the original SARS-CoV-1 and cow corona virus is airborne.[17] Now there is a vast number of studies showing that this is also the case for SARS-CoV-2.[18]

Thus, any measures reducing the amount of virus inhaled, like the use of facemasks, should be considered essential. Even if facemasks do not always protect from infection, as neither do vaccines, they may help to protect from severe disease and indeed prevent further spread.[19]

Antiviral compounds and vaccines

Early in 2020 virus research laboratories, and the pharmaceutical industry companies, started to develop antiviral compounds to prevent and treat SARS-CoV-2 virus production. Today there are at least two very promising SARS-CoV-2 specific antiviral drugs which can be administered orally.[20] One, Paxlovid, developed by Pfizer, is a virus proteinase inhibitor, and one by Merck and Company is the ribonucleoside analogue inhibitor Molnuvirapir, first developed as an influenza virus inhibitor. Drugs inhibiting virus replication will have to be administered early in the infection. When the SARS-CoV-2 infection induces the viscious inflammatory circle in the lungs, described earlier, it will be too late for any effective antiviral treatment.

There are now also several vaccines for prophylaxis of infection.[21] Mostly, viral vaccines do not totally prevent infection (i.e., they are not sterilising, but protect from disease from the infection). Historically, vaccines have been either attenuated live virus vaccines like those for measles, mumps and rubella; killed whole virus vaccines like the Salk polio vaccine; virus protein subunit vaccines or recombinant virus vaccines, where for instance a gene for a virus protein has been inserted in the genome of a virus vector (i.e., another carrier-virus like adeno virus). The Covid-19 vaccine of AstraZeneca is an example of the latter.[22] In December of 2020 and in January of 2021 a new type of vaccine was introduced by the two pharmaceutical companies BioNTech/Pfizer and Moderna, respectively, based on mRNA coding for the spike protein of SARS-CoV-2 virus.[23] Both vaccines have proven to be very efficacious. As mentioned, mRNAs are short-lived in the cell. However, in the Pfizer and Moderna vaccines, one of the nucleosides (U) has been chemically modified to increase the mRNA's longevity in the cell. A problem with all corona virus vaccines, however, is that the protective immune response to the virus is relatively short lived, for reasons we do not yet fully understand.

Virus diagnostics

How do we determine or diagnose a SARS-CoV-2 infection? In the acute phase we can detect either the presence of virus proteins in swab material from the throat and/or nose or in saliva, with an antigen test detecting virus proteins or detecting viral genetic material (RNA) from the same type of test material. The latter is done with a semi-quantitative reverse transcription polymerase chain reaction (rtPCR).[24] Antigen tests are less sensitive and specific than rtPCR tests but are rapid and can be performed by a layperson. In the rtPCR, a part of the viral RNA is first transferred to its complementary DNA by what we call reverse transcription, and then this DNA is amplified in cycles where the amount of DNA is doubled in every cycle until the amount of DNA is high enough to be detected. Hence, a bonus with the rtPCR tests used is that one gets a conception of how much virus an infected person is excreting in the upper respiratory tract. It was discovered early that the amount of virus RNA in patient samples could differ by more than a factor of a million.[25] Obviously, an infected person is more infectious than another infected person if he or she excretes one million times more virus. In fact, in the first wave of Covid-19 with the first variant (Wuhan) of SARS-CoV-2, it was estimated that only every fifth infected person transmitted the virus.

SARS-CoV-2 and children

Already in late February of 2020 (i.e., two months after the discovery of the virus), it was known that the virus could infect children and that they could excrete very high amounts of virus, and thus they were mostly, probably highly, infectious. A young couple with a healthy infant girl was hospitalised in Singapore with Covid-19. Since the infant did not have another caretaker than her mum and dad, she accompanied her parents to the hospital. Samples for rtPCR were taken daily also from the infant. It turned out that the child was excreting much more virus than either of her parents, both in her upper respiratory tract and in her intestine.[26] From this and other studies we learned early that the virus could effectively infect children,[27] that the infection could be asymptomatic and that infected children most likely could be infectious. All this was denied by the Swedish FHM. Also consecutively taken rtPCR tests from other diseased patients showed that peak virus amounts were always in the first day or days of illness and then decreased exponentially.[28] It was not likely that the amount of virus, and thus infectiousness, went from zero to the highest amounts in a matter of hours. So, already in February of 2020 we also knew that the infection could spread pre-symptomatically. This understanding was supported by the finding that, although the incubation time was considered to be five to six days, the serial interval (i.e., the time from someone got infected till the time he or she infected another person) was only three to four days and is shorter for the Omicron variant of SARS-CoV-2.[29] Also, early in the spring of 2020 there were scientific publications describing pre-symptomatic and asymptomatic spread of SARS-CoV-2 infections.[30]

So why were the representatives of the FHM saying that children did not get infected and that you only spread the infection if you were sick or at least had symptoms? It is true that the WHO previously had sent people to Wuhan interrogating those engaged in tracing contacts to infected people and had said that they were not aware of any child spreading the infection to adults.[31] But since the children most probably were asymptomatically infected how likely is it that they would be aware of children spreading the disease? Like other human corona viruses this was obviously a respiratory-spread virus. So, why should it avoid infecting children? Were the people at FHM just ignorant? To answer these questions, let us look at the history of the FHM.

The history of FHM and how the expert agency lost its experts

From the beginning of the last century until 1993, Sweden had an agency for surveillance of infectious diseases called *Statens Bakteriologiska Laboratorium* (SBL). It was located in Solna just north of Stockholm. SBL had diagnostic laboratories for bacteria, viruses, parasites and immunology. It also had a department for epidemiology and a facility for vaccine production. Each unit was led by a physician, a specialist senior consultant, having the title of Professor. In 1993 the Government decided that SBL should be closed and instead Sweden was to form a new agency called *Smittskyddsinstitutet* (SMI) or in English: The Swedish Institute for Infectious Disease Control. It was relocated to the north campus of the Karolinska Institute. The vaccine production facility was sold but the departments of bacteriology, virology, parasitology, immunology, epidemiology and vaccine research were maintained. The senior consultants of SBL were offered to become full professors of the Karolinska Institute with the combination of a senior consultancy at the SMI. The routine diagnostic activity, except for rare and dangerous infections, ceased. New research laboratories were built, and each professor/consultant was given 300 square meters (approximately 3,000 square feet) of space. Besides free rent of the laboratory space, the Government also provided each professor with a basic grant, providing salary not only for the professor him/herself but also enough money for a secretary and for a post-doctorial position. Usually, each professor had a research group of approximately ten people; thus there were up to 60 people actively performing research at the SMI. The two first director generals were Erik Nordenfeldt (1994 to 2000), a professor of clinical virology at the University of Lund, and Ragnar Norrby (2000 to 2009), a professor of infectious diseases at the same university.

In 2009 the associate professor of infection epidemiology Johan Carlson, a civil servant at the National Board of Health and Welfare, was appointed as director general for SMI. At the same time a governmental investigation advised that research not directly applicable to infectious disease control should not be performed at SMI. The year after, 2010, Johan Carlson decided to terminate the SMI consultant employment of the six professors. They had to choose to either let the director general decide what research to perform or leave the premises together with their research groups, and to be fully employed only by the Karolinska Institute. At the end, all professors and their research groups left SMI. Four years later again SMI was restructured to take over environmental health and other public health issues from the National Board of Health and Welfare and from a smaller agency which thereupon ceased to exist. The SMI now changed its name to Public Health Agency of Sweden (FHM). Johan Carlson was appointed as Director-General of FHM. This agency should now not only consider infectious disease control, but the general health at large. The Director-General interpreted this as to when to recommend measures to be taken to reduce the spread of the SARS-CoV-2 virus causing the Covid-19 pandemic; he should also consider the impact such actions would have on other aspects of the society. Disease control interventions could be considered to have possible negative psychological effects on individuals and families, domestic violence, the economy at large and so forth (i.e., in my view in fact to be political decisions).

So, when the Covid-19 pandemic reached Sweden in February of 2020, the Swedish expert agency for handling infectious disease control did not have the necessary staff with the required and high-level expertise! Albeit that the agency had employed microbiologists and epidemiologists, none of them were internationally renowned active scientists of the same calibre as were those professor/consultants working at the agency before 2010. To compensate for the lack of expertise, on

March 31, 2020, the agency formed a pandemic advisory group with four senior consultants in clinical virology, three of whom are full university professors, and two retired county infectious disease control officers. I asked one of the virologists how often they met with the agency, and he told me they met once a month and that they only discussed diagnostics and testing procedures and never the general strategy for dealing with the pandemic. In reality, the strategy was formed by the state epidemiologist Anders Tegnell, a specialist in infectious diseases also holding a PhD. Before joining the SMI in 2012 he had, like the Director-General Johan Carlson, been at the National Board of Health and Welfare where previously the two had worked together. In 2014 he was appointed state epidemiologist, a position at the FHM, by its Director-General Johan Carlson.

As I mentioned in the beginning of this chapter, FHM did nothing when the pandemic hit Europe in the beginning of 2020. They even said that it was very unlikely that the infection should spread to Sweden.[32] And when it did, it would only be a few cases and nothing to worry about. Sweden was not alone in having this attitude early on (e.g., England and Norway initially had the same attitude about the pandemic), but learning from what happened in northern Italy, the other European countries soon changed their strategies. Why didn't Sweden? Did Tegnell and his colleagues at FHM have a plan to let the virus slowly spread in the population to create herd immunity? Emil J. Bergholtz's chapter in this book will deal with this in detail. Was the reason for their strategy that they judged that infection control measures like quarantining infected individuals or even public lockdowns (i.e., shutting up major parts of the society like they did in other European countries) would be worse for the general health of the population than the virus infection itself? If so, how did they reach these conclusions?

Earlier, I have described how the FHM was established and how it lost its science experts and now was staffed with civil servants, albeit some with basic training in medicine and microbiology. Their mistake most probably was that they did not consult with those that were active scientists and who could follow the scientific literature. They were missing scientific information and the knowledge of consultant virologists who were, or had been, engaged in research on virus infection in experimental animals, and thus could make educated guesses. There was an absence of knowledge to practise what I would term *common sense medicine*. As it turns out this did not happen. Tegnell made a point of how he consulted with his international colleagues in the same position as he. But they were also civil servants and not active researchers in virology. However, leaders in the other European countries decided to take the safe way and tried to control the infection as well as possible, with testing, tracing and isolating infected individuals, and applying public constriction measures. In fairness, Tegnell was not alone in the medical society who early on thought that there was no point in trying to control the spread of the virus and all that one should aim at was to reduce its spread, so that the health care system could cope with the patients needing hospital care. His confidants were, among others, Johan von Schreeb, a surgeon who also is a professor of global disaster medicine, and Jonas Ludvigsson, a paediatrician who is also a professor of epidemiology. Another was Johan Giesecke, one of his predecessors as state epidemiologist and former boss. They all recommended going for herd immunity by letting the virus slowly spread in the population.

With this strategy, did they deliberately disinform the public on how the virus infection could be transmitted from one person to another? Did they ignore any scientific data showing asymptomatic and pre-symptomatic viral spread, that it was an airborne disease, that facemasks could protect from serious illness, that children could get infected and could transmit the virus? When more and more convincing evidence of this was published in the scientific literature, Tegnell and the other officials of the agency were still in denial. The answer is probably to be searched for, among others, in the personality of Tegnell himself. He has a reputation of never changing his mind once he has set it. Perhaps he thinks that if the agency changes its recommendations or its information on how the virus is spread, the agency would lose the public's confidence and trust. Maybe he thinks it would create chaos in the society? For instance, it has been impossible for the agency to admit that facemasks, particularly FFP2 and FFP3 masks, have any significant role in controlling the spread of SARS-CoV-2 despite overwhelming scientific data that this is the case.[33] Only this stubbornness has cost thousands of lives in Sweden.[34]

What still disappoints and surprises me is the lack of reaction to the FHM's lax attitude to the pandemic from most of the Swedish medical community. Why did my colleague physicians not protest and demand action from the authorities? Why did they defend the FHM when the death rates in Sweden rapidly deteriorated to reach magnitudes higher than our neighbouring countries? Why was there not an outrage from my fellow physicians when older infected people were left to die and were given morphine and sedatives instead of oxygen and necessary medical care? I cannot understand why many of them still have a venial attitude towards the FHM. I suppose I shall never get an answer.

Lessons to be learned

How can we remedy the Swedish response to future pandemics? First, political decisions should be made by politicians and not by civil servants. During the present Covid-19 pandemic, the Swedish Government, as it seems, has based all its decisions, as regards to how to handle Covid-19, entirely on the recommendations from the civil servants employed at FHM. Not only the Government, but also the politicians of the opposition parties, have declared that they trust their expert agency, the FHM. Hence, in Sweden the politicians have handed over the responsibility for the Swedish Covid-19 strategy to non-politicians. In reality, and as I have already described, this Swedish so-called expert agency dismissed its experts in virology, immunology, epidemiology and vaccine research 12 years ago. Neither was an outside group of experts consulted by the FHM before making strategic decisions on how to handle this or indeed any future pandemic. The advice given by the Royal Swedish Academy of Sciences[35] was ignored by the agency. Therefore, in my opinion, the FHM should be shut down and an expert agency much like the former SMI should be formed, where top-notch scientists doing active research should be employed. Also, scientific advisory groups for emergencies like those of the United Kingdom (SAGE) and Germany (Expertenrat)[36] should be formed, manned with both national and international experts from academia. Such expert advisory groups and experts of the new agency should only make recommendations on how to best control infectious diseases and leave decisions on possible negative effects of their recommendations on the society at large to the politicians. For example, weighing infection control measures against the economy is a political consideration. The decision-making then becomes transparent and those responsible can be held accountable.

Notes

1 www.dn.se/nyheter/sverige/folkhalsomyndigheten-barn-smittar-inte-i-samma-utstrackning-som-vuxna/ . Still in March 2021 Tegnell withholds this, www.svd.se/anders-tegnell-liten-risk-att-barn-drabbas .
2 Cf. www.expressen.se/debatt/nar-tar-fhm-hojd-for-att-symtomfria-kan-smitta/ .
3 Cf. www.mabra.com/halsa/anders-tegnell-munskydd-corona/6513922 .
4 Das, Ankur, R. Ahmed, S. Akhtar, K. Begum, and S. Banu. "An Overview of Basic Molecular Biology of SARS-CoV-2 and Current COVID-19 Prevention Strategies", *Gene Reports* 23 (2021): 101122; Jackson, C.B., M. Farzan, B. Chen, and H. Choe. "Mechanisms of SARS-CoV-2 Entry into Cells", *Nature Reviews Molecular Cell Biology* 23:1 (2022): 3–20; Ou, X., Y. Liu, X. Lei, P. Li, D. Mi, L. Ren, L. Guo, R. Guo, T. Chen, J. Hu, Z. Xiang, Z. Mu, X. Chen, J. Chen, K. Hu, Q. Jin, J. Wang, and Z. Qian. "Characterization of Spike Glycoprotein of SARS-CoV-2 on Virus Entry and Its Immune Cross-Reactivity with SARS-CoV", *Nature Communications* 11:1 (2020): 1620; Hartenian, E., D. Nandakumar, A. Lari, M. Ly, J.M. Tucker, and B.A. Glaunsinger. "The Molecular Virology of Coronaviruses", *Journal of Biological Chemistry* 295:37 (2020): 12910–12934.
5 Kirtipal, N., S. Kumar, S.K. Dubey, V.D. Dwivedi, K. Gireesh Babu, P. Malý, and S. Bharadwaj. "Understanding on the Possible Routes for SARS CoV-2 Invasion Via ACE2 in the Host Linked with Multiple Organs Damage", *Infection, Genetics and Evolution* 99 (2022): 105254.
6 Das et al. "An Overview of Basic Molecular Biology", 101122; Jackson et al. "Mechanisms of SARS-CoV-2 Entry into Cells", 3–20; Ou et al. "Characterization of Spike Glycoprotein", 1620; Hartenian et al. "The Molecular Virology of Coronaviruses", 12910–12934.
7 Gu, W., H. Gan, Y. Ma, L. Xu, Z.J. Cheng, B. Li, X. Zhang, W. Jiang, J. Sun, B. Sun, and C. Hao. "The Molecular Mechanism of SARS-CoV-2 Evading Host Antiviral Innate Immunity", *Virology Journal* 19:1 (2022): 49; Wong, N.A., and M.H. Saier. "The SARS-Coronavirus Infection Cycle: A Survey of Viral Membrane Proteins, Their Functional Interactions and Pathogenesis", *International Journal of Molecular* Sciences 22:3 (2021): 1308; Oh, S.J., and O.S. Shin. "SARS-CoV-2-Mediated Evasion Strategies for Antiviral Interferon Pathways", *Journal of Microbiology* 60:3 (2022): 290–299.
8 Buchrieser, J., J. Dufloo, M. Hubert, B. Monel, D. Planas, M.M. Rajah, C. Planchais, F. Porrot, F. Guivel-Benhassine, S. Van der Werf, N. Casartelli, H. Mouquet, T. Bruel, and O. Schwartz. "Syncytia Formation by SARS-CoV-2-Infected Cells", *EMBO Journal* 39:23 (2020): e106267; Santana, M.F., R.A.A. Pinto, B.H. Marcon, L.C.A.S. Medeiros, T.B.D.N. Morais, L.C. Dias, L.P. Souza, G.C. Melo, W.M. Monteiro, M.V.G. Lacerda, F.A. Val, P.J. Lalwani, and L.C.L. Ferreira. "Pathological Findings and Morphologic Correlation of the Lungs of Autopsied Patients with SARS-CoV-2 Infection in the

Brazilian Amazon Using Transmission Electron Microscopy", *Journal of the Brazilian Society of Tropical Medicine* 54 (2021): e0850; Stadlmann, S., R. Hein-Kuhnt, and G. Singer. "Viropathic Multinuclear Syncytial Giant Cells in Bronchial Fluid from a Patient with COVID-19", *Journal of Clinical Pathology* 73:9 (2020): 607–608.

9 Upadhya, S., J. Rehman, A.B. Malik, and S. Chen. "Mechanisms of Lung Injury Induced by SARS-CoV-2 Infection", *Physiology (Bethesda)* 37:2 (2022): 88–100.

10 Welker, C., J. Huang, I.J.N. Gil, and H. Ramakrishna. "2021 Acute Respiratory Distress Syndrome Update, with Coronavirus Disease 2019 Focus", *Journal of Cardiothoracic and Vascular Anesthesia* 36:4 (2022): 1188–1195.

11 Hanff, T.C., A.M. Mohareb, J. Giri, J.B. Cohen, and J.A. Chirinos. "Thrombosis in COVID-19", *American Journal of Hematology* 95:12 (2020): 1578–1589; Vinayagam, S., and K. Sattu. "SARS-CoV-2 and Coagulation Disorders in Different Organs", *Life Sciences* 260 (2020): 118431; Rajan, Ashna, Ganesh Keshav Thirunavukkarasu, Richard F. Lockey, and Narasaiah Kolliputi. "Is the Mechanism of COVID-19 Coagulopathy Still a Rabbit's Hole?" *Cell Communication and Signaling* 16:1 (2022): 1–3; Bussani, R., E. Schneider, L. Zentilin, C. Collesi, H. Ali, L. Braga, M.C. Volpe, A. Colliva, F. Zanconati, G. Berlot, F. Silvestri, S. Zacchigna, and M. Giacca. "Persistence of Viral RNA, Pneumocyte Syncytia and Thrombosis Are Hallmarks of Advanced COVID-19 Pathology", *eBioMedicine* 61 (2020): 103104; Adelborg, K., J.B. Larsen, and A.M. Hvas. "Disseminated Intravascular Coagulation: Epidemiology, Biomarkers, and Management", *British Journal of Hematology* 192:5 (2021): 803–818; Lorini, F.L., M. Di Matteo, P. Gritti, L. Grazioli, A. Benigni, L. Zacchetti, I. Bianchi, F. Fabretti, and L. Longhi. "Coagulopathy and COVID-19", *European Heart Journal – Supplements* 23: Suppl E (2021): E95–E98; Savla, S.R., K.S. Prabhavalkar, and L.K. Bhatt. "Cytokine Storm Associated Coagulation Complications in COVID-19 Patients: Pathogenesis and Management", *Expert Review* of *Anti-Infective Therapy* 19:11 (2021): 1397–1413; Boussier, J., N. Yatim, A. Marchal, J. Hadjadj, B. Charbit, C. El Sissy, N. Carlier, F. Pène, L. Mouthon, P.L. Tharaux, A. Bergeron, D.M. Smadja, F. Rieux-Laucat, D. Duffy, S. Kernéis, V. Frémeaux-Bacchi, and B. Terrier. "Severe COVID-19 Is Associated with Hyperactivation of the Alternative Complement Pathway", *Journal of Allergy and Clinical Immunology* 149:2 (2022): 550–556.e2.

12 Page, E.M., and R.A.S. Ariëns. "Mechanisms of Thrombosis and Cardiovascular Complications in COVID-19", *Thrombosis Research* 200 (2021): 1–8.

13 Savla et al. "Cytokine Storm Associated Coagulation Complications in COVID-19 Patients", 1397–1413; Boussier et al. "Severe COVID-19 Is Associated with Hyperactivation of the Alternative Complement Pathway", 550–556.e2.

14 Haidar, M.A., Z. Shakkour, M.A. Reslan, N. Al-Haj, P. Chamoun, K. Habashy, H. Kaafarani, S. Shahjouei, S.H. Farran, A. Shaito, E.S. Saba, B. Badran, M. Sabra, F. Kobeissy, and M. Bizri. "SARS-CoV-2 Involvement in Central Nervous System Tissue Damage", *Neural Regeneration Research* 17:6 (2022): 1228–1239; Gwenaëlle, Douaud, Soojin Lee, Fidel Alfaro-Almagro, Christoph Arthofer, Chaoyue Wang, Paul McCarthy, Frederik Lange, Jesper L.R. Andersson, Ludovica Griffanti, Eugene Duff, Saad Jbabdi, Bernd Taschler, Peter Keating, Anderson M. Winkler, Rory Collins, Paul M. Matthews, Naomi Allen, Karla L. Miller, Thomas E. Nichols, and Stephen M. Smith. "SARS-CoV-2 Is Associated with Changes in Brain Structure in UK Biobank", *Nature*, 7 March 2022; Wei-Bin, Shen, James Logue, Penghua Yang, Lauren Baracco, Montasir Elahi, E. Albert Reece, Bingbing Wang, Ling Li, Thomas G. Blanchard, Zhe Han, Matthew B. Frieman, Robert A. Rissman, and Peixin Yang. "SARS-CoV-2 Invades Cognitive Centers of the Brain and Induces Alzheimer's-Like Neuropathology", *bioRxiv* (3 February 2022): 01.31.478476.

15 Montani, D., L. Savale, N. Noel, O. Meyrignac, R. Colle, M. Gasnier, E. Corruble, A. Beurnier, E.M. Jutant, T. Pham, A.L. Lecoq, J.F. Papon, S. Figueiredo, A. Harrois, M. Humbert, and X. Monnet (COMEBAC Study Group). "Post-Acute COVID-19 Syndrome", *European Respiratory Review* 31:163 (2022): 210185; Bussani et al. "Persistence

of Viral RNA", 103104; Xie, Y., E. Xu, B. Bowe, and Z. Al-Aly. "Long-Term Cardiovascular Outcomes of COVID-19", *Nature Medicine* 28:3 (2022): 583–590.

16 Tellier, R. "COVID-19: The Case for Aerosol Transmission", *Interface Focus* 12:2 (2022): 20210072; McNeill, V.F. "Airborne Transmission of SARS-CoV-2: Evidence and Implications for Engineering Controls", *Annual Review of Chemical and Biomolecular Engineering*, 17 February 2022.

17 Wang Chia, C., Kimberly A. Prather, Josué Sznitman, Jose L. Jimenez, Seema S. Lakdawala, Zeynep Tufekci, and Linsey C. Marr. "Airborne Transmission of Respiratory Viruses", *Science* (27 August 2021): 373(6558): eabd9149; Niskanen, R., A. Lindberg, and M. Tråvén. "Failure to Spread Bovine Virus Diarrhoea Virus Infection from Primarily Infected Calves Despite Concurrent Infection with Bovine Coronavirus", *Veterinary Journal* 163:3 (2002): 251–259.

18 Tellier. "COVID-19", 20210072; McNeill. "Airborne Transmission of SARS-CoV-2".

19 Negin, Shaterian, Fatemeh Abdi, Zahra Atarodi Kashani, Negar Shaterian, and Mohammad Darvishmotevalli. "Facemask and Respirator in Reducing the Spread of Respiratory Viruses: A Systematic Review", *Archives of Academic Emergency Medicine* 9:1 (2021): e56; Seo, Kim Min et al. "Comparative Effectiveness of N95, Surgical or Medical, and Non-Medical Facemasks in Protection Against Respiratory Virus Infection: A Systematic Review and Network Meta-Analysis", *Reviews in Medical Virology* (26 February 2022): e2336.

20 Painter, W.P., W. Holman, J.A. Bush, F. Almazedi, H. Malik, N.C.J.E. Eraut, M.J. Morin, L.J. Szewczyk, and G.R. Painter. "Human Safety, Tolerability, and Pharmacokinetics of Molnupiravir, a Novel Broad-Spectrum Oral Antiviral Agent with Activity Against SARS-CoV-2", *Antimicrobial Agents and Chemotherapy* 65:5 (2021): e02428–20; Fischer, W., J.J. Eron, W. Holman, M.S. Cohen, L. Fang, L.J. Szewczyk, T.P. Sheahan, R. Baric, K.R. Mollan, C.R. Wolfe, E.R. Duke, M.M. Azizad, K. Borroto-Esoda, D.A. Wohl, A.J. Loftis, P. Alabanza, F. Lipansky, and W.P. Painter. "Molnupiravir, an Oral Antiviral Treatment for COVID-19", *medRxiv* (17 June 2021): 2021.06.17.21258639; Wen, W., C. Chen, J. Tang, C. Wang, M. Zhou, Y. Cheng, X. Zhou, Q. Wu, X. Zhang, Z. Feng, M. Wang, and Q. Mao. "Efficacy and Safety of Three New Oral Antiviral Treatment (Molnupiravir, Fluvoxamine and Paxlovid) for COVID-19: A Meta-Analysis", *Annals of Medicine* 54:1 (2022): 516–523; Marei, H.E., A. Althani, N. Afifi, G. Pozzoli, T. Caceci, F. Angelini, and C. Cenciarelli. "Pandemic COVID-19 Caused by SARS-CoV-2: Genetic Structure, Vaccination, and Therapeutic Approaches", *Molecular Biology Reports* 48:9 (2021): 6513–6524.

21 Yap, C., A. Ali, A. Prabhakar, A. Prabhakar, A. Pal, Y.Y. Lim, and P. Kakodkar. "Comprehensive Literature Review on COVID-19 Vaccines and Role of SARS-CoV-2 Variants in the Pandemic", *Therapeutic Advances in Vaccines and Immunotherapy* (24 November 2021): 25151355211059791; Szabó, G.T., A.J. Mahiny, and I. Vlatkovic. "COVID-19 mRNA Vaccines: Platforms and Current Developments", *Molecular Therapy* (19 February 2022): S1525–0016(22)00099–5; Patel, R., M. Kaki, V.S. Potluri, P. Kahar, and D. Khanna. "A Comprehensive Review of SARS-CoV-2 Vaccines: Pfizer, Moderna & Johnson & Johnson", *Human Vaccines & Immunotherapeutics* 18:1 (2022): 2002083.

22 Merryn, Voysey, Sue Ann Costa Clemens, Shabir A. Madhi, Lily Y. Weckx, Pedro M. Folegatti, Parvinder K. Aley, Brian Angus, Vicky L. Baillie, Shaun L. Barnabas, Qasim E. Bhorat, Sagida Bibi, Carmen Briner, Paola Cicconi, Andrea M. Collins, Rachel Colin-Jones, Clare L. Cutland, Thomas C. Darton, Keertan Dheda, Christopher J.A. Duncan, Katherine R.W. Emary, Katie J. Ewer, Lee Fairlie, Saul N. Faust, Shuo Feng, Daniela M. Ferreira, Adam Finn, Anna L. Goodman, Catherine M. Green, Christopher A. Green, Paul T. Heath, Catherine Hill, Helen Hill, Ian Hirsch, Susanne H.C. Hodgson, Alane Izu, Susan Jackson, Daniel Jenkin, Carina C.D. Joe, Simon Kerridge, Anthonet Koen, Gaurav Kwatra, Rajeka Lazarus, Alison M. Lawrie, Alice Lelliott, Vincenzo Libri, Patrick J. Lillie, Raburn Mallory, Ana V.A. Mendes, Eveline P. Milan, Angela

M. Minassian, Alastair McGregor, Hazel Morrison, Yama F. Mujadidi, Anusha Nana, Peter J. O'Reilly, Sherman D. Padayachee, Ana Pittella, Emma Plested, Katrina M. Pollock, Maheshi N. Ramasamy, Sarah Rhead, Alexandre V. Schwarzbold, Nisha Singh, Andrew Smith, Rinn Song, Matthew D. Snape, Eduardo Sprinz, Rebecca K. Sutherland, Richard Tarrant, Emma C. Thomson, M. Estée Török, Mark Toshner, David P.J. Turner, Johan Vekemans, Tonya L. Villafana, Marion E.E. Watson, Christopher J. Williams, Alexander D. Douglas, Adrian V.S. Hill, Teresa Lambe, Sarah C. Gilbert, Andrew J. Pollard, and Oxford COVID Vaccine Trial Group. "Safety and Efficacy of the ChAdOx1 nCoV-19 Vaccine (AZD1222) Against SARS-CoV-2: An Interim Analysis of Four Randomised Controlled Trials in Brazil, South Africa, and the UK", *The Lancet* 397:10269 (2021): 99–111.

23 Szabó et al. "COVID-19 mRNA Vaccines".

24 Dhar, B.C. "Diagnostic Assay and Technology Advancement for Detecting SARS-CoV-2infections Causing the COVID-19 Pandemic", *Analytical and Bioanalytical Chemistry* 414:9 (2022): 2903–2934.

25 Lirong, Zou, Feng Ruan, Mingxing Huang, Lijun Liang, Huitao Huang, Zhongsi Hong, Jianxiang Yu, Min Kang, Yingchao Song, Jinyu Xia, Qianfang Guo, Tie Song, Jianfeng He, Hui-Ling Yen, Malik Peiris, and Jie Wu. "SARS-CoV-2 Viral Load in Upper Respiratory Specimens of Infected Patients", *New England Journal of Medicine* 382:12 (2020): 1177–1179.

26 Kam, K.Q., C.F. Yung, L. Cui, R. Tzer Pin Lin, T.M. Mak, M. Maiwald, J. Li, C.Y. Chong, K. Nadua, N.W.H. Tan, and K.C. Thoon. "A Well Infant with Coronavirus Disease 2019 With High Viral Load", *Clinical Infectious Diseases* 71:15 (2020): 847–849.

27 J.M. Patel. "Multisystem Inflammatory Syndrome in Children (MIS-C)", *Current Allergy and Asthma Reports*, 22 March 2022; Anusrita, Kundu, Swagata Maji, Suchismita Kumar, Shreya Bhattacharya, Pallab Chakraborty, and Joy Sarkar. "Clinical Aspects and Presumed Etiology of Multisystem Inflammatory Syndrome in Children (MIS-C): A Review", *Clinical Epidemiology and Global Health* 14 (March–April 2022): 100966.

28 Kim, J.Y., J.H. Ko, Y. Kim, Y.J. Kim, J.M. Kim, Y.S. Chung, H.M. Kim, M.G. Han, S.Y. Kim, and B.S. Chin. "Viral Load Kinetics of SARS-CoV-2 Infection in First Two Patients in Korea", *Journal of Korean Medical Science* 35:7 (2020): e86.

29 Backer, J.A., D. Eggink, S.P. Andeweg, I.K. Veldhuijzen, N. van Maarseveen, K. Vermaas, B. Vlaemynck, R. Schepers, S. van den Hof, C.B. Reusken, and J. Wallinga. "Shorter Serial Intervals in SARS-CoV-2 Cases with Omicron BA.1 Variant Compared with Delta Variant, the Netherlands, 13 to 26 December 2021", *Euro Surveillance* 27:6 (2022): 2200042.

30 Rothe, C., M. Schunk, P. Sothmann, G. Bretzel, G. Froeschl, C. Wallrauch, T. Zimmer, V. Thiel, C. Janke, W. Guggemos, M. Seilmaier, C. Drosten, P. Vollmar, K. Zwirglmaier, S. Zange, R. Wölfel, and M. Hoelscher. "Transmission of 2019-nCoV Infection from an Asymptomatic Contact in Germany", *New England Journal of Medicine* 382:10 (2020): 970–971; Kimball, A., K.M. Hatfield, M. Arons, A. James, J. Taylor, K. Spicer, A.C. Bardossy, L.P. Oakley, S. Tanwar, Z. Chisty, J.M. Bell, M. Methner, J. Harney, J.R. Jacobs, C.M. Carlson, H.P. McLaughlin, N. Stone, S. Clark, C. Brostrom-Smith, L.C. Page, M. Kay, J. Lewis, D. Russell, B. Hiatt, J. Gant, J.S. Duchin, T.A. Clark, M.A. Honein, S.C. Reddy, J.A. Jernigan, Public Health – Seattle & King County, and CDC COVID-19 Investigation Team. "Asymptomatic and Presymptomatic SARS-CoV-2 Infections in Residents of a Long-Term Care Skilled Nursing Facility – King County, Washington, March 2020", *Morbidity and Mortality Weekly Report* 69:13 (2020): 377–381; Lai, C.C., Y.H. Liu, C.Y. Wang, Y.H. Wang, S.C. Hsueh, M.Y. Yen, W.C. Ko, and P.R. Hsueh. "Asymptomatic Carrier State, Acute Respiratory Disease, and Pneumonia Due to Severe Acute Respiratory Syndrome Coronavirus 2 (SARS-CoV-2): Facts and Myths", *Journal of Microbiology, Immunology and Infection* 53:3 (2020): 404–412; Hwang, H., J.S. Lim, S.A. Song, C. Achangwa, W. Sim, G. Kim, and S. Ryu. "Transmission Dynamics of the Delta Variant of SARS-CoV-2 Infections in South Korea", *Journal of the Infectious Diseases* 225:5 (2022): 793–799.

31 "Report of the WHO-China Joint Mission on Coronavirus Disease 2019 (COVID-19)", www.who.int/docs/default-source/coronaviruse/who-china-joint-mission-on-covid-19-final-report.pdf .

32 "Att vi skulle få en stor spridning i Sverige är inte troligt." [It is not likely that we should get a large spread in Sweden.] Anders Tegnell, 20 January 2020, www.aftonbladet.se/nyheter/a/WbBgwL/kinesiska-viruset-har-spridits-till-flera-lander–aven-via-manniskor .

33 Tegnell admitted that his and the agency's doubt about facemasks has influenced the people's attitude, www.dn.se/sverige/tegnell-svart-att-andra-attityden-till-munskydd/ .

34 Experts calculate that ca 3,000 lives could have been saved if Sweden would have used facemasks, www.gp.se/debatt/obegripligt-att-munskyddskrav-inte-inf%C3%B6rs-mot-omikron-1.63685437 .

35 www.kva.se/sv/vetenskap-i-samhallet/halsa/akademien-och-covid-19 .

36 Cf. www.gov.uk/government/organisations/scientific-advisory-group-for-emergencies and https://de.wikipedia.org/wiki/Corona-Expertenrat_der_Bundesregierung .

4

THE COVID-19 PANDEMIC AND THE SWEDISH STRATEGY

Central aspects of the strategy in relation to evidence and evidence-based medicine criteria

Martin Lindström

Introduction

The Covid-19 pandemic reached a societal spread in many European countries in late February and early March 2020, although singular individuals may have already become infected in late 2019. The first seriously affected country in Europe was Italy, but soon Spain, France, Belgium, the United Kingdom, the Netherlands and other countries became affected with just a short time lag. On 11 March 2020, the World Health Organization (WHO) Director General declared the outbreak as a pandemic.[1] The WHO recommended important measures such as physical distancing, mass testing and contact tracing.[2]

The Government policies and restrictions in Europe generally followed the WHO recommendations. Still, the policy measures implemented by Governments differed between European countries. A thorough reading of the timeline of events in different countries as well as the Oxford Government Response Tracker index for different countries over time clearly demonstrates that there were different forms of policies and physical distancing measures in the early spring of 2020.[3] Despite often decisive restrictions, quarantines, border closures, testing and contact tracing, the lack of tempo, early policy measures and most importantly weak public health institutions and institutional structures to protect population health in Europe have been criticized. These weaknesses may have resulted in comparatively high infection rates and mortality particularly compared to the countries in East Asia first affected by the pandemic.[4]

Sweden adopted to an important extent a different strategy to handle the pandemic than the other Nordic countries and most European countries. The official Swedish strategy consisted of six aims. The two first and major aims were to decrease the infection rate in order not to overload the healthcare system, while at the same time protecting the elderly and other risk groups. The other four

DOI: 10.4324/9781003289364-5

aims entailed to reduce negative effects on vital societal functions, to reduce the consequences of the pandemic for the public and the enterprises, to reduce anxiety and to enact correct measures with correct timing.[5] In early 2020, the Social Democrat-led coalition Government delegated full control over the handling of the pandemic to the Public Health Agency (*Folkhälsomyndigheten*, FHM) from the beginning. For a description of the history of FHM and its predecessors see Anders Vahlne's chapter in this book. The Swedish strategy in the spring of 2020 in its official definition and the Swedish strategy in its unofficial application was thus designed by the FHM. The strategy and its implementation strongly deviated from the previously cautious approach to public health and preventive measures practiced in Sweden for centuries described in the chapter by Gunnar Steineck.

The unofficial Swedish strategy included a strong, although not officially stated and mostly not openly stated, belief in the comparatively rapid achievement of natural herd immunity (i.e. herd immunity through natural infection of a major part of the population). The belief was openly stated already in an interview in the business newspaper *Dagens Industri* on 2 April 2020 and other interviews by the former state epidemiologist Johan Giesecke (1995–2005), who had been commissioned as an expert adviser by the FHM and who was without doubt one of the masterminds behind the strategy.[6] Herd immunity was expected to be achieved by natural spread in the population following deliberately relaxed restrictions and the partial stop of testing and contact tracing for other groups than in-hospital patients and risk groups after the second week of March.[7] The unofficial Swedish strategy also included a very strong belief in individual responsibility in handling the pandemic, almost to an extent that the Government and the FHM were supposed to be relieved from their responsibility. There was also a distinctly stated reference to evidence-based medicine, which is the focus of this chapter. Finally, the unofficial strategy (in part indirectly) included a neglect to cooperate internationally with the WHO, the EU, the European Centre for Disease Prevention and Control (ECDC) and the neighbouring Nordic countries.[8] In fact, Sweden was criticized internationally for the outcomes following from the main components of the strategy.[9]

The tax-financed Swedish public service television company seemingly supported even the unofficial parts of the strategy without too many critical questions, and uncritically informed the public that 50% of the population was expected to be infected by the end of April 2020.[10] This would have meant a rapid achievement of natural herd immunity, because the company also uncritically informed the public that natural herd immunity would be achieved when 50–60% of the population had been infected,[11] not mentioning how many deaths would occur as a result (with a 0.5–1.0% mortality, probably 25,000–50,000 deaths in the spring). Later in the spring when it became completely apparent that the spread of the contagion was clustered and considerably slower, the public service television company reported that 40% of the population infected would suffice for herd immunity under certain conditions of heterogeneity in the population.[12] Swedish news outlets and journalists in general also mostly "informed" the population concerning the strategy rather than critically questioning it in the spring of 2020.[13]

The former State Epidemiologist Johan Giesecke stated in the interview on 2 April 2020 that all other countries were wrong and that the Swedish strategy would result in Swedish society probably going back to normal at some point in May 2020.[14]

When the FHM was consulted regarding protective measures and other preventive measures against SARS-CoV-2 the answer was often that there was a lack of evidence, a position based on the concept of evidence-based medicine. Most countries in Europe and many countries globally sought to eradicate the virus by physical distancing, mass testing and contact tracing. In clear contrast, Swedish regions responsible for the healthcare system ended full-scale testing and contact tracing in the end of the second week of March and only targeted in-hospital patients and risk groups following an active recommendation from the FHM. This recommendation was also implemented in regions in southern Sweden with very low infection rates in the spring of 2020.[15] The FHM also displayed a consistent resistance to facemasks in crowded public places, including public transport in intense commuting hours, despite severe criticism from different sources including *Kungliga Vetenskapsakademien*.[16] The former State Epidemiologist, commissioned as expert adviser by the FHM from January until May 2020, explained in an interview with CNN on 17 April, 2020:

> We, or the Swedish Government, decided early, in January, that the measures we should take against the pandemic should be evidence-based. And when you start looking around at the measures being taken now by different countries, you'll find that very few of them have a shred of evidence. . . .
>
> But we know of one that has been known for 150 years or more, that washing your hands is good for you and good for others when you're in an epidemic. But the rest, border closures, school closings, social distancing . . . there's almost no science behind most of this.[17]

At the initially daily press conferences, together with representatives from other public state and regional healthcare authorities, the State Epidemiologist Anders Tegnell and other officials from the FHM often referred to "evidence" and "evidence-based" medicine as the scientific basis of the FHM's decisions and recommendations.

The results of the initial Swedish strategy during the first wave in the spring (March–June) of 2020 showed high mortality compared to the other Nordic countries and most countries in Europe.[18] Only later would Swedish Covid-19 mortality approach the European average. At the end of June 2020, the three Nordic countries, Denmark, Finland and Norway, had registered 605, 328 and 249 deaths with Covid-19, respectively, while Sweden reported 5,310 deaths.[19] The per capita death toll in Sweden was thus approximately ten times higher than in Finland and Norway.

Given the claim by the FHM and its commissioned former State Epidemiologist adviser that the Swedish strategy in the spring of 2020 was evidence-based, the question is to what extent this claim is valid. The aim is to discern to what extent the central tenets of the Swedish strategy during the spring of 2020 outlined earlier were in accordance with principles of evidence-based medicine and evidence available at the time.

Evidence-based medicine

The ideas of evidence-based medicine started to develop in the 1970s and 1980s. Evidence-based medicine integrates clinical experience, the aim to achieve the best possible outcome for the patient, and available scientific evidence and empirical facts of high quality in order to create the best possible basis for decision-making in order to solve medical problems. Evidence-based medicine concerns "the use of mathematical estimates of the risk of benefit and harm, derived from high-quality research on population samples, to inform clinical decision-making in the diagnosis, investigation and management of individual patients",[20] but the basic principles may also be applied to epidemiological problems in public health and population health.

Epidemiological studies can be divided broadly into intervention (or experimental) studies and observational studies. Intervention studies entail some form of intervention in the study design and study set-up, including comparisons between, for example, pharmacologically active medical treatment versus placebo, new medical treatment versus established (traditional) medical treatment, different new medical treatments, treatment versus non-treatment or combinations of more than two of these. Practically, intervention studies are mostly randomized clinical trials (RCTs). In RCTs, the patients are randomly assigned to any of the two or more treatment alternatives or to placebo (the patient not knowing that the placebo does not include any pharmacologically active substance). A major strength of randomization in RCTs is that both known and unknown confounders are adjusted for. A confounder is a factor associated with the exposure that also has an effect on the outcome. For instance, age and sex are regarded as natural confounders because they are associated with most exposures and have an effect on most outcomes. RCTs are mostly also double-blinded (i.e. both the doctor (MD) and the patient are unaware of the exact content of the treatment given to the specific patient). Intervention studies can also be conducted without randomization. Such intervention studies are generally regarded to have lower quality than randomized intervention studies. The ethical pre-conditions for conducting intervention studies include that experts should have differing opinions regarding the outcome and that the expected differences between different treatments or prevention strategies should be comparatively small. It should be noted that intervention studies may also be conducted at the societal level or any level of social setting instead of the individual, although individual level studies are much more common.[21]

Observational studies, in contrast, contain no components of active intervention and are solely based on data to observe and analyze. Observational studies include a wide array of study designs including cross-sectional and longitudinal studies.

Longitudinal studies fulfil the temporality criterion for causation (i.e. the strongest criterion for the judgement of causality in epidemiological studies). Prospective cohort studies, retrospective cohort studies, case-control studies, case-crossover studies and panel data studies are examples of longitudinal observational studies.[22] For discussion of the Swedish strategy in relation to epidemiology, see the chapter by Nele Brusselaers, and also the detailed report edited by her and others.[23]

A major principle of evidence-based medicine is that a hierarchy of scientific evidence and epidemiological study designs exists. Beginning in the late 1980s, several organizations have elaborated systems for grading the quality and validity of evidence. In 1989, the US Preventive Services Task Force (USPSTF) constructed a system hierarchy with RCTs at the top (Level I), followed by well-designed controlled trials lacking randomization (Level II-1). In this system, Level II-2 entails evidence-based well-designed cohort studies or case-control studies, preferably from several study centres or research groups. Level II-3 consists of time series designs including or excluding the intervention. Finally, Level III entails judgements of authorities, based on descriptive studies, reports from expert committees or clinical or other experience.[24]

Evidence-based medicine was first used as a defined concept in 1990. In 1992 the evidence-based medicine working group suggested a "new paradigm" in clinical medicine[25] as an attempt to formulate a basis for systematic assessments of medical evidence beyond the previous less systematic evidence base which also included elements of tradition, anecdote and theoretical reasoning.[26] Systematic reviews and meta-analyses are often considered to have the highest position in this original hierarchy,[27] although this position as well as their inclusion in the hierarchy of evidence-based medicine has been increasingly questioned.[28] Systematic reviews and meta-analyses are then followed in the hierarchy by intervention studies with particular emphasis on RCTs, followed by observational studies in the form of (particularly prospective) cohort studies, followed by case-control studies and subsequently followed by case series and case reports at the lowest level in the hierarchy of validity. Other less common versions of the hierarchy include elements of external validity (applicability)[29] and separation of internal (risk of bias) and external validity.[30]

The evidence-based medicine approach has its own weaknesses that have been increasingly discussed. First, the "quality mark" of evidence-based medicine has to some extent been distorted and misappropriated by vested interests in the pharmaceutical and medical equipment industry. These interests decide the tests to be performed, the treatments to be tested and the outcome measures to be evaluated. Furthermore, their RCTs are sometimes overpowered to make certain that small differences become statistically significant. In other instances they are underpowered. The inclusion criteria may be defined in ways favourable to the expected outcomes, doses of both intervention and control drugs may be controlled, surrogate endpoints may be used and the process may be subject to publication bias. The checklists and risk of bias tools developed in accordance with evidence-based medicine may be unable to detect increasingly subtle biases in industry-sponsored studies. Some policy recommendations following from evidence-based medicine results also seem to be based largely on political conviction. Second, the sheer volume of evidence in terms of clinical guidelines has become almost unmanageable. Third, evidence-based medicine is increasingly claimed to be a science approach with marginal gains. Large trials conducted in already well-researched fields of science run a risk to overestimate potential benefits and a corresponding risk to underestimate potential harms. Correspondingly, a shift from disease to the risk concept may be discerned. Fourth, well-intended efforts to automatize evidence through computerized decision support schemes may marginalize local, individualized and patient-initiated elements of the clinical consultation process. Such systems may also contribute to the tendency of increasing managerialism and politicization of clinical practice, which tends to be an increasingly driven technocratic exercise. Finally, study designs such as RCTs often have a poor fit for comorbidity. The process of aging of many populations worldwide results in an increasing prevalence of comorbidity (i.e. several parallel diseases and medical conditions in the same individual). Applying RCTs to such individuals may be highly and increasingly problematic.[31]

The evidence-based medicine criteria obviously have both pros and cons. Furthermore, the relative balance between these pros and cons also seem to have changed over time. This chapter neither defends nor challenges the use and practice of the principles of evidence-based medicine to evaluate scientific studies and research results. Instead, it assesses whether or not the Swedish strategy to handle the first wave of the pandemic in the spring of 2020 adhered to and followed the principles of evidence-based medicine and available evidence, as claimed by the FHM and its commissioned expert adviser themselves. Following the preceding exposition of the hierarchical system of evidence with regard to the status of studies and study designs, a ranking order of studies may be listed based on validity following evidence-based medicine:

1 Systematic reviews and meta-analyses (sometimes not included in the hierarchy).
2 Randomized controlled trials (RCTs).
3 Other not randomized intervention studies.
4 Cohort studies (particularly prospective cohort studies).
5 Case-control studies.
6 Multiple time series designs, cross-sectional data, ecological (aggregate) data.
7 Opinions of respected authorities based on clinical experience and descriptive studies or reports from expert committees.

Empirical evidence and practical experience in early 2020

During the earliest part of the Covid-19 outbreak and in the early part of the pandemic declared on 11 March 2020, Governments and health authorities were forced to make often very rapid decisions based on ecological observational data and group-level summaries rather than individual data. Apart from mathematical models, politicians and other decision-makers as well as their scientific advisers were confined to aggregate observational data such as incidence data at country, regional or municipal levels in order to make decisions concerning physical distancing, school closures, business closures, public transport closures, public places closures, mask wearing and other non-pharmaceutical interventions. Intervention studies such as RCTs but also non-randomized intervention studies were not available and are mostly not ethically defensible in this context. Natural experiments comparing different outcomes of physical distancing and lockdown measures in different countries or regions appeared useful. Still, such studies were only possible to analyze after preventive policy measures had been implemented, after some time had elapsed and after data comparable across countries and regions could be compiled.

Early observational studies included designs such as pre-post studies (a pre- versus post-implementation of measures comparison, in most studies without a control group), interrupted time series studies (a pre- versus post-implementation of measures comparison with extended time mostly without control group) and difference in differences designs (a pre- versus post-implementation of measures comparison with control group).[32] However, such studies were only possible after substantial time had elapsed. Most countries in Europe delayed the implementation of non-pharmaceutical physical distancing measures, which resulted in rapid virus transmission.[33] In a natural experiment study including 149 countries or regions, incidence rate ratios (IRRs) of Covid-19 before and after implementation of physical distancing interventions between 1 January and 30 May 2020 were analyzed. The physical distancing measures included closures of schools, workplaces and public transport, restrictions on mass gatherings and public events, and restrictions on movements/lockdowns. The results indicated that physical distancing interventions until 30 May or until 30 days post-intervention were associated with reductions in the incidence of Covid-19 globally. No additional effect of public transport closure was observed when the other four physical distancing measures were implemented. Earlier implementation of lockdown was significantly associated with a larger reduction in the IRRs of Covid-19. These results may be very helpful for planning and implementation of future measures, but the analyses of the non-pharmaceutical measures to implement physical distancing during the first wave in the spring of 2020 were only possible to assess after the first wave had elapsed.[34]

An overview of systematic reviews was conducted by the International Network of Coronavirus Disease 2019 (InterNetCovid-2019) regarding the validity of systematic reviews until the beginning of the pandemic on 11 March 2020. These systematic reviews concerned basic empirical, mostly descriptive findings regarding previously unknown information such as clinical symptoms; severe symptoms; shock reactions; prevalence at varying points in time; increased death rates among men, elderly and risk groups; health risks connected with pregnancy; risk of infection across the placenta; pharmacological and non-pharmaceutical treatments; diagnostics; test assessment; laboratory and radiological findings. This overview that analyzed evidence from the first 18 systematic reviews published after the emergence of Covid-19 until March 2020 concluded that confidence in the results of all reviews was "critically low" and of questionable usefulness. The authors of the overview of the systematic reviews characterized the results of the systematic reviews as "research waste".[35] Only one of the 18 systematic reviews concerned intervention studies with RCT design (the other systematic reviews included no intervention studies). This overview concluded that the current diagnostic and therapeutic alternatives, including rapid diagnostics and vaccines, are essential to limit transmission of respiratory infectious diseases such as the novel SARS-CoV-2 virus. Possible diagnostic approaches suggested included RT-PCR, serological assays and point-of care testing.[36] The other of the systematic reviews in the overview included observational studies and case reports. The percentage of cases with severe symptoms of all infected cases and case fatality rates was, for example, the subject of these reviews.[37] Almost none of the studies in the 18 systematic reviews in the overview were longitudinal cohort studies or case-control studies. The overview of systematic reviews concluded that even during public health emergencies such as the appearance of the pandemic, studies and systematic reviews should adhere to established methodological standards.[38]

At least in January until well into March of 2020, decision-makers were mainly confined to cross-sectional data, incidence data, ecological data, mathematical modelling (all point 6) and opinions of respected authorities based on clinical experience and descriptive studies or reports from expert committees (point 7). This begs the question how the official and unofficial Swedish strategies fared during the first wave in the spring of 2020 when the FHM openly defied several of the WHO recommendations. Since little was known about the SARS-CoV-2 virus in early 2020, the fact that most virus agents have different (not identical) mechanisms of transmission pointed to early detection and prompt implementation of infection control to avoid transmission in hospital settings and elsewhere,[39] which was also confirmed later.[40]

The Swedish strategy in the spring of 2020 in relation to evidence and evidence-based medicine

The Swedish strategy practiced during the first wave of the pandemic may be assessed in relation to available evidence at the time and the evidence-based medicine hierarchy of studies. The two main aims of the official Swedish strategy to decrease the infection rate in order not to overload the healthcare system and at the same time to protect the elderly and other risk groups was assessed already by the first of the Government and Parliament (*Riksdag*)-associated Corona Commission reports presented on 15 December 2020. The main conclusion is that the aim to protect the elderly in the municipality and private care homes failed for two main reasons. First, the care homes for the elderly lacked adequate and sufficient protection equipment, a serious shortage that was also observed throughout the healthcare system. Second, the lack of general testing, contact tracing and the aim to only decrease the infection rate instead of eradicating it led to high infection rates in the general population. Especially in combination with the lack of protection equipment, the high infection rates led to comparably high infection rates also in the care homes for the elderly, because the staff in the care homes is a part of the general population.[41] The decision by the FHM (with delegation from the Government) to allow comparably high infection rates in the population during the spring of 2020 without full-scale testing and contact tracing in the general population was also specifically criticized in the second Corona Commission report published on 29 October 2021.[42] This decision by the FHM not only contradicted evidence outlined earlier but probably also violated the law against communicable diseases (SFS, 2004) from 2004. The lax recommendations regarding physical distancing and the downsizing of testing and contact tracing in the general population were thus not in accordance with evidence and the recommendations from the WHO and previous experience from infectious disease prevention formalized as law. For an analysis of the time-scale and load on the healthcare system that would have been required to achieve natural herd immunity, see the chapter by Emil J. Bergholtz.

The officially stated Swedish strategy also made the claim to have good timing of the implementation of measures. Still, the Oxford Government Response Tracker indicates that the average level of Government interference and restrictions did not differ to any important extent between Sweden, Finland and Norway over the entire period mid-March to the end of June 2020. The index value 0 of the Oxford Government Response Tracker indicates no Government interference in general and no restrictions, and the index value 100 indicates total Government interference.[43] In fact, Sweden's average index for the period (average of eight measure points from mid-March to the end of June) was 56.7, while the average for Finland was a somewhat lower 52.6, for Norway 60.6 and for Denmark 64.8. The main difference between Sweden and particularly Finland and Norway (and to some extent Denmark) is not the average over the period but the timing of Government response over the period. The low index numbers for Sweden in March and early April indicate a lax and slow Government response. On 16 March, Sweden's index was 22.20, Denmark's 65.74, Finland's 57.41 and Norway's 60.19. In contrast, the high indexes for Sweden in late May and June indicate problems of relaxed Government interference due to the much more extensive and uncontrolled spread. On 30 June, Sweden's index was 59.26, Denmark's 57.41, Finland's 35.19 and Norway's 40.74.[44] The fact that Sweden in the spring (March to June) of 2020 had an average index close to those of Finland and Norway but more than ten times higher per capita mortality indicates a distinctly poor timing of implementation in the early part of the spring. The officially stated aim to handle the pandemic with good timing was simply not met during the first wave in the spring of 2020.[45]

These conclusions regarding the official Swedish strategy lead to the unofficial version of the Swedish strategy in the spring of 2020.

The belief in the possibility to relatively rapidly achieve natural herd immunity in the first wave of the pandemic also appeared uncertain given the important lack of knowledge regarding characteristics of the immunity from SARS-CoV-2 and the duration of immunity over time. There was a general lack of longitudinal serological and other studies regarding the characteristics of immunity and duration of immunity after infection with SARS-CoV-2: "Longitudinal serological studies are urgently needed to determine the extent and duration of SARS-CoV-2 immunity" (Kissler et al., 2020).[46] There was thus almost a complete lack of empirical evidence in the spring of 2020 that it would be possible to achieve natural herd immunity, particularly in a relatively short reach of time.

The strong reliance on individual responsibility in solving a global pandemic was not in accordance with early evidence. Evidence in early 2020 suggested that community-centred approaches in countries with strong infrastructures were successful. Evidence from early affected East Asian countries including South Korea[47] and Taiwan[48] suggested community-centred strategies including rapid expansion of diagnostic capacities, widespread testing, screening programs, and extensive efforts to isolate infected cases, tracing and putting contacts in quarantines. Effective measures in somewhat poorer countries with more limited capacity for testing such as Vietnam[49] included case identification, case isolation, extensive contact tracing, mass masking (facemasks) with the aim to reduce community transmission and quarantine of suspected cases. There was thus no evidence from earlier affected countries in East Asia for a strategy instead emphasizing individual decision-making (often based on unclear messages from the FHM).

The relative lack of international cooperation and coordination was also a trait of the unofficial Swedish strategy during the first wave in the spring of 2020. This weak international orientation inevitably followed from the belief in the relatively rapid achievement of natural herd immunity and the belief in individual responsibility. An honest interview statement that "All other countries are wrong"[50] was probably coloured by a strong sense of Swedish exceptionalism. This poor international orientation and possible sense of national superiority clearly defied previously existing empirical evidence and the principles of evidence-based medicine. In fact, international cooperation and coordination in matters of public health started with the International Sanitary Conference in Paris in 1851. The aim of this conference was exclusively to control and restrict the spread of communicable diseases such as plague, yellow fever, smallpox and particularly cholera across borders through international cooperation and the signing of international conventions regarding appropriate preventive measures such as quarantines. In total, 14 such conferences were held in 1851–1938, exclusively focused on prevention of communicable infectious diseases. The WHO was founded in 1948. In 1951, the WHO issued the International Sanitary Regulations (ISR) regarding the handling and prevention of infectious diseases. The ISR were later revised and expanded in 1969 into the International Health Regulations (IHR).[51] The sanitary conferences before the Second World War and the post-war ISR issued by the WHO focused on communicable infectious diseases, but international cooperation was later widened to non-communicable diseases and other public health issues and redefined as international health. Later, the new post-war concept of international health was developed further, most importantly promoted by the Alma-Ata Declaration

(1978), into the broader concept of global health. Global health as a basis for international cooperation incorporates a broader definition of health as complete physical, mental and social well-being. Global health further incorporates equality, health as a socioeconomic issue and as a human right, considerations regarding the role of public institutions and organizations regarding health issues, and the incorporation of primary healthcare into healthcare systems and international cooperation,[52] but international cooperation began with cooperation concerning communicable infectious diseases. The lack of coordination with other countries clearly defied this unquestionable historical experience.

The Swedish strategy in the spring of 2020 was to an important extent not in accordance with available evidence. The FHM seems to have put low or no requirements on evidence supporting the strategy. In sharp contrast, the FHM set up very high demands on evidence regarding protective measures. The FHM for instance displayed active resistance against facemasks in public spaces at the public press conferences throughout the first pandemic year 2020, often claiming lack of evidence even regarding crowded places such as public transport during commuting hours. The FHM was criticized for this stance by *Kungliga Vetenskapsakademien*.[53] Already in the spring of 2020, systematic international reviews and meta-analyses clearly suggested protective effects of facemask both in public places in general and in hospitals to a similar extent.[54] Similar studies published just somewhat later confirmed these results.[55] The resistance from the FHM against facemasks in crowded public places is only comprehensible given the in-official strategy to achieve natural herd immunity. It is an illustration of the pronounced imbalance between the low requirements of evidence for decisions following from the strategy, in contrast to the very high requirements on evidence for protective measures.

Conclusions

The FHM claimed to be following best evidence and the principles of evidence-based medicine during the first wave of the pandemic in March to June 2020 (and even later). However, accumulated knowledge regarding the effects of physical distancing, mass testing and contact tracing was scarce and based on empirical data and observational studies with low ranking in the hierarchy of studies as defined according to the principles of evidence-based medicine. Systematic reviews produced at this point in time were in later assessments classified as "research waste". Intervention studies were almost non-existent, and had at this point in time not been conducted with regard to non-pharmaceutical interventions and non-laboratory research. Intervention studies with regard to physical distancing would also have required ethical permissions, which would have been particularly hard to obtain, and studies based on natural experiments were only possible to conduct in retrospect in order to formulate recommendations concerning how to handle future waves. Comparatively high-ranking observational studies with longitudinal study designs such as cohort studies and case-control studies were also very scarce or non-existing. Consequently, political and administrative decision-makers were confined to multiple time series designs, cross-sectional data, ecological (aggregate) data and opinions of respected authorities based on clinical experience and descriptive studies or reports from expert committees, based on crude data and practical experience (i.e. the lowest ranking levels in the evidence-based medicine hierarchy). In order to follow evidence, the major reasonable path would have been to follow the recommendations from the WHO regarding physical distancing, general testing and contact tracing based on crude observational studies and experience. Following the recommendations from a respected expert authority would have been the appropriate decision based on scarce evidence and principles of evidence-based medicine.

In the late winter and early spring of 2020, the characteristics and the duration of immunity against SARS-CoV-2 were essentially unknown and there was a call for longitudinal serological studies internationally. The unofficially stated claim in national and international interviews that Sweden would return to normal at some point in time in May 2020 (following the achievement of natural herd immunity) was thus essentially unsubstantiated. Furthermore, the belief in comparatively rapid achievement of natural herd immunity was particularly hazardous and scientifically unsupported given the nearly complete lack of protection equipment in the care homes for the elderly and disabled and in the general healthcare system, a fact that was particularly strongly criticized in the first Corona Commission report. The decision to give up mass testing and contact tracing for all except in-hospital patients and certain risk groups in the second week of March 2020 was not only directly contrary to the principles of evidence-based medicine in defying recommendations by the WHO based on crude empirical data from earlier affected countries. It probably also defied the law regarding infectious disease control (SFS, 2004) which states that accurate necessary measures should be taken to protect the public. The belief that people below risk age should be given a major responsibility in handling a global pandemic and make individual decisions to protect the elderly and other risk groups seems to have lacked evidence at the time.

The lack of cooperation with the WHO, the EU and neighbouring Nordic countries was also directly contrary to available evidence.

This chapter has mainly focused on some of the most crucial traits of the Swedish strategy during the spring of 2020. In some instances evidence supporting protective measures was downplayed or neglected. One example is the resistance against facemasks in crowded places and the claim by the FHM during most of 2020 that facemasks would divert users' attention from other recommendations such as physical distancing, which essentially lacks scientific support.[56] The lack of evidence from high-ranking studies such as RCTs does not exclude strong protective measures, including the dissuasion or rather prohibition of jumping from airplanes at high altitude without a parachute involving absolute death risk from strong gravitational forces.[57] The initial Swedish strategy involved no or low demands in terms of evidence on the components of the strategy itself, but very high demands on evidence for protective measures.

In sum, the FHM, which was commissioned by the Government to lead the handling of the pandemic during the first wave in the spring of 2020 and until some time had elapsed into the second wave in the autumn of 2020, did not sufficiently follow evidence or adhere to the principles of evidence-based medicine, as claimed. The FHM constructed its strategy based on other principles and hypotheses involving rapid achievement of natural herd immunity. In contrast, evidence-based public health policy should take all epidemiological, medical, clinical and practical circumstances into account.

Notes

1 World Health Organization. *WHO announces COVID-19 outbreak a pandemic*, Geneva: World Health Organization, 2020.
2 United Nations. "'You Cannot Fight a Fire Blindfolded': WHO Chief Blasts Slow Virus Testing Response", *UN News*, Global Human Stories, UN, 16 March (2020), https://news.un.org/en/story/2020/03/1059552 (accessed 10 January 2022).
3 Hale, T., N. Angrist, R. Goldszmidt, B. Kira, A. Petherick, T. Phillips, S. Webster, E. Cameron-Blake, L. Hallas, S. Majumdar, and H. Tatlow. "A Global Panel Database of Pandemic Policies" (Oxford COVID-19 Government Response Tracker), *Nature Human Behavior* 5 (2021): 529–538.
4 Shokoohi, M., M. Osooli, and S. Stranges. "COVID-19 Pandemic: What Can the West Learn from the East?" *International Journal of Health Policy and Management* 9:10 (2020): 436–438.
5 Regeringskansliet. *Regeringens arbete med coronapandemi: Strategi med anledning av det nya coronaviruset*, Stockholm: Regeringskansliet, 7 April 2020, www.regeringen.se/regeringens-politik/regeringens-arbete-med-coronapandemin/strategi-med-anledning-av-det-nya-coronaviruset/ .
6 Grundberg Wolodarski, K. "Johan Giesecke: Alla andra länder gör fel", *Dagens Industri*, 2 April 2020, https://weekend.di.se/intervjuer/alla-andra-lander-gor-fel .
7 Karlsson, P. "Nya strategin-slutar räkna exakta antalet coronafall", *Aftonbladet*, 13 March (updated 17 March), 2020, www.aftonbladet.se/nyheter/samhalle/a/70GQRV/nya-strategin-slutar-rakna-exakta-antalet-coronafall; Lindström, M. "The COVID-19 Pandemic and the Swedish Strategy: Epidemiology and Postmodernism", *SSM Population Health* 11 (2020): 100643; Lindström, M. "A Commentary on 'The Trouble with Trust: Time-Series Analysis of Social Capital, Income Inequality, and COVID-19 Deaths in 84 Countries'", *Social Science and Medicine* 263 (2020): 113386.
8 Lindström. "The COVID-19 Pandemic and the Swedish Strategy".
9 Standard Ethics. *Sweden Standard Ethics Downgrading*, London: Standard Ethics, 21 May 2020, www.reddit.com/r/svepol/comments/gp1aj0/press_release_sweden_standard_ethics_rating/ .
10 SVT. "Halva Sveriges befolkning smittad i april", 1 April 2020 (updated 6 April 2020), www.svt.se/nyheter/inrikes/halva-sveriges-befolkning-smittad-i-april .
11 SVT. "Så fungerar flockimmunitet", 20 April 2020 (updated 21 April 2020), www.svt.se/nyheter/inrikes/sa-fungerar-flockimmunitet .
12 SVT. "Ny uppskattning: 40% smittade kan ge immunitet", 9 May 2020 (updated 14 May 2020), www.svt.se/nyheter/tegnell-vi-kommer-med-besked .
13 Andersson, U., M. Bergman, G. Bohlin, F. Brounéus, P. Dahlgren, E. Ekdahl, M. Ghersetti, B. Johansson, D. Morton, E. Starke Sundén, A. Widholm, E. Östlund, and L. Truedson (eds.). *Journalistik i coronans tid*, Stockholm: Institutet för Mediastudier, 2021, https://mediestudier.se/wp-content/uploads/2021/02/Journalistik-i-coronans-tid_sammanslagen_webb.pdf; Ghersetti, M., and T. Odén. *Coronapandemin våren 2020. En undersökning om nyheter och opinion*, Göteborg, Karlstad: Göteborgs Universitet,

Myndigheten för samhällsskydd och beredskap, March 2021, https://rib.msb.se/filer/pdf/29525.pdf; Lindström, M. "The New Totalitarians: The Swedish COVID-19 Strategy and the Implications of Consensus Culture and Media Policy for Public Health", *SSM Population Health* 14 (2021): 100788.

14 Grundberg Wolodarski. "Johan Giesecke: Alla andra länder gör fel".

15 Karlsson. "Nya strategin- slutar räkna exakta antalet coronafall".

16 Kungliga Vetenskapsakademien. *Ny rapport om munskydd och ventilation från vetenskapsakademiens expertgrupp om COVID-19*, Stockholm: Kungliga Vetenskapsakademin, 19 November 2020, www.kva.se/sv/pressrum/pressmeddelanden/ny-rapport-om-munskydd-och-ventilation-fran-vetenskapsakademiens-expertgrupp-om-covid-19 .

17 Sayers, F. "Swedish Expert: Why Lockdowns Are the Wrong Policy – The Post", *UnHerd*, 17 April 2020.

18 World Health Organization. *Coronavirus Disease 2019 (COVID-19). Situation Report-162*, Geneva: World Health Organization, 2020.

19 *Ibid.*

20 Greenhalgh, T. *How to Read a Paper: The Basics of Evidence-Based Medicine*, Chichester, West Sussex, UK and Hoboken, NJ: Wiley-Blackwell, 2010.

21 Aschengrau, A., and G.R. Seage III. *Epidemiology in Public Health*, 3rd ed., Boston, MA: Jones & Bartlett Learning, 2014.

22 *Ibid.*

23 Brusselaers, Nele, David Steadson, Kelly Bjorklund, Sofia Breland, Jens Stilhoff Sörensen, Andrew Ewing, Sigurd Bergmann, and Gunnar Steineck. "Evaluation of Science Advice During the COVID-19 Pandemic in Sweden", *Humanities and Social Sciences Communications* 9, Article number: 91 (2022), www.nature.com/articles/s41599-022-01097-5 .

24 US Preventive Services Task Force. *Guide to Clinical Services: Report of the US Preventive Services Task Force*, Darby, PA: DIANE Publishing, 1989.

25 Guyatt, G., J. Cairns, D. Churchill, D. Cook, B. Haynes, J. Hirsh, J. Irvine, M. Levine, M. Levine, J. Nishikawa, D. Sackett, P. Brill-Edwards, H. Gerstein, J. Gibson, R. Jaeschke, A. Kerigan, A. Neville, A. Panju, A. Detsky, M. Enkin, P. Frid, M. Gerrity, A. Laupacis, V. Lawrence, J. Menard, V. Moyer, C. Mulrow, P. Links, A. Oxman, J. Sinclair, and P. Tugwell (Evidence Based Medicine Working Group). "Evidence Based Medicine. A New Approach to Teaching the Practice of Medicine", *JAMA* 268:17 (1992): 2420–2425.

26 Greenhalgh, T., J. Howick, and N. Maskrey. "Evidence Based Medicine: A Movement in Crisis?" *British Medical Journal* 348 (2014): g3725.

27 Paul, M., and L. Leihove. "Systematic Review or Meta-Analysis? Their Place in the Evidence Hierarchy", *Clinical Microbiology and Infection* 20 (2014): 97–100.

28 Murad, M.H., N. Asi, M. Alsawas, and F. Alahdab. "New Evidence Pyramid", *Evidence Based Medicine* 21:4 (2016): 125–127.

29 Agoritsas, T., P. Vandvik, I. Neumann, B. Rochwerg, R. Jaeschke, R. Hayward, G. Guyatt, and K.A. McKibbon. "Finding Current Best Evidence", in Guyatt, G., D. Rennie, M.O. Meade, and D.J. Cook (eds.). *Users' Guide to the Medical Literature: A Manual for Evidence-Based Clinical Practice*, 3rd ed., New York, NY: McGraw-Hill, 2015: 29–50.

30 Tomlin, G., and B. Borgetto. "Research Pyramid: A New Evidence-Based Practice Model for Occupational Therapy", *American Journal of Occupational Therapy* 65 (2011): 189–196.

31 Greenhalgh et al. "Evidence Based Medicine".

32 Digitale, J.C., K. Stojanovski, C.E. McCulloch, and M.A. Handley. "Study Designs to Assess Real-World Interventions to Prevent COVID-19", *Frontiers in Public Health* 9 (2021): 657976.

33 Nanda, M., Aashima, and R. Sharma. "Review of COVID-19 Epidemiology and Public Health Response in Europe in 2020", *Clinical Epidemiology and Global Health* 12 (2021): 100882.

34 Islam, N., S.J. Sharp, G. Chowell, S. Shabnam, I. Kawachi, B. Lacey, J.M. Massaro, R.B. D'Agostino Sr, and M. White. Physical distancing interventions and incidence of coronavirus disease 2019: natural experiment in 149 countries. *British Medical Journal* 370 (2021): m2743.

35 Borges do Nascimento, I.J., D.P. O'Mathuna, T.C. von Groote, H.M. Abdulazeem, I. Weerasekara, A. Marusic, L. Puljak, V.T. Civile, I. Zakarija-Grkovic, T. Poklepovic Pericic, A.N. Atallah, S. Filoso, N.L. Bragazzi, and M. Soriano Marcolino (The International Network of Coronavirus Disease 2019 (InterNetCovid-19)). "Coronavirus Disease (COVID-19) Pandemic: An Overview of Systematic Reviews", *BMC Infectious Diseases* 21 (2021): 525.

36 Pang, J., M.X. Wang, I.Y.H. Ang, S.H.X. Tan, R.F. Lewis, J.I.P. Chen, R.A. Gutierrez, S.X.W. Gwee, P.E.Y. Chua, Q. Yang, X.Y. Ng, R.K. Yap, H.Y. Tan, Y.Y. Teo, C.C. Tan, A.R. Cook, J.C.H. Yap, and L.Y. Hsu. "Potential Rapid Diagnostics, Vaccine and Therapeutics for 2019 Novel Coronavirus. (2019-nCoV): A Systematic Review", *Journal of Clinical Medicine* 9:3 (2020): 623.

37 Sun, P., S. Qie, Z. Liu, J. Ren, K. Li, and J. Xi. "Clinical Characteristics of Hospitalized Patients with SARS-CoV-2 Infection: A Single Arm Meta-Analysis", *Journal of Medical Virology* 92:6 (2020): 612–617.

38 Borges do Nascimento et al. "Coronavirus Disease (COVId-19) Pandemic".

39 Bonvehi, P.E., and E.R. Temporiti. "Transmission and Control of Respiratory Viral Infections in the Healthcare Setting", *Current Treatment Options in Infectious Diseases* 10 (2018): 182–196.

40 Havers, S.M., E.K. Martin, A. Wilson, and L. Hall. "A Systematic Review and Meta-Analysis of Policy Intervention Characteristics That Influence the Implementation of Government-Directed Policy in the Hospital Setting: Implications for Infection Prevention and Control", *Journal of Infection Prevention* 21:3 (2020): 84–96.

41 Melin, M., S. Ahlbäck Öberg, A. Enander, V. Jovic, C. Lif, T. Persson, G. Stiernstedt, M. Thorslund, J. Sonnergård, E. Björkegran, M. Bedelius, P. Jansson, M. Neijnes, S.E. Wånell, H. Ziobro, and O. Östergren. *Coronakommissionen. Äldreomsorgen under pandemin*, Stockholm: Delbetänkande av Coronakommissionen, Statens Offentliga utredningar, SOU, 2020: 80, https://coronakommissionen.com/wp-content/uploads/2020/12/sou_2020_80_aldreomsorgen-under-pandemin_webb.pdf .

42 Melin, M., S. Ahlbäck Öberg, A. Enander, V. Jovic, C. Lif, T. Persson, G. Stiernstedt, M. Thorslund, J. Sonnergård, E. Björkegran, M. Bedelius, P. Jansson, M. Neijnes, S.E. Wånell, H. Ziobro, and O. Östergren. *Coronakommissionen. Sverige under pandemin. Volym 1. Smittspridning och smittskydd*, Stockholm: Delbetänkande av Coronakommissionen, Statens Offentliga utredningar, SOU, 2021: 89, https://coronakommissionen.com/wp-content/uploads/2021/10/sverige-under-pandemin-volym-1_webb.pdf .

43 Hale et al. "A Global Panel Database of Pandemic Policies".

44 *Ibid.*

45 Melin et al. *Coronakommissionen. Sverige under pandemin. Volym 1.*

46 Kissler, S.M., C. Tedijanto, E. Goldstein, Y. Grad, and M. Lipsitch, M. "Projecting the Transmission Dynamics of SARS-CoV-2 Through the Post-Pandemic Period", *Science* 368:6493 (2020): 1–17.

47 Normile, D. "Coronavirus Cases Have Dropped Sharply in South Korea. What's the Secret to Its Success?" *Science*, 17 March 2020; Park, S., G.J. Choi, and H. Ko. "Information Technology-Based Training Strategy in Response to COVID-19 in South Korea-Policy Controversies", *JAMA* 323:21 (2020): 2129–2130.

48 Wang, C.J., C.Y. Ng, and R.H. Brook. "Response to COVID-19 in Taiwan: Big Data Analytics, New Technology, and Proactive Testing", *JAMA* 323:14 (2020): 1341–1342.

49 Trevisan, M., L.C. Le, and A.V. Le. "The COVID-19 Pandemic: A View from Vietnam", *American Journal of Public Health* 110:8 (2020): 1152–1153.

50 Grundberg Wolodarski. "Johan Giesecke: Alla andra länder gör fel".

51 Birn, A.E. "The Stages of International (global) Health: Histories of Success or Successes of History?" *Global Public Health* 4:1 (2009): 50–68.
52 Holst, J. "Global Health – Emergence, Hegemonic Trends and Biomedical Reductionism", *Globalization and Health* 16:1 (2020): 42.
53 Kungliga Vetenskapsakademien. *Ny rapport om munskydd och ventilation från vetenskapsakademiens expertgrupp om COVID-19*, Stockholm: Kungliga Vetenskapsakademin, 19 November 2020, www.kva.se/sv/pressrum/pressmeddelanden/ny-rapport-om-munskydd-och-ventilation-fran-vetenskapsakademiens-expertgrupp-om-covid-19 .
54 Chu, D.K., E.A. Akl, S. Duda, K. Solo, S. Yaacoub, and H.J. Schunemann (Covid-19 Systematic Urgent Review Group Effort (SURGE) Study, 2020). "Physical Distancing, Facemasks, and Eye Protection to Prevent Person-to-Person Transmission of SARS-CoV-2 and COVID-19: A Systematic Review and Meta-Analysis", *The Lancet* 395 (2020): 1973–1987.
55 See, for example, Howard, J., A. Huang, Z. Li, Z. Tufekci, V. Zdimal, H.M. van der Westhuizen, A. von Delft, A. Price, L. Fridman, L.H. Tang, V. Tang, G.L. Watson, C.E. Bax, R. Shaikh, F. Questier, D. Hernandez, L.F. Chu, C.M. Ramirez, and A.W. Rimoin. "An Evidence Review of Facemasks Against COVID-19", *PNAS* 118:4 (2021): e2014564118 (1–12); Matuschek, C. et al. "Facemasks: Benefits and Risks During the COVID-19 Crisis", *European Journal of Medical Research* 25:32 (2020): 1–8; Li, Y., M. Liang, L. Gao, M.A. Ahmed, J.P. Uy, C. Cheng, Q. Zhou, and C. Sun. "Facemasks to Prevent Transmission of COVID-19: A Systematic Review and Meta-Analysis", *American Journal of Infection Control* 49 (2021): 900–906.
56 Kungliga Vetenskapsakademien. "Ny rapport om munskydd och ventilation från vetenskapsakademiens expertgrupp om COVID-19".
57 Smith, G.C.S., and J.P. Pell. "Parachute Use to Prevent Death and Major Trauma Related to Gravitational Challenge: Systematic Review of Randomized Controlled Trials", *British Medical Journal* 327 (2003): 1459–1461; Yeh, R.W., L.R. Valsdottir, M.W. Yeh, C. Shen, D.B. Kramer, J.B. Strom, E.A. Secemsky, J.L. Healy, R.M. Domeier, D.S. Kazi, and B.K. Nallamother. "Parachute Use to Prevent Death and Major Trauma When Jumping from Aircraft: Randomized Control Trial", *British Medical Journal* 363 (2018): k5094.

5

THE SWEDISH COVID-19 RESPONSE

From poorly judged utilitarianism to history revisionism and the tragedy of the commons

Emil J. Bergholtz

Prologue

There is an eerie similarity between the Swedish Covid-19 strategy and the four-stage strategy described in the 1980s British political satire *Yes, Prime Minister*:[1]

- In stage one we say nothing is going to happen.
- In stage two we say maybe something is going to happen, but we shall do nothing about it.
- In stage three we say maybe there is something we should do about it, but there is nothing we can do.
- In stage four we say maybe there is something we could have done, but it is too late now.

At the time of writing, Sweden is in December 2021 encountering the fourth wave of the Covid-19 pandemic whereby the Delta variant is joined by Omicron.[2] The fourth wave, like the first three, was greeted with denial by state epidemiologist Anders Tegnell.[3] Tegnell's public denials persisted long after evidence from other countries was available and being used internationally to prepare for a new wave of infection. Sweden's leaders largely downplayed risks in spite of the overwhelming evidence.

There are many possible ways of explaining the anomalous Swedish response to the pandemic, and it will likely remain a controversial topic of social science research for a long time ahead. Perhaps the simplest plausible explanation involves lack of relevant competence,[4] normalcy bias, and an inability to admit errors by the leaders both at FHM, including Tegnell and General Director Johan Carlson, and in the Government including Prime Minister Stefan Löfven and Minister of social affairs Lena Hallengren. The hunt for herd immunity underpinned the actions

DOI: 10.4324/9781003289364-6

during the first wave, while sunk cost fallacy, plan continuation bias,[5] and the inability to admit errors and to learn from failures[6] hindered self-correction during the following (so far) three waves.

From the start, FHM did much to downplay the threats posed by the pandemic. Tegnell opined on January 16, 2020:

> For a large outbreak it is necessary for the virus to be good at being transmitted from human to human. This does not seem to be the case.[7]

Even late in February, after large outbreaks in countries like Italy and Iran, Tegnell remained confident that it was not going to be followed by a major outbreak in Sweden.[8] On March 2, FHM General Director Johan Carlson claimed that, in the worst-case scenario, Sweden could get 10 000–15 000 cases.[9] On March 8, facing an increasing number of new cases in Sweden (203 confirmed at that point), Tegnell said that his prediction of just a few days earlier that the spread should already have peaked was a bit too optimistic and he instead predicted that Sweden would peak in a day or two,[10] on March 9 or 10.

Just a few days later, a remarkably abrupt change of attitude occurred. On March 13, FHM signalled that widespread testing was no longer desirable:[11] instead of almost no infections, almost the entire population was suddenly expected to get infected. In fact, this became the strategy; in an email correspondence on March 15 with (former) infection doctor Peet Tüll, Tegnell confirmed the choice of aiming for herd immunity.[12] In *Aftonbladet* on March 16 he praised the UK strategy that was at the time still openly advocating for herd immunity by mass infection.[13] Tegnell also stated that it was the only way to control the spread of infection. On the same day, the UK abruptly changed strategy. Already by then, these ideas had been condemned by numerous experts and by the WHO,[14] but a report from Imperial College London[15] estimating the disastrous implications of a mitigation strategy aiming for herd immunity via infection seemed to have been the last straw for the UK. Suddenly, Sweden stood alone.[16]

Thus, it seems that at some point in time between March 8 and 13, 2020, a decision was made that the best option was to let the disease spread throughout the society in a "controlled manner" only aiming to "flatten the curve" so that health care would not be overwhelmed.[17] Although passivity and an unwillingness to admit that they should have acted earlier likely played a role, the argumentation was utilitarian[18] (based on a calculation supposedly leading to an optimal common outcome): the chosen path was claimed to be more scientific and rational.

Löfven stated:

> We have chosen the strategy of flattening the curve . . . this means that we will have more seriously ill people who must be cared for in intensive care, we will have significantly more deaths. We will count the deaths in thousands.

This was on April 3, 2020, long before it had gone that far.[19] In contrast, for example, Prime Minister of New Zealand Jacinda Arden stated that resolute interventions were necessary to not risk the lives of (tens of) thousands of New Zealanders.[20] These turned out to be self-fulfilling prophecies, for both countries.

Former state epidemiologist and influential FHM advisor Johan Giesecke said that "powerful interventions that are visible on TV are only important for politicians," and that "if we let the disease spread relatively undisturbed we will get a great immunity in the population that will eventually stop the epidemic, and in a second wave we will be considerably better protected."[21] One may have fundamental ethical concerns about such a strategy, but from an utilitarian viewpoint it could at least in principle be warranted, for instance if one would have known with a decent degree of confidence that the disease would have been harmless and that it would spread so efficiently that trying to stop it would require overly costly interventions. This was clearly not the case and we now know that "flattening the curve" has been a disastrous strategy. It led to worse outcomes in all regards, as compared to pursuing a strategy aiming to eliminate the disease: for health, for the economy, and for the civil liberties.[22]

This outcome was glaringly obvious to many including the author of this chapter in the early spring of 2020. To illuminate this, we will now critically revisit the basic assumptions of the Swedish strategy in the light of what was known in February 2020 about the original strain of the virus.

The Fata Morgana of herd immunity: the issues of timescales and a false dichotomy

It was commonly accepted early on during this pandemic that at least 60% of the population would have to become infected to reach herd immunity; according to Tegnell and his peers, it was the only thing that could stop the pandemic.[23] It was claimed by FHM and the proponents of the Swedish strategy that this state could be reached within a few months, perhaps even a few weeks, without overwhelming the health care capacity. At the same time, early 2020, it was also estimated that around 2% of all infected would require intensive care treatment and that each such patient would spend on average about 15 days in an ICU. Sweden, with a population of slightly over 10 million, had around 500 ICU beds in total, the second lowest amount per capita in Europe.[24] Let us assume that all these beds would be used exclusively for Covid-19 (in practice, extra beds would obviously be needed for, say, people involved in traffic accidents and patients suffering organ failure, sepsis, heart attacks, or strokes), and (also unrealistically)[25] that precisely all ICU beds, but no more, would be filled at all times. We thus arrive at a minimal time needed to reach herd immunity of approximately $0.6 \times 0.02 \times 15 \times 10\,000\,000/500 = 3600$ days (i.e. around 10 years!). It would also imply thousands of deaths each year. With the fatality rate of 0.6% as estimated by FHM based on the young population of Stockholm during the spring of 2020, there would be a total of 36 000 deaths before reaching the desired (mirage of) herd immunity. More realistic estimates based on the age profile of Sweden as a whole lead to even higher estimates for the death toll as discussed in the chapter by Rodney Edvinsson.

Clearly, there was significant uncertainty in these early numbers. However, although the average time spent in an ICU later turned out to be somewhat shorter outside of China,[26] the estimate of several years or even decades until reaching potential herd immunity – rather than a few weeks or months – remains robust. FHM themselves estimated that 5% (!) of all infected would require ICU care.[27] Moreover, corona viruses generally have short-lived immunity lasting months rather than decades, which has now been confirmed for SARS-CoV-2 as re-infections are becoming ever more prevalent.[28] Even worse, as we will return to later in this chapter, the virus is mutating. SARS-CoV-2 has become increasingly more infectious throughout the pandemic, posing an ever-greater challenge to humanity. While the original strain was relatively easy to stop, the new variants Delta and Omicron proved to be much more formidable opponents.

As has been painfully documented, Sweden did not provide adequate care for its weakest.[29] Without physical examination and without consulting the sick or their relatives, many elderly were routinely directed to palliative care and provided, for example, morphine instead of life-saving care and oxygen.[30] While at the same time temporarily doubling the number of ICU beds, it was proclaimed that Sweden had managed to retain sufficient health care capacity at all times. Furthermore, the number of cancelled planned surgeries were many more in Sweden compared to, for example, Denmark.[31] This, together with inadequate non-pharmaceutical interventions (NPIs),[32] accelerated the pandemic in Sweden, yet after the first wave was over, the number of infected was only about a tenth of what would have been necessary for hypothetical herd immunity. All this took place at a price of over 5000 dead and many more long-term ill with unclear future prospects, many of whom still suffer terribly.[33] Long-term sequelae have never been taken into account within the Swedish strategy. At a press conference in January 2021, Tegnell answered that post Covid "is primarily a healthcare issue" to the question of whether post Covid (a.k.a. long-Covid or long-hauler Covid) is a public health issue.[34] The first references to post Covid appeared on the website of FHM as late as in April 2021 (!).

One wonders, are there loopholes? Could we have missed something crucial in these considerations? Could there be another way of arriving at herd immunity, that is much quicker while at the same time actually protecting the vulnerable?

The impossibility of selective containment

Is there anything we could have done to reach herd immunity quickly without overburdening the health care capacity and/or sacrificing elderly and risk groups? The much-debated "Great Barrington Declaration" (GBD), which was signed at the headquarters of the libertarian think-tank American Institute for Economic Research (AIER), asserts that this is the case.[35] The signers claim that people who are at risk should be shielded while the disease spreads more or less freely through the rest of the society. They do not specify how this "focused protection," as they call it, should be practically achieved.

The Declaration and the Swedish approach are incredibly similar in both ideology and policy. The Declaration calls for, and Sweden delivered, a strategy which selectively puts in place strong restrictions only for at-risk groups, in particular people above 70 years of age[36] and in long-term residential care homes.[37] In the meantime, younger people were repeatedly told that they are in no danger and children were deemed to be essentially immune (cf. the chapter by Johanna Höög). In practice, this failed to prevent the infection spread in the risk groups, as is evident from Sweden's much higher death toll compared to its Scandinavian neighbours. In fact, the death toll in care homes has closely followed the overall spread of the disease in society, as has been shown in detailed studies of many countries around the world.[38] The Swedish Corona Commission, appointed by the Government to investigate the Covid response concluded:

> Most likely . . . the single most important factor behind the major outbreaks and the high number of deaths in residential care is the overall spread of the virus in the society.[39]

Thus, the outcome of the Swedish strategy was the worst possible for our most vulnerable: they were forced into isolation but did not benefit from a reduced spread of infection that such measures would have entailed if done in solidarity by society at large. Instead they perished, often alone.

It should have been clear to almost anyone, and particularly Swedish public health officials, that this outcome was inevitable, as any basic understanding of the dynamics of epidemic spread makes clear:[40] synchronisation is a generic phenomenon of coupled dynamical systems. In this case, it implies that a major outbreak in one part of a society (e.g. in the group with assumed low personal risk) necessarily entails an outbreak in all other parts of the same society (including those with high personal risk) at a rate proportional to that of the initial outbreak.[41] It is worth noticing that while the "experts" were enthusiastically calculating overly optimistic herd immunity thresholds and immune population percentages, it was left to "hobby epidemiologists"[42] such as the author of this chapter to clarify this undeniable mathematics of why the GBD and the Swedish approach could never work as advertised.

It is furthermore important to point out that, while age and pre-existing health conditions fairly reliably predict the risk of acute life-threatening illness, there is no easy way to predict risk of long-Covid,[43] a suffering which also affects the previously young and healthy, even children, to a significant extent.

It is easier to protect the population than to protect the health care capacity

Would it not be easier if we accept an amount of cases in the society to match health care capacity rather than keeping it close to zero? To analyse this, it is helpful to note that regardless of which level of ambition you settle for, one needs to reach a situation where the effective reproduction number, R, equals one (or less). Otherwise, there will be a continued exponential increase of cases and eventually a breakdown of health care. At time *t*, the reproduction number is $R(t) = N(t)/N(t-1)$, where N(t) is the number of new cases (per unit of time, e.g. 5 days) at time *t* and $N(t-1)$ is the corresponding number of cases one generation earlier in the chain of transmissions.[44]

Now notice that we can express $N(t) = N_0(t) - N_{TTI}(t)$ where $N_0(t)$ is the number of new cases that would occur if society had not implemented a *test-trace-isolate* (TTI) strategy as advised by WHO, while $N_{TTI}(t)$ is the number of cases that the TTI eliminates. We can thus write $R(t) = [N_0(t)/N(t-1)] - [N_{TTI}(t)/N(t-1)]$. The first term, $N_0(t)/N(t-1)$, reflects our interactions in society. It is proportional to both how many potential encounters we have, on average, where we could potentially transmit the disease, and to the probability that the transmission would indeed occur at such an encounter. Active interventions to lower this term would usually limit social life and also, one may argue, our freedom.

The second term, $N_{TTI}(t)/N(t-1)$, however, is qualitatively different. Most of society is unaffected by organised TTI-activities, because they do not influence the vast majority of inhabitants (namely those who are neither working as contact tracers nor are subject to an active TTI-investigation). The capacity of TTI is, however, finite, making its effect significant only when the incidence, i.e. N, is low.

Let us consider a couple of simple examples to see how this may play out in practice. Let us assume that we have a situation in which each person would on average infect two others in absence of any non-pharmaceutical interventions (NPIs) and that the maximal number of cases that could be prevented by TTI per unit time is 2000. In absence of TTI the society would need to introduce NPIs that cut half of the transmission, that is, reducing it by 50% in order to reach a stable situation with $R(t) = 1$.

Example 1: We have a case number corresponding to $N(t-1) = 1000$. At this moderate prevalence we might be able to eliminate half of the new cases, that is, $N_{TTI}(t) = 2 \times 1000/2 = 1000$. Thus the TTI would completely alleviate the need for NPIs (unless we would like to go for zero cases) in order to maintain a stable situation since $R(t) = N_0(t)/N(t-1) - N_{TTI}(t)/N(t-1) = 2 - 1000/1000 = 1$.

Example 2: We have a case number corresponding to $N(t-1) = 10000$. At this high prevalence we might be able to eliminate more cases, since they are easier to find, but with the assumed finite resources, there is invariably a limit at $N_{TTI}(t) = 2000$. In this case $N_{TTI}(t)/N(t-1)$ is only 0.2. We would thus need other significant NPIs to reduce the probability of transmission by 40% on average ((2 − 1.2)/2 in %), such that $N_0(t)/N(t-1) = 1.2$, in order to maintain a stable situation with $R(t) = 1.2 - 0.2 = 1$.

Example 3: We have a case number corresponding to $N(t-1) = 100\ 000$. At this extremely high prevalence, we are still limited by $N_{TTI}(t) = 2000$, hence $N_{TTI}(t)/N(t-1) = 0.02$ and we would need even more significant NPIs to reduce the probability of transmission by about 49% ((2 − 1.02)/2 in %)

such that $N_0(t)/N(t-1) = 1.02$, in order to maintain a stable situation with $R(t) = 1.02 - 0.02 = 1$.

In examples 2 and 3, it becomes evident that the effect of *test-trace-isolate* becomes progressively negligible as the number of cases increases, while it was facilitating an essentially undisturbed social society at low incidence as in example 1. As trivial as it seems, this message does not appear to have reached, or has at least not been appreciated by the leaders in charge. It also explains why the population of countries aiming for elimination, a.k.a. zero Covid, have enjoyed great freedom during most of the pandemic.[45]

In other words, neither in theory nor in practice is there any dichotomy between freedom on the one hand and proactive infection control measures on the other. Acting early, keeping levels low at all times, is beneficial in all respects – even before adding the unnecessary pain and sorrow that the disease casts upon those affected by it. Waiting too long, however, leads to the need for much more invasive measures such as lockdowns, the non-pharmaceutical analogue of amputation.

Moving goalposts and the denial

The first wave: how it played out during the spring of 2020

Despite the absurdity of the estimates of quick herd immunity – in glaring conflict with data coming in from other countries[46] – Swedish officials and local scientists continuously pushed this narrative and media provided them with nearly unlimited limelight.

The scene had been set, if not earlier, once Carlson in the beginning of March 2020 compared critical scientists with an indigenous (Sámi) weather forecaster predicting future weather by looking at fish intestines.[47] Around the same time Tegnell insinuated that critical researchers were after research funding rather than having sincere concerns.[48] The debate climate deteriorated and became polarised and national chauvinistic tendencies, exceptionalism, and aspects of outright xenophobia became evermore evident, as we shall highlight in the following.

Giesecke, the former state epidemiologist who called Tegnell and Carlson "my boys,"[49] has acted as a godfather of the Swedish strategy. He was a frequent feature in national[50] and international media[51] during spring 2020 with statements like "All other countries are doing it wrong" and "Sweden is doing the right thing. Everyone else does it wrong." In an interview with *Unherd* on March 13, 2020, Giesecke explained,

> The people who are frail and old will die first. And when that group of people is sort of thinned out, you will get fewer deaths as well.[52]

During the time (after March 23, 2020) when he appeared as an independent expert in the media, promising a rapid arrival of herd immunity, it was later revealed that he was on a paid contract with FHM.[53] In April, once there was a substantial growth in Sweden's death toll, Tegnell turned this fact around and used it as an opportunity to further fuel the Swedish exceptionalism, stating that "Deaths from the corona virus are measured in different ways around earth, but nobody can measure it as exactly as in Sweden."[54] Playing further on the nationalistic tendencies Tegnell repeatedly blamed immigrants for Sweden's high death tolls[55] and Hallengren declared that "we do not have that tradition, that culture" regarding facemasks.[56]

Agnes Wold, a professor of bacteriology at Gothenburg University and omnipresent in both social and traditional media, claimed:

> But many authoritarian leaders have this thing that they want to be like the military, they want to block off, they want to close borders, they want control, they want to stuff away women and children somewhere. It is patriarchal infection policy. Thankfully, Sweden has a public health authority that understands this.[57]

Apparently she did not reflect on the fact that, in contrast to Sweden, all of Sweden's neighbouring countries had female leaders – who all did what Wold interpreted as "You want to show that you are a bit macho and can make tough decisions."[58] When people warned about mutations Wold tweeted,

> [I] do not understand this obsession with mutations and that it would have [anything] to do with danger and contagion. There must be some Hollywood movies that the young people have seen that did not exist in my time.[59]

While these particular statements are from March and April 2020, Wold has persisted as a source of disinformation.[60] She nevertheless remains extremely popular as she tends to say what people want to hear, namely that Sweden is superior and there is nothing to worry about.

Johan von Schreeb, a professor of global disaster medicine at prestigious Karolinska Institutet, wrote arguably the most destructive article during the pandemic.[61] He furiously attacked Peter Wolodarski, the chief editor of Sweden's premiere newspaper *Dagens Nyheter*, who had been a rare voice of reason by questioning the Swedish strategy and the slow response once it became clear that it was at odds with the rest of the world. Wolodarski was accused of propagating dangerous disrespect for Swedish science, knowledge, and authorities. Other media followed in full force, leaving many critics like Wolodarski silenced. (Instead von Schreeb himself became influential as responsible for educating Swedish health care workers about Covid – an occasion that was used for propagating unscientific and erroneous claims about how Covid spreads.)[62]

With this discussion climate the scene was open for FHM and their allies to propagate theories and numbers in glaring conflict with international data and even with basic principles of epidemiological spread. The early estimates of hospital capacity needed to meet Covid demands, released on March 20 and updated on

March 27, compared to Wuhan and implicitly assumed that they had reached herd immunity.[63] Thus although it should have been obvious to anyone at that time that the very stringent NPIs enforced in Wuhan had an effect, FHM ignored this in their considerations. That Tegnell himself did not understand basic epidemiological concepts such as the reproduction number, R, has become clear from public email conversations, but apparently such ignorance must have been widespread also at the analysis department at FHM. Still they publicly praised their own competence and declared it meaningless to take in help from the outside.[64]

The debacle with analyses at FHM continued. At the press conference on April 21, 2020, the main claim, triumphantly announced, was that there were about 1000 cases undetected for each detected case.[65] When it was pointed out that this would imply over 6 million cases in Stockholm county – more than twice the total number of inhabitants – FHM referred to the head of the analysis department who said it was just a typo on the PowerPoint. But it was not just a typo. The factor 1000 was, in fact, the best fit they obtained in their detailed report. Later on, they came up with a new analysis suggesting 75 hidden cases for each observed one[66] – apparently with no justification or new input data, but again in support of the narrative of an approaching herd immunity, only this time not leading to equally and obviously absurd conclusions.

Local scientists were on the same track: on the news show *Aktuellt* on April 20, 2020, Jan Albert, a professor of microbiology and infection prevention at Karolinska Institutet, presented fresh research results which showed that 11 out of 100 blood donors tested had developed antibodies.[67] In the same program, Tom Britton, a professor of mathematics at Stockholm University, estimated an immunity level of 30% in the general population. Both Albert and Britton were completely confident that the true level in the population was much higher than the measured 11%. Again, the embarrassment came quickly. The day after the announcement, Jan Albert had to return to *Aktuellt* to announce that they had mixed up the tests, which may have partly been from Covid patients.[68] Remarkably, however, no conclusions were altered despite this. Instead, Albert completed the argumentation circle by saying that FHM had calculated numbers agreeing with Britton's, showing at least one-quarter, possibly one-third of the population should have developed antibodies. The belief in rapid herd immunity was unshakable.

Tom Britton was omnipresent in Swedish media with his predictions of enormous infection numbers and upcoming herd immunity. In early April, he predicted half of the Swedish population to be immune already in April,[69] then by mid-April that the 50% level and herd immunity was due in mid-May (now only in Stockholm),[70] then in May that the herd immunity was to be reached in June, now according to his new calculations instead at around 40% immunity.[71] In spring 2020, herd immunity was always a month away.

In a debate article on March 31, 2020, Anders Björkman, a professor of infectious diseases at the Karolinska Institutet, promised that Sweden would reach herd immunity after at most 1000 deaths.[72] Soon thereafter, on April 28, he instead suggested at most 3000 deaths,[73] which he had changed to 7000 deaths already on May 9.[74] In each article he delivered fierce critique of those questioning the herd immunity strategy, claiming that they were incompetent and unable to make correct predictions. The irony was seemingly unintentional. Björkman is still active in the debate and being regularly interviewed by some of the main Swedish media outlets. Matti Sällberg and Anna-Maria Ekström are two more professors at the Karolinska Institutet who promised that herd immunity, "with no doubt," would occur before any vaccines would become available.[75]

Martin Kulldorff wrote in *Dagens Nyheter* on May 4, 2020, that "It is better to have somewhat higher death tolls now if we get closer to herd immunity."[76] Kulldorff is one of the three main authors of the GBD. Being originally Swedish, he was interviewed several times by the Swedish press,[77] and published opinion articles.[78] It emerged that during the time he was also in email contact with Tegnell, praising the Swedish strategy as a model to the world. Kulldorff has now left academia and joined the Brownstone Institute, the spiritual child of the GBD.

Jonas Ludvigsson, a paediatrician and yet another professor at the Karolinska Institutet, advocated for infecting children in order to reach herd immunity in a public lecture on March 16, 2020, notably at a time when nothing was known about long-term effects on children.[79] He also gave the false promise that no children would die from Covid. Ludvigsson has been in close contact with the authorities and is one of the 47 original signatories of the GBD. He has worked actively to tone down the risks of Covid for kids with a methodology that has been fiercely criticised internationally, including twice (!) in the leading scientific journal *Science*.[80] In Sweden, however, Ludvigsson has enjoyed compact support from the establishment. He was also acquitted from all allegations of research misconduct. Together with Kulldorff, Ludvigsson praised the Swedish strategy with such statements as: "Herd immunity is not unscientific" and "Stockholm has the lowest number of deaths per person with antibodies."[81] While actively advocating for infecting children with Covid, Ludvigsson was promoted and appointed national scientific expert in paediatrics at the National Board of Health and Welfare.[82]

In contrast, critical scientists were scolded over their tone and irrelevant details. The early attempts from the scientific community to influence the strategy included a letter with more than 2000 signatories, mostly doctors and researchers, including many prominent professors, urging the FHM to take action.[83] On April 14, 2020, after all of these had been ignored, a group of 22 researchers and doctors penned an opinion article in *Dagens Nyheter* (the most prestigious debate platform in Swedish newspapers). This article has became the most-read ever, but instead of focusing on the urgently important message of the article, the focus was on a) the tone and b) a single number: the average number of deaths per day which, according to the official statistics reported by Sweden to Worldometer and ECDC and quoted by the 22 critics had reached 105 per day. This number was much higher than that of our Scandinavian neighbours and was reaching the levels of Italy (per capita), which was famously one of the earliest European countries to suffer a major Covid-19 wave.

Tegnell dismissed the article and claimed that the numbers were completely wrong.[84] He claimed instead that the true number of deaths per day was around 60, and that the researchers misunderstood the difference between reported and actual deaths – and that Sweden was already experiencing the positive effects of herd immunity.[85] Swedish media, including many Swedish science journalists, deemed the 22 researchers and doctors completely incompetent and repeatedly painted them as a shame for Sweden.[86]

It later turned out that the 22 critics were remarkably accurate: the actual deaths during the discussed period (April 7–9) converged to 104, according to the official numbers based on death certificates[87] (April 8–10 was also mentioned in the debate article and then the average number of deaths were 108/day). Thus the 22 researchers were remarkably close to the actual outcome, while Tegnell was far off by over 40%. Half a year later, in a very rare instance of official critique, the state-run public service (Sveriges Radio) was found guilty by The Swedish Press and Broadcasting Authority of not being objective, when on April 15 reporting on this dispute in favour of FHM.[88]

On April 27, 2020, deputy state epidemiologist Anders Wallensten claimed, "the drawback with lockdowns is that there won't be much disease transmission and then you have the problem remaining when you ease up."[89] In the beginning of May this message was repeated by Tegnell: "complete lockdowns have had a big effect, it actually stopped the epidemic in many countries"[90] and he mentioned Austria and Finland as examples that had the problem that very few had been infected.[91]

On May 8, 2020, Giesecke made the self-assured prediction that all other Nordic countries would have caught up with Sweden's death toll in one year's time.[92] His prediction proved to be off by multiple factors. On May 8, 2021, the number of deaths per million (the 2020 numbers in parenthesis)[93] were: Sweden 1395 (313), Denmark 430 (90), Finland 166 (47), Norway 140 (40), and Iceland 84 (29). Thus, Sweden remained by far the worst, continued to have many times more deaths, and the claims that its immunity from previous infection would protect it clearly did not materialise.

As Sweden's exceptionally high death numbers drew increasing international attention, Löfven hosted a press conference in English mid-May, 2020, bluntly stating,

> The casualties in Sweden are mostly in elderly homes and the older people. That has nothing to do with people walking in the city.[94]

While many more examples of denialism related to the first wave could be added, one can get a feeling about the mentality in Sweden during the pandemic following the books by political scientist Gina Gustavsson[95] and writer and virologist Lena Einhorn,[96] as well as the thorough podcast on the Swedish strategy by Martin

Norlin,[97] and Martin Lindström's sharp essay on "The New Totalitarians."[98] In summary: it was the support from all parts of society that enabled grossly incorrect statements to propagate and turn into the perceived reality of the majority.

The denial, part 1

Although it was obvious to anyone following international data, as described in the chapter by Rodney Edvinsson, the first more serious antibody test results[99] from FHM hit as a bomb on May 20, 2020. Stockholm had the highest positivity rate in Sweden with 7.3%, in Västra Götaland (including Gothenburg) it was 3.7%, and in Skåne (including Malmö) 4.2%. The results were thus one order of magnitude lower than promised!

The denial was compact. The only clear exception was Britton who admitted that he had been wrong.[100] Instead T-cells became the red herring of the season.[101] It was argued by the herd immunity crowd that people had been infected in large amounts albeit without developing antibodies, but instead protective T-cells. Again, in stark contrast to international consensus not linking T-cells in absence of antibodies to SARS-CoV-2 exposure but more likely to common colds,[102] Carlson claimed that Stockholm should have around 40% immunity.[103] This, invoking Britton's mathematical results, would prevent any second wave. Already from early June 2020, both the Government and FHM spoke about Sweden entering a "late pandemic phase."[104]

In his much-celebrated *Sommarprat* (*Summer Talk*) – a popular program on public service radio – Tegnell, still very proud of the Swedish way, declared on June 24, 2020, that "it was like the whole world went mad."[105] Swedish journalists looked forward to disaster in neighbouring countries assuming that they would be jealous.[106] Meanwhile, the public narrative shifted from "we need to protect the old and vulnerable" (which is impossible at high prevalence) towards "it is just the old and vulnerable that die anyway."

Various prizes and awards started pouring over the faithful. Tegnell was named "the straight back man of the year"[107] as well as distinguished "Alumni of the year" at Linköping University.[108] To name just one out of many more: Kulldorff, the lead author of the GBD, was awarded an honorary doctorate by Umeå University in northern Sweden.[109] By contrast, the GBD has been widely condemned internationally.[110]

The denial, part 2 and beyond

During the late fall of 2020 and the winter 2020/2021 it became even more apparent that the promise of herd immunity stemming from the first wave was a monumental miscalculation. Sweden experienced a second wave that was again far worse than in the other Scandinavian countries. Instead of admitting error almost all aforementioned key players chose to double down once again. Again the exception was Tom Britton who admitted thousands of lives could have been saved with a different strategy.[111] He, however, kept on providing unrealistic predictions[112] although by now they presumably had less devastating implications.

Much less honourable was the action of the people in charge, including Minister Hallengren. In fact this went as far as the Government's online description of the pandemic strategy being crucially changed in the beginning of 2021: "The overall goal of the Government's work is to reduce the rate of the spread of infection, i.e. to flatten the curve so that not many people get sick at the same time" became "The overall goal of the Government's work is to reduce the spread of infection in society."[113] This change – which precisely echoed the defence strategy of Hallengren, Carlson, and Tegnell when criticised by the Corona Commission appointed by the Government, in TV questionings, and in the Constitutional Committee's (KU) hearing – was made without indicating that it had changed at all. Once confronted, Hallengren claimed that it was changed by mistake.[114] In the KU interrogation Hallengren went on to say that "No, we did not have a formally decided strategy" and "We did everything we could to reduce the spread of infection and to get protective equipment."[115] This happened in a country that still today does not recommend general use of facemasks and where state epidemiologist Tegnell declared in April 2020, "It is dangerous to believe that protective equipment stops anything" and "In our strategy it does not matter much since we have never said that we should stop all transmission."[116] Adding to the web of assertive but self-contradicting statements, Carlson claimed on January 9, 2021, that "It is impossible to close a society in such a way that the disease transmission does not continue."[117] PM Löfven, as did several of the other key players, went as far as denying that there is a clear causal connection between interventions and outcomes in February 2021.[118]

An expert group of the Royal Swedish Academy of Sciences concluded in November 2021:[119]

> The strategy that FHM chose to implement was to "flatten the infection curve." . . . Although the WHO and the European Agency for Communicable Disease Control (ECDC) recommended that the countries of the world minimise the spread of infection by all means, this goal was not part of the strategy presented by FHM. The extensive morbidity and high mortality Sweden experienced during the first two pandemic waves was primarily due to too mild and delayed measures to prevent the initial spread of infection.

The expert group also identified the science denial at FHM which was set during the initial stages and which they have still not abandoned:

> The information has been contradictory and unreasonable. One example is FHM's objection to the use of facemasks, as well as the early disregard for the risk that individuals with presymptomatic or asymptomatic infection could be infectious.[120]

Similarly the Corona Commission has delivered fierce critique. Refuting Löfven's statements about a lack of connection between the society and deaths in elderly care homes, the Commission concluded that the latter is a consequence of high community spread of the disease.[121] The harsh critique has, however, had only a minor influence on the local debate. The media have remained defensively patriotic, politicians continue to deny the failure, and FHM carries on with their dogmatic, or even nihilistic, approach to public health.

Remarkably, while FHM and politicians alike continuously ridiculed the use of facemasks, claiming that they do not belong to our culture (Hallengren) and that they may even increase the spread of the disease (FHM on multiple occasions), facemasks were in fact recommended, and even mandatory, in the Parliament during times of high community spread,[122] and also in the Governmental Offices.[123]

The tragedy of the commons and parallels with climate change

One might ponder on how to reconcile humanity's remarkable development and success in science and technology with our inability to handle global crises such as the Covid pandemic and climate change. Part of the answer may lie in the following simple observation: progress and innovation is driven by the "best," by brilliance and ingenuity. Individual failures become irrelevant. The opposite is true for collective failures, for Covid and the climate catastrophe. These are driven by the "worst," those that won't even try, and those that refuse to cooperate. The good cannot compensate.

At the beginning of the pandemic, decision makers indeed appeared to face something akin to the prisoner's dilemma (or its multi-partite generalisation leading to the tragedy of the commons): while the obviously best option globally would be to aim for elimination, it would only work if all cooperated and not cooperating could (naively) be seen as a chance of obtaining a competitive advantage. That was the game that FHM and Sweden gambled on. In essence, it unleashed the tragedy of the commons.

Sweden is certainly not the only nation that handled the pandemic disastrously, although we are certainly extreme given our favourable preconditions. The fatal Swedish influence is well documented[124] with officials promoting "do nothing" and herd immunity based strategies around the world, notably including countries such as Brazil, the UK, South Africa, and India, which have later fostered new virus mutations. Before spearheading the GBD, Kulldorff praised Tegnell in emails stating that he would also like to see the Swedish strategy as a model for the world, and it is obvious that Sweden influenced the GBD. The propaganda on schools, Covid, and children pushed by Swedish officials as well as GBD-signee Ludvigsson, have also most likely had devastating implications far beyond the borders of Sweden.[125]

In a weird twist, Swedish public service television pushed the narrative that Covid NPIs imply a lack of solidarity with developing countries in their science program *Vetenskapens värld*. They went as far as saying that interventions against

Covid have caused more deaths than the disease itself,[126] and Anna-Maria Ekström claimed in the same program that "because of school closings at least 13 million girls have been forced into marriage." With these erroneous claims the public was reinforced in the belief that Sweden has done the right thing. It promoted *Sverigebilden*, the self-perception of Sweden as a "moral superpower."[127] When it really matters, however, Sweden has shown a very different attitude remaining among the few countries actively blocking the temporary patent waiver for Covid vaccines.[128] Again, the attitude hits back: while the waiver initiative was taken by India and South Africa, these countries have, in part due to low vaccination rates, been fertile grounds for potent new virus variants.

The analogy between Covid and climate change goes beyond the tragedy of the commons.[129] It is no coincidence that signers of the GBD are backed by climate change deniers.[130] The same crowd used the same argumentation for the need to "live with climate change," "flattening the curve," and now "live with Covid." Each of these statements has the same components. It sounds reasonable and realistic at first. It obfuscates that there is an alternative. Most importantly, it does not account for tipping points and their concomitant non-linear feedback loops (further changes driven by the change itself). Instead, the statements are based on inadequate linear and short timescale logic.

It is sadly no surprise that economists often embrace such ideas. William Nordhaus received the 2018 Nobel prize in Economics for his calculations suggesting that an increase of Earth's temperature by 3.5°C until 2100 would be optimal.[131] Fortunately, there are climate scientists with a broad spectrum of backgrounds that understand dynamical systems, and thus that Nordhaus's estimate is dangerously incorrect.[132] There are non-linear and long-term effects missed by Nordhaus and others. Tipping points include melted glaciers, changed ocean currents, deforestation, etc. beyond which it is qualitatively harder to bring Earth back to normalcy.[133] For example, melted glaciers imply that less sunlight is reflected away from Earth, more is absorbed and hence heats the planet: this thus leads as a feedback loop since further heating is induced by the heating itself. It is now consensus that 3.5°C is far too high, possibly threatening our entire existence.[134]

For Covid the tipping points are the emergence of new mutated variants that are harder to control due to either higher transmissibility or immune escape.[135] The number of new mutations is proportional to the number of replications, which in turn reflects the total amount of transmission. Thus a new variant further increases the probability of further ones. It unleashes a feedback loop.

"Living with Covid" is the equivalent of continuing to burning enormous amounts of fossil fuel, it invites the emergence of new tipping points and feedback loops at ever greater cost to humanity. Here one should note three crucial things: first, while the timing of tipping points of climate change to a certain degree are predictable, the tipping points of Covid occur stochastically with a probability proportional to the amount of circulating viruses. The probability of new virus variants therefore is proportional to the volume of the infection spread. It is thus key to limit this as much as possible. Second, while the climate disaster has played out over many decades and the basic process was known[136] already to the Swedish Nobel laureate Svante Arrhenius in 1895, the evolution of the Covid disaster is much more rapid. This is yet another reason to act fast. Third, contrary to initial hopes, there is no clear tendency yet that the virus mutates to become milder.[137] This is likely due to the lack of selection pressure on a virus exhibiting significant asymptomatic transmission: there is no immediate evolutionary loss if the host is killed once the virus has already been transmitted. The only significant selection pressure is to make the virus more transmissive and immune evading. Thus the laws of evolution are not on our side. Relying on luck is not a viable strategy.

An independent panel[138] commissioned by the WHO has concluded that the pandemic could have been ended in the beginning of 2020 given an adequate pro-active response. Humanity, in particular Western society, has failed spectacularly. The victims include millions of dead and (at least) tens of millions of long-term sick. Sweden has become an example of how science denial and short-sighted nationalistic populism can impact public health and costs lives.[139] But the pandemic is not over yet. There is time for change. The central challenge is to drop the prestige, embrace the science on airborne and asymptomatic transmission, and admit past failure. The science of what needs to be done is unambiguous.[140]

Notes

1 "A Victory for Democracy" episode from *Yes, Prime Minister*, first aired February 13, 1986. The relevant clip can be seen here, youtube.com/watch?v=nSXIetP5iak .
2 https://ourworldindata.org/explorers/coronavirus-data-explorer?zoomToSelection=true&facet=none&pickerSort=asc&pickerMetric=location&hideControls=true&Metric=Confirmed+cases&Interval=7-day+rolling+average&Relative+to+Population=true&Align+outbreaks=false&country=~SWE .
3 https://twitter.com/EmilBergholtz/status/1400500795875934213?s=20 .
4 Cf. the chapter by Anders Vahlne.
5 https://en.wikipedia.org/wiki/Sunk_cost#Fallacy_effect .
6 Cf. Sigurd Bergmann's Chapter 6 in this book.
7 www.folkhalsomyndigheten.se/nyheter-och-press/nyhetsarkiv/2020/januari/nytt-coronavirus-upptackt-i-kina/ .
8 https://aftonbladet.se/nyheter/a/qLMB1e/tror-inte-pa-ett-stort-utbrott-i-sverige .
9 https://dn.se/nyheter/sverige/folkhalsomyndigheten-10000-15000-kan-bli-sjuka-i-varsta-fall/ .
10 https://aftonbladet.se/nyheter/a/9vdbWd/tegnell-backar-coronakulmen-pa-mandag-eller-tisdag .
11 https://aftonbladet.se/nyheter/samhalle/a/70GQRV/nya-strategin–slutar-rakna-exakta-antalet-coronafall .
12 www.expressen.se/nyheter/varningen-till-tegnell-innan-valet-av-strategi/ .
13 www.aftonbladet.se/nyheter/a/6j7vaO/anders-tegnell-hyllar-brittisk-tanke-kring-flockimmunitet-dit-vi-beh .
14 www.aftonbladet.se/nyheter/a/qLdrBE/brittisk-expert-vill-stoppa-corona–genom-att-40-miljoner-smittas .
15 N.M. Ferguson et al. "Impact of Non-Pharmaceutical Interventions (NPIs) to Reduce COVID-19 Mortality and Healthcare Demand", 2020, https://www.imperial.ac.uk/media/imperial-college/medicine/sph/ide/gida-fellowships/Imperial-College-COVID19-NPI-modelling-16-03-2020.pdf .

16 Caracciolo, B. et al. "How the Mitigation Strategy Tempted Northern Europe and Convinced Only Sweden", 2020, https://medium.com/@barbara_c/how-the-mitigation-strategy-tempted-northern-europe-and-convinced-only-sweden-f6fb9197d49a. On the unethical method of aiming at natural herd immunity see Bergmann, Sigurd, www.abc.net.au/religion/the-ethics-of-swedens-herd-immunity-strategy/12764868 .
17 See, for example, the collection of emails published on Emanuel Karlsten's blog, https://emanuelkarlsten.se/tegnell-mejlen-sa-fick-flockimmuniteten-faste-hos-folkhalsomyndigheten/ .
18 Cf., for example, Lapo Lappin's chapter and his article "The Justice of Gold: The Philosophical Roots of Sweden's Pandemic Strategy", *Macrina Magazine*, 2021, https://macrinamagazine.com/issue-6-general/guest/2021/02/20/the-justice-of-gold-the-philosophical-roots-of-swedens-pandemic-strategy/; Bergmann, Sigurd. "Navigating Ethics in a Pandemic – Contempt for the Weak Versus Love of Neighbor in a Swedish Lens", *Dialog* 60:4 (2021): 421–431, https://onlinelibrary.wiley.com/doi/epdf/10.1111/dial.12697, as well as *Filosofi och pandemi*. Gavelin, Åke, and Lapo Lappin (eds.), Skellefteå: Norma, 2021.
19 www.dn.se/nyheter/sverige/stefan-lofven-tusentals-kommer-att-do/ .
20 www.researchprofessionalnews.com/rr-news-new-zealand-2020-3-ardern-announces-nz-lockdown-to-stop-spread-of-coronavirus/ .
21 www.svt.se/nyheter/inrikes/fd-statsepidemologen-kraftfulla-atgarder-som-syns-pa-tv-ar-bara-viktigt-for-politiker .
22 www.thelancet.com/journals/lancet/article/PIIS0140-6736(21)00978-8/fulltext#articleInformation .
23 www.nature.com/articles/d41586-020-01098-x .
24 https://en.wikipedia.org/wiki/List_of_countries_by_hospital_beds .
25 It is extremely hard, not to say impossible, to precisely calibrate the rate such that the hospital capacity would be close to maximal but not overrun. This is particularly so with exponential processes with a long delay between infection and hospitalisation and when one navigates in the dark as we did without proper testing.
26 https://bmcmedicine.biomedcentral.com/articles/10.1186/s12916-020-01726-3 .
27 www.folkhalsomyndigheten.se/contentassets/1887947af0524fd8b2c6fa71e0332a87/skattning-av-vardplatsbehov-folkhalsomyndigheten.pdf .
28 www.nature.com/articles/d41586-022-00438-3 .
29 See, for example, the article "Why did the elderly have to die without doctors treatment?" by Maciej Zaremba, www.dn.se/kultur/varfor-fick-de-aldre-do-utan-lakarvard/ and the official investigation by the Inspection for Health and Social Care (IVO), www.ivo.se/publicerat-material/nyheter/2020/ingen-region-har-tagit-fullt-ansvar-for-individuell-vard/ .
30 See, for example, https://sverigesradio.se/artikel/7561304 and age researcher Håkan Jönsson on why this represents "one of our time's worst healthcare scandals", www.lu.se/artikel/en-av-var-tids-storsta-vardskandaler .
31 www.svt.se/nyheter/inrikes/danmarks-minskade-vardskuld-opererade-tidigare-an-sverige . January 25, 2022, it has been estimated that one has carried out 169 000 less surgeries in the pandemic and that tens of thousands patients are queueing, https://tt.omni.se/tiotusentals-svenskar-koar-for-operation/a/g6KOVJ .
32 Emails between Tegnell and local scientists, which are public according to Swedish law, reveal that they were aware that "herd immunity will occur if our applied actions are not too efficient."
33 https://covidforeningen.se/ .
34 https://www.altinget.se/vard/artikel/debatt-braadskande-vaard-forsenas-nar-statistik-om-laangtidsCovid-saknas .
35 https://en.wikipedia.org/wiki/Great_Barrington_Declaration .
36 www.folkhalsomyndigheten.se/nyheter-och-press/nyhetsarkiv/2020/mars/personer-over-70-bor-begransa-sociala-kontakter-tills-vidare/ .

37 www.folkhalsomyndigheten.se/nyheter-och-press/nyhetsarkiv/2020/september/forslag-om-att-besoksforbudet-pa-sarskilda-boenden-ska-upphora/ .
38 Comas-Herrera et al. “Mortality Associated with COVID-19 in Care Homes: International Evidence”, 2021, Article in LTCCovid.org, International Long-Term Care Policy Network, CPEC-LSE, https://ltccovid.org/2021/02/02/updated-international-report-mortality-associated-with-Covid-19-in-care-homes-data-up-to-26th-january-2021/ .
39 https://coronakommissionen.com/publikationer/delbetankande-1/ .
40 A discussion in Swedish is available here, www.youtube.com/watch?v=9wHMvaIlafM .
41 Budich, J.C., and E.J. Bergholtz. “Synchronization in Epidemic Growth and the Impossibility of Selective Containment”, *Mathematical Medicine and Biology: A Journal of the IMA* 38:4 (December 2021): 467–473, https://academic.oup.com/imammb/article/38/4/467/6409757 .
42 www.gp.se/debatt/tegnell-kvalificerar-sig-inte-ens-som-hobbyepidemiolog-1.39302498 .
43 https://en.wikipedia.org/wiki/Long_COVID .
44 This generation time has often been assumed to be around five days although the new variants are associated with a shorter generation time, and its numerical value is irrelevant for the argument made here.
45 www.thelancet.com/journals/lancet/article/PIIS0140-6736(21)00978-8/fulltext .
46 Cf. the chapter by Rodney Edvinsson for details.
47 www.svd.se/virolog-resenarer-fran-italien-borde-stanna-hemma .
48 www.dn.se/nyheter/sverige/statsepidemiolog-anders-tegnell-sverige-har-valdigt-svart-att-acceptera-risker/ .
49 www.sjukhuslakaren.se/jag-tror-vi-klarar-den-har-utmaningen/ .
50 www.di.se/nyheter/giesecke-alla-andra-lander-gor-fel/ .
51 www.dagbladet.no/nyheter/sverige-gjor-riktig-alle-andre-gjor-feil/72296080 .
52 www.youtube.com/watch?v=bfN2JWifLCY&t=597s .
53 www.dn.se/nyheter/sverige/giesecke-har-miljonavtal-med-folkhalsomyndigheten-nu-dras-faktura-tillbaka/ .
54 www.aftonbladet.se/nyheter/a/0nyOrE/tegnell-darfor-har-sverige-hogre-dodstal .
55 https://kvartal.se/artiklar/skyll-inte-dodstalen-pa-invandrarna/ .
56 www.expressen.se/tv/nyheter/coronaviruset/hallengren-s-i-sverige-fattar-vi-inte-politiska-beslut-nar-det-galler-skyddsutrustning-/ .
57 www.expressen.se/nyheter/wold-om-politiska-besluten-vill-visa-att-man-ar-macho/ .
58 *Ibid.*
59 https://twitter.com/AgnesWold/status/1236411368644972545?s=20 .
60 https://kvartal.se/artiklar/wold-i-stallet-for-vetenskap/ .
61 www.svd.se/johan-von-schreeb-wolodarski-bidrar-till-kunskapsforaktet .
62 www.biblioteksbladet.se/ideer/essa/vadan-av-blind-kalltillit/?fbclid=IwAR3c_TXhtaR3qT0l7AB8CQpWyVtDR0035-q5GVWBwQjzu4sde06HglqQPdc .
63 www.folkhalsomyndigheten.se/contentassets/1887947af0524fd8b2c6fa71e0332a87/skattning-av-vardplatsbehov-folkhalsomyndigheten.pdf .
64 https://sverigesradio.se/avsnitt/1475828 .
65 https://emanuelkarlsten.se/folkhalsomyndigheten-om-siffrorna-det-blev-alldeles-galet/ .
66 *Ibid.*
67 www.svt.se/nyheter/inrikes/11-procent-av-stockholmarna-har-antikroppar-mot-Covid-19 .
68 www.svt.se/nyheter/inrikes/nya-antikroppstestet-baserat-pa-osakert-underlag .
69 www.aftonbladet.se/nyheter/a/K3mzq7/halva-sveriges-befolkning-smittad-i-april .
70 www.svd.se/professor-stockholm-kan-na-flockimmunitet-i-maj .
71 www.svd.se/ny-berakning-stockholm-kan-na-immunitet-i-juni .
72 www.dn.se/debatt/skrackprognoser-om-corona-forsvarar-for-beslutfattare/ .

73 https://lakartidningen.se/opinion/debatt/2020/04/dodligheten-i-Covid-19-svar-att-berakna-och-drabbar-olika/ .
74 www.svd.se/flockimmunitet-pa-lagre-niva-kan-hejda-smittan/i/senaste .
75 https://twitter.com/ar_covid/status/1447105883390062592?s=20 .
76 www.dn.se/debatt/hog-dodlighet-i-dag-kan-ge-farre-doda-pa-sikt/ .
77 www.dn.se/sverige/svensk-bakom-forskarupprop-mot-nedstangningar/ , www.dn.se/vetenskap/hammaren-och-dansen-en-strategi-som-kom-av-sig/ .
78 www.dn.se/debatt/flockimmunitet-ar-inte-en-ovetenskaplig-scientism/ , www.dn.se/debatt/hog-dodlighet-i-dag-kan-ge-farre-doda-pa-sikt/ .
79 www.youtube.com/watch?v=NXCcSF1IYQk .
80 www.science.org/content/article/how-sweden-wasted-rare-opportunity-study-coronavirus-schools and https://www.science.org/content/article/critics-slam-letter-prestigious-journal-downplayed-Covid-19-risks-swedish .
81 www.dn.se/debatt/flockimmunitet-ar-inte-en-ovetenskaplig-scientism/ .
82 https://news.ki.se/jonas-f-ludvigsson-appointed-national-scientific-expert-in-pediatrics-at-the-national-board-of .
83 https://lakartidningen.se/aktuellt/nyheter/2020/03/forskarupprop-regeringen-maste-ta-till-striktare-atgarder/ .
84 www.expressen.se/nyheter/coronaviruset/tegnell-darfor-har-forskarna-totalt-fel-om-svenska-dodsfallen/ .
85 www.aftonbladet.se/nyheter/a/b5vr65/tegnell-borjar-se-effekt-av-en-flockimmunitet .
86 For a contemporary description, see www.aftonbladet.se/debatt/a/kJr5b6/jag-anklagar-er-for-att-tysta-coronadebatten .
87 https://www.socialstyrelsen.se/statistik-och-data/statistik/statistik-om-covid-19/ .
88 www.svd.se/vetenskapsradion-falls-for-osaklighet .
89 www.youtube.com/watch?v=Ql36S61C3io&t=2252s .
90 https://youtu.be/x8J9CvgB1AE?t=2415 .
91 Summary at with both statements, www.youtube.com/watch?app=desktop&v=a_7nuG0ctBk&feature=share .
92 www.dn.se/nyheter/sverige/giesecke-om-ett-ar-ar-ovriga-norden-i-kapp-sveriges-dodstal/ .
93 https://ourworldindata.org/explorers/coronavirus-data-explorer?zoomToSelection=true&facet=none&pickerSort=asc&pickerMetric=location&hideControls=true&Metric=Confirmed+deaths&Interval=Cumulative&Relative+to+Population=true&Align+outbreaks=false&country=NOR~SWE~FIN~DNK~ISL .
94 www.expressen.se/tv/nyheter/coronaviruset/har-pressas-lofven-av-utlandska-journalister-om-corona/ .
95 Gustavsson, Gina. *Du stolta, du fria: om svenskarna: Sverigebilden och folkhälsopatriotismen*, Stockholm: Kaunitz & Olsson, 2021.
96 Einhorn, Lena. *Bland hobbyepidemiologer och expertmyndigheter: En resa i pandemins Sverige*, Stockholm: Norstedts, 2022.
97 https://floderochtekoppar.blogspot.com/2021/09/sveriges-hantering-av-coronapandemin.html .
98 Lindström, Martin. "The New Totalitarians: The Swedish COVID-19 Strategy and the Implications of Consensus Culture and Media Policy for Public Health", *SSM – Population Health* 14 (2021): 100788, www.sciencedirect.com/science/article/pii/S235282732100063X .
99 www.folkhalsomyndigheten.se/nyheter-och-press/nyhetsarkiv/2020/maj/forsta-resultaten-fran-pagaende-undersokning-av-antikroppar-for-Covid-19-virus/ .
100 www.aftonbladet.se/nyheter/a/rAw99A/matteprofessorn-kan-betyda-att-dodligheten-ar-hogre .
101 https://news.ki.se/immunity-to-covid-19-is-probably-higher-than-tests-have-shown .
102 www.science.org/doi/full/10.1126/science.abd3871 .

103 www.dn.se/nyheter/sverige/fhm-stockholm-kan-ha-40-procents-immunitet/ .
104 https://sverigesradio.se/artikel/7488433 .
105 https://sverigesradio.se/artikel/7501940 .
106 See, for example, https://twitter.com/juanitafranden/status/1308316823234936833?s=20 .
107 https://corren.se/bli-prenumerant/artikel/7jnv96nl .
108 https://liu.se/en/news-item/rustad-med-talamod-mot-gackande-coronavirus-alumn-2020 .
109 www.umu.se/en/news/harvard-statistician-appointed-honorary-doctor-at-the-faculty-of-science-and-technology_9277314/ .
110 www.theguardian.com/world/2020/oct/12/who-chief-says-herd-immunity-approach-to-pandemic-unethical , Public health organizations condemn herd immunity scheme for controlling spread of SARS-CoV-2, https://apha.org/news-and-media/news-releases/apha-news-releases/2020/public-health-orgs-condemn-sars-Covid2-plan .
111 www.thelocal.se/20201020/sweden-could-have-prevented-4000-deaths-with-spring-lockdown-maths-expert/ .
112 www.svd.se/britton-efter-felen–har-ar-hans-nya-prognos .
113 https://emanuelkarlsten.se/kartlaggning-vad-hande-nar-regeringskansliet-andrade-en-formulering-i-coronastrategin/ .
114 www.expressen.se/nyheter/lena-hallengren-avfardar-kritik-om-andrad-coronamening/ .
115 www.svt.se/nyheter/inrikes/hallengren-forsvarade-svenska-strategin-i-ku .
116 www.svt.se/nyheter/inrikes/virologidoktorn-folkhalsomyndighetens-strategi-ar-farlig .
117 www.svt.se/nyheter/carlson-finns-en-overtro-pa-nedstangningar .
118 www.youtube.com/watch?v=bBrZ0k-vYbQ&t=1966s .
119 www.kva.se/sv/publicerat/sammanfattning-vad-kan-vi-lara-av-pandemin .
120 *Ibid.*
121 https://coronakommissionen.com .
122 www.riksdagen.se/sv/aktuellt/2021/feb/25/rekommendation-om-munskydd-i-kammare-och-kammarfoaje/ .
123 www.dn.se/debatt/dubbelmoral-fran-politiker-om-behovet-av-munskydd/ .
124 An excellent summary has been compiled by Virpi Flyg, https://twitter.com/VirpiFlyg/status/1452765297581113346?s=20 .
125 www.science.org/content/article/how-sweden-wasted-rare-opportunity-study-coronavirus-schools .
126 https://kvartal.se/artiklar/svts-spektakulara-pastaende-kan-forsvara-smittskyddsarbete/ .
127 www.ft.com/content/71c8a636-4d40-4d0e-947f-af8de9b6b82c .
128 www.nature.com/articles/d41586-021-01242-1 .
129 www.politico.eu/article/climate-change-coronavirus-global-tipping-points/ .
130 https://bylinetimes.com/2020/10/09/climate-science-denial-network-behind-great-barrington-declaration/ .
131 https://foreignpolicy.com/2018/12/06/the-nobel-prize-for-climate-catastrophe/ .
132 https://liu.se/en/news-item/liu-forskare-riktar-skarp-kritik-mot-ekonomipristagare .
133 www.nature.com/articles/d41586-019-03595-0 .
134 www.ipcc.ch/report/ar6/wg1/ .
135 Cf. our article, www.politico.eu/article/climate-change-coronavirus-global-tipping-points/ .
136 https://libris.kb.se/bib/12447617 .
137 Katzourakis, A. "COVID-19: Endemic Doesn't Mean Harmless", *Nature* 601:485 (2022), www.nature.com/articles/d41586-022-00155-x .
138 The Independent Panel for Pandemic Preparedness & Response, https://theindependentpanel.org/mainreport/ .

139 Brusselaers, Nele, David Steadson, Kelly Bjorklund, Sofia Breland, Jens Stilhoff Sörensen, Andrew Ewing, Sigurd Bergmann, and Gunnar Steineck. "Evaluation of Science Advice During the COVID-19 Pandemic in Sweden", *Humanities and Social Sciences Communications* 9, Article number: 91 (2022), www.nature.com/articles/s41599-022-01097-5 .

140 www.bmj.com/content/376/bmj.o1 .

6

LEARNING FROM FAILURE

Mastering a pandemic in the triad of science, politics and trust

Sigurd Bergmann

The demise of a moral superpower

Allow me to start with some personal words. Having offered the reader a rather objective description of Sweden's experiment in the first chapter, this chapter will not separate emotion and reason but entangle compassionate and reflexive thinking.

When the SARS-CoV-2 virus entered Europe late in the winter of 2019/2020, and we all wondered what to think, to feel and to do, I lived off the information flows in all my three *Heimaten* (home countries): Germany, Sweden and Norway. Attending one of the first Swedish daily live transmitted press conferences, where many citizens for a long time gathered daily around the Agency's comforting campfire, it took me only ten minutes before I felt qualmish. My intuition immediately fired up all the engines of my critical reason (trained in countless academic expert evaluations in local, national and international bodies). The apparently emotionally disengaged state epidemiologist's mix of cherry-picked facts and quasi-scientific explanations became obvious to me in these minutes. I felt certain that the country was doomed. Others spoke about sleep disturbance during these weeks, due to anxiety, not so much with regard to the virus but to the national response. How could such a civil servant administrate all power in Sweden's pandemic emergency, and why did so many, including many friends, rely on him and the Agency as confidence inspiring?

The moral indignation about such a leadership pretending expertise[1] and at the same time refusing all dialogue with learned scientists has raised serious aspects of research ethics and law. This exasperation has served as a central driving force for my and many others' attempts to deepen the public debates with reliable scientific knowledge and to turn the national strategy into a life-enhancing process.

At the same time I started my "hobby epidemiologist"[2] education by listening to the daily radio-transmitted podcasts by acknowledged virologist Christian Drosten

DOI: 10.4324/9781003289364-7

in conversation with top-educated science journalists from my home region in Northern Germany.[3] Together with 40 million (!) careful listeners we learnt in detail about the virus, its microbiology, mobility and infectiousness, the need for testing and tracing and whatnot.[4] While political decision-makers in Berlin and the Federal States also followed his and many other wise scientists' advice, the Government in Stockholm chose to blindfold themselves, abdicate and hand over all power to Johan Carlson and Anders Tegnell. When the Agency's Director-General (GD, *generaldirektör*) Carlson in March 2020 declared criticism (of Tegnell) to be indecent and degrading ("*ovärdigt*"),[5] I became painfully aware that not only the health and life of fellow human beings was in danger, but also the community of shared values, the welfare system and the formerly proud country's democracy, trust and solidarity.

After that I had to revise my understanding of what kind of a country I have been living in since 1976. The gap between the imagined national identity and its practical appearance, which Gina Gustavsson has excellently explored,[6] became for me an open wound. While a majority of friends and colleagues either lapsed into silence or attacked me and other critics as traitors, I found some comfort in sharing such strange experiences with new colleagues and friends in the academy and media. Friends, journalists and scholars in the international sphere also approached me with worry and questions.[7] In analogy to the quickly evolving disaster in Sweden's pandemic response, the network of interconnected critical voices grew rapidly stronger. The critical mass started in small groups at the margins, and was unconcerned with ideological, scientific or cultural differences. After the first debate article published by the so-called 22 scientists,[8] it is legitimate to speak of a social movement that interpenetrates many spheres of society. Its history is still to be written in detail, in a national context but also with regard to international widespread alliances of scientists, politicians and media writers all around the planet. Associations such as Science Forum Covid-19, Save Sweden, Doctors to Doctors, Association Covid-19 School and Children, and others, as well as many individual voices, have been bravely swimming against the stream and preventing society from turning into one monistic conformist herd that followed its leaders blindly into whatever deadly waters. My participation in the Science Forum Covid-19 offered me a new home in this odd pandemic alienation. Critical compassionate thinking and learning about pandemic, virology, epidemiology and virus politics and ethics could flourish here. Whereas I lost some friends, who asked me to either shut my mouth or emigrate, I met many new friends at the barricades against the nation's stock "bunker mentality".[9]

Of course, not everything went wrong in the mystery of Sweden responding to the pandemic emergency. In a Christian tradition, human beings are always capable of failing and committing more or less fatal sins while simultaneously doing well and loving and caring for each other. Martin Luther's belief in the human as both "justified and sinner" has always offered a practical belief and also a good reason for me to strive to do what one can do, leaving the whole in God's hands, not passively but actively in synergy between men/women and the Creator.

Moreover, Sweden is deeply shaped historically by Catholicism and the Reformation's values and views of life, even if today it is among the world's most secularised countries. Given this long history, it felt even more painful to experience how central beliefs, including in their secularised forms – such as love for the neighbour and especially for the most vulnerable – solidarity and dignity of life[10] were deactivated in the pandemic, not by the virus but by some kind of mysterious navigating into a collective "shipwreck",[11] a horrible "failure"[12] without any analogy in Sweden's history since the Thirty Years' War and its loss of being a European military superpower in the battle of Poltava in 1709. It might be worth remembering in our context that between 1620 and 1720 the Empire's attempts to defend its power caused the loss of 300,000 young men's lives (in a population of 2 million).

It might also be worth remembering that the unique political separation of power between the Government and the Agencies, often declared as a specific reason (and apology) for the country's politically passive pandemic response, was established by Chancellor Axel Oxenstierna, who led the Empire as war strategist after Gustaf II Adolf's death in action, and substantially contributed to prolonging the disastrous Thirty Years' War. It will be interesting to see if Swedes after the pandemic will continue to adore Oxenstierna's equipment of the Agencies with nearly autocratic power,[13] or if Sweden will be able to learn lessons for its long-term political structure. In modern times the country successfully buried its military ambitions and instead developed into a peace-making force in international diplomacy. It invested heavily in welfare systems. But now, not only in the eyes of the prominent German television moderator Markus Lanz but also in the observations of other countries, the aspiration to perform as a moral superpower has definitively come to an end in Sweden's failed pandemic *Sonderweg*.[14]

In the following I will try out tools from cultural analysis to uncover clues to the mystery of why a majority of the population for almost a year followed its national leadership into the "politosomatic pandemonium",[15] into the place where all demons gather fuelling the fear of pain in individual and social bodies. Has this conceivably to do with shame within conformism? What role does a high level of trust play when confidence is shaken? What does it mean for the conditions of restoring trust when responsible leaders time and time again deny that they have failed? Can one restore the legal system so that civil servants and politicians can be held accountable for violations of the law?

I cannot promise to provide comprehensive answers but would be happy if I could convince my readers of the relevance of such problem formulation. Finally I will offer a hypothetical model for analysing the pandemic interplay in the triad of science, politics and trust. This might allow more comprehensive comparison of countries' different responses in future research.

Anticipating my conclusion: Sweden is distinguished from others in a *unique asymmetry* of a) a high level of trust in politics,[16] b) no trust from politics in science,[17] and c) an ambiguous high-and-low level of trust from politics (Government and Authorities) in the people (trust in individual responsibility and distrust of citizens' acceptance of tough measures).

After ten months, however, the people's original high level of trust declined in the second wave but increased slowly again after the third wave in 2021.[18] It remains unclear how the national management of the pandemic had impacted on (the traditionally high level of) trust between citizens. At this stage one should also mention the trust between individuals as a significant counterbalancing force where many tried to do their best to minimise the spread from below, even if it remains unclear to what sense the media's often uncritical messages impacted on this individual force. Politics' distrust of (institutionalised) science still continues but the media have become more careful to include different voices from science and Tegnell is no longer presented by them as the main expert. As of January 2022 the people's confidence in him and FHM had dropped to circa 50%.[19]

After circa 15 months the triad came into motion. Might experiences of broken trust, lack of shame, waning emotional security (*trygghet*) and the sin of the national state's infallibility work as a deeper driving power in what Gina Gustavsson has analysed as blind public health patriotism?[20] Has the first year of patriotism, as she suggests, turned into the second year of denial,[21] and might something good in the third year come out of the National Commission's sharp and etching criticism on the one side and the responsible leaders' refusal to accept this on the other?

Conformism, freedom, infallibility: excavating the cultural dimension

Swedes usually identify themselves as citizens in one of the best-developed and best-functioning modern welfare societies of the world. The country's history, though, offered a rather monistic and less pluralistic culture until the process of globalisation entered and transformed Sweden. Developing an all-embracing welfare system impacted on the population's emotional security, where *trygghet* (safety and comfort) represents a central value in the Swedish cultural soul. Instructions from the national authorities for how to clean our homes meticulously, what and how to eat and drink, how to care for children and one's body and health, and much more were obeyed and internalised favourably by most citizens from the thirties onwards when the arts of social engineering rose to new pinnacles. Inhabitants proudly experienced their national leadership and social system as *trygg*,[22] comfortable, safe and exceptional.

Comparing oneself to other countries did not make any sense. In fact it rather felt unpleasant and unnecessary as one expected others to follow Sweden's pioneering model. Religious beliefs were displaced into so-called "private religiosity",[23] and Sweden became one of the world's most secularised countries. So-called "state individualism"[24] characterises the people where the state acts as guarantee to protect and preserve its citizens' individual liberal rights of freedom, even if the individual remains rather powerless with regard to the welfare state and its institutions in spite of his or her eager attitudes to it.[25] One cultural principle that grew strong at this time was *to leave each other in peace* and *not to bother others in cases of need*.[26] Disappointingly for citizens, the FHM also practises such a principle of do-not-bother-us in contact with worried citizens.[27] To this day, health coaches can preach the mantra of *everyone as architect of his/her own fortune*.[28] While on the one side individuals should be responsible for their own fortune, the national welfare system on the other side is expected to take care of all kinds of miseries. Solidarity is praised as foundational value but not really internalised in daily life. Although the Swedish constitution clearly demands that public power be executed "with respect to all humans' equal value" and "for the individual human's freedom and dignity (*värdighet*)" (§ 2), one might wonder why the Swedish language does not offer a word for the dignity of humankind (German *Menschenwürde*) but only offers *människovärde*, the value of a human (*Menschenwert*), a quality that one can easily interpret quantitatively in a reductionist way, whereas the essence of dignity should never be quantified.[29]

At the same time as liberal individualism achieved a maximum of freedom for the individual, conformism was internalised in analogy. On interwoven conformism, shame and alienation, Karl Ove Knausgård tells a striking story in his *Min kamp* of when he and his daughter are invited to a kids' birthday party where the daughter, born in Norway, wonders why not "sausages, ice cream and soda? Lollipops? Jell-O? Chocolate pudding?" To her great disappointment others are proudly celebrating the day with "dip", that is healthy dishes of carrot sticks and cucumber sticks. For the author, painfully following his daughter's modes of trying to cope with the ambiguity of the situation, an outstanding experience of strange- and otherness emerges compared to the Swedes being so modern and healthy, mixed with feelings of shame of not knowing and not practising the conformist codes of Swedish behaviour and lifestyle.[30]

Philosopher Per Bauhn points to the late history of the society's urbanisation: it was not until the thirties that a majority of people lived in urban contexts, and older value systems, such as rural collectivism in village life, moved and survived in the cities. The one who dared to oppose and criticise was regarded as a problem. Conflicts are in such a culture solved in consensus, and the demand for consensus is high so that everyone can move into the same direction. All move forward and one should not speak up critically. Conformism and liberal individualism coalesced in this way in a unique and deeply internalised synergy. Gustavsson traces the roots in the cultural history and reminds us about the Lutheran state church and its powerful unification and education of the people. Can we understand Tegnell and the uncritical media following him as a kind of secularist continuation of this history, where the spiritual authority demands loyalty and understanding of why we should wash our hands and keep at distance?[31]

Writer Göran Rosenberg also considers convincingly the Swedish consensus culture in terms of its weakness at including, respecting and dignifying otherness and its tendency to avoid conflicts rather than to solve them.[32] In the pandemic, it was alleged that Swedes were collectively choosing freedom instead of safety, Locke instead of Hobbes, the individual instead of the community. The striving for consensus fuels the fear of conflict. But there is every indication that it was not freedom but rather the striving for the previously mentioned *trygghet*, the feeling of collective safety and comfort, that was at stake.[33]

Peter Baldwin highlights a curious contradiction, where Swedes on the one hand were relied on for "taking responsibility themselves", as Foreign Minister Ann Linde explained loudly for the international audience,[34] but on the other could not really be relied on as politicians could not rely on them accepting and sustaining an endured lockdown.[35] How should we understand such asymmetry of a high level of trust in the Government and the Government's lack of trust in its subjects? Tegnell describes Sweden's approach explicitly as "trust-based" but does not mention that he and his Agency must appropriately deserve the people's trust. By not admitting any of his many misjudgements, failures and disinformation he instead betrayed the people's trust.[36] Blind trust and patriotism, accompanied by the politicians' passivity and denial of their many failures, rather erodes than enhances the fruitful interplay of trust, science and politics. What Tegnell calls "trust-based measures" implied his and the Government's failure to take responsibility for implementing the best possible course of action instead of placing all responsibility on the individuals' shoulders.[37] One of the worst examples was when the Agency simply asked all people over 70 to stay at home, for more than seven months (!).

Martin Lindström explores how Swedish top-down consensus culture in connection with the media's financial dependence on the state can explain the lack of a critical dialogue at the Agency's press conferences. He raises the question about the emergence of a "new totalitarian" political and media culture in the country.[38] In analogy, early in the pandemic Finnish writer Jari Ernrooth raised similar serious questions about an underlying totalitarian tendency in Sweden's strategy, and I have followed him in analysing the "underlying pathology" of the country's virus politics by applying Vilhelm Moberg's older term of "democrature" (that is a mix of democracy and soft dictatorship).[39]

Obviously something went wrong with the basic cultural codes in the times of the pandemic, in a country that often claims to be a prototype of a society where welfare and equity are at the core. Did this imply the "collapse of the Swedish model" and the end of the Swedish welfare state, as prominent political scientist Bo Rothstein asked provokingly?[40] Even long before the pandemic, Sweden was known among the other European nations for being worst at being modernist, and in suppressing the past for the sake of the future.[41] Swedes are, as Susan Sontag pointed out, well known for being proud of their "uniqueness" and "their accomplishments (i.e. their modernity)".[42] Acknowledged poet Hans Magnus Enzensberger, in his chapter "Swedish autumn" in the classic work *Ach Europa!* (1987), aptly characterises Sweden as a country that is so preoccupied with its care for its citizens that it ends up seeing the population as immature and needing to be led. The historylessness, where the whole of life is harshly restructured from top to bottom, the author observes as only one of various symptoms of the country's condition. A common saying that has often made my German post-war soul feel uncomfortable goes like this: Let's leave that behind us now and look forward,

forward, forward. The "myth of progress" (Georg Henrik von Wright) seems to be deeply rooted in the Swedes' national identity.

Peter Weiss, in his famous *Aesthetics of Resistance* (1975–81), explicitly develops the historical-philosophical demand to let memories contribute to "the self-liberation of the oppressed".[43] He draws on his observations as a German immigrant to Stockholm and depicts in a similar way a situation where the self-righteous bourgeoisie in Sweden separates itself from the mal-adjusted in the 1950s welfare society. As a former German, Weiss probably appreciated the advantages of the informal society, where families, friends, allies and partners help each other if needed, while in Sweden the significance of informal neighbourhoods has been reduced in favour of the nationally structured welfare system. Modernist power has been moved to the system in its "colonization of the lifeworld", to put it in Jürgen Habermas' famous words.

In the context of the ongoing pandemic, one will most probably find ethnographic reasons for the overwhelming conformist response to the Agency's monopolising all information about the virus's spread. The quick turn into what was called *folkhälsonationalism* (popular health nationalism),[44] also described as legitimating *särartsnationalism* (exceptionalist nationalism),[45] was surprising many abroad as Swedish exceptionalism went against all voices worldwide,[46] including in science. This can scarcely be explained by only the Agency's harsh top-down crisis communication policy, applying military methods from psychological defence. The feeling of being exceptional obviously also relied on the belief in the good state and the supporting deeper cultural codes that Swedes were not able to question and transform. Many other Agency directors-general had to leave due to comparably small frailties (PM Löfven replaced several of them in the time of his regime), but surprisingly FHM GD Carlson was not questioned a single time by anyone publicly about his responsibility for thousands of avoidable deaths. Instead PM Löfven twice awarded him an extension of his mandate beyond his age of retirement.

Social scientists Staffan Andersson and Nicholas Aylott point out four reasons why Sweden did not change course in spite of sharply rising deaths: the structure of national public administration, an outburst of nationalism in parts of the media, the uneven impact of the virus and a political leadership that was willing to delegate responsibility for policy almost entirely.[47] In addition, one might wonder if the rapidly emerging public health nationalism might be anchored in a kind of territorial "inverted xenophobia",[48] although the only political criticisms against the Public Health Agency's power were expressed by the nationalist populist right-wing party Sverigedemokraterna, who usually delve most into the depths of xenophobia.[49] Similarly to other controversial debates, the so-called "opinion corridor" in Sweden during the time of the pandemic has been oppressively narrow, so that only views that respectable people hold have been allowed, mostly in favour of the official management, while criticism has been pushed to the margins.[50]

How a majority of Swedes hold fast to their image of the good welfare state that takes care of its people is a mystery for me. Germany's well-informed journalist at the prestigious *Der Spiegel* summarised the situation when it accelerated at its worst as a national "*ättestupa*", that is, the premodern ritual where the oldest are pushed over an edge to die.[51] Ageism, that is contempt for the weak elderly, was practised nationally on the state's mandate in a country that had already for a long time scored below the weakest with regard to respect and dignity for the elderly; in the World Values Survey in 2015, Sweden took second position from the bottom.[52]

Besides the elderly, children's rights were also violated. In June 2021 the governmental Agency The Ombudsman for Children in Sweden (*Barnombudsmannen*) departed from the UN convention on children's rights and presented its investigation of what has happened to children in the pandemic,[53] with regard to their rights to survival, life and health but also to education, protection and care. The Government was still in September 2021 proudly declaring how it was right not to close schools, while at the same time it refused to take into account how many more children have suffered and died than in neighbouring countries and how circa 35% of all school children and circa 50% of all teachers have been infected in a country that just recently in late October 2021, as the last one in Europe, decided to start to vaccinating children over 12. Johanna Höög's chapter will deepen the question of what children can teach us about mastering a pandemic.

Another unbelievable contempt for the most vulnerable was practised by the FHM in the fourth wave. Since risk groups, among them people with Downs and those in the care system for the disabled (LSS) were vaccinated primarily in spring 2021, their vaccine protection faded away in September. Nevertheless, the FHM refused to provide a third booster dose for these groups with much higher Covid risks, and did not even answer the Swedish National Association for People with Intellectual Disability (FUB) and The Swedish National Down Syndrome Association's open letters in September and November.[54] Has solidarity with the most vulnerable faded away? Why did Tegnell's agency execute such an unethical and illegal contempt for the weak?[55] Does Social Democratic welfare only include the strong? Has this to do with bureaucrats enjoying power to decide over others' life . . . and death? After three months, in late November 2021, the Government finally decided to offer them booster vaccines, which were distributed after three more weeks. The Agency keeps silent about how many innocent have suffered because of their unwillingness. Does this offer an example of *ableism* (discrimination against people with disabilities) in analogy to the first year's *ageism*?

Not only did a feeling of danger and anxiety emerge in the unexpected crisis, but the preservation of people's image of good life in a good society was also threatened in the pandemic's first spring. When critical voices appeared publicly, these were, along the well-known older codes of rural conformism, perceived as nest befouling, and later on even distrusted as politically dangerous, influencing and threatening the state through alleged disinformation.[56] Threats and hate naturally became a part of the strong reaction against those who dared to pipe up. In this situation, speaking up critically was regarded as "hysterical" and "un-Swedish" and was met with personal attack.[57] Enemies of national security damaged democracy fatally when opinion formations were treated and mistrusted by both the Agency and the Swedish national Radio as so-called "political influencing", state hostile propaganda, and a technical term that is common in the context of psychological warfare operations.[58] For the first time in late modern times, methods of psychological warfare were used by the national state against its own citizens, through the FHM's press office[59] and Sveriges Radio's science section. The method was to let an alleged expert[60] verify that the critics of Sweden's *Sonderweg* qualify as political enemies of the state executing dangerous *informationspåverkan*, and to attack one's own citizens who dared to criticise. The right to express one's opinion freely was crucially violated hereby. Trust in the politically controlled national media was broken once more. The leader responsible for the Radio's science section, Ulrika Björkstén, was again (after her former false blaming of critics' use of statistics) snowed under by several reports to the National Media Commission. One can certainly wonder how much the previously mentioned highly valued liberal rights of free speech and opinion were handled herein, "when free opinion turned into a threat" as *Kvartal* columnist Staffan Dopping strikingly put it.[61]

Exceptionalism grew even stronger when the worried voices, together with many in the international public, criticised and questioned Sweden's approach. Probably the worst scenario took place when scholars in the Science Forum published an article where they described the disaster and encouraged the USA not "to follow Sweden's example",[62] an article that was shared widely and together with many other voices contributed to the USA's critical overcoming of Trump's deadly corona management. Unfortunately it did not lead to any debate or change in Sweden itself.

Accordingly one must ask if the majority of citizens in 2020, in a kind of blind, uncritical patriotism,[63] preferred to adhere to their image of the good welfare state and its all-embracing care for all rather than questioning their leaders and their own longstanding and deeply entrenched social order. Cultural scientists have tried to explain this as a kind of herd mentality that was fuelled by the Agency's intense biased crisis communication on its high-risk strategy and the marginalisation and condemnation of all critical voices in science and the public.

The silent patriotism among a majority of scholars in the life sciences and among practising doctors especially demands a deeper explanation. From Germany's history I am well aware of the academic establishment's bandwagon effect, its cowardice and delusion. Bertolt Brecht strikingly talked about scientists as "a family of inventive *dwarfs* who can be hired for any purpose",[64] and one can only wonder for what purpose a majority of scholars decided to let the power constellation hire and delude them. This is even difficult to ask, as at the beginning of the crisis we saw an overwhelming 2300 life scientists signing a petition that demanded from the Government a more efficient and strong response.[65] The demand was ignored and most of the scholars and doctors decided to stay silent or to actively support the state at any price.

Instead the 22 authors of the first critical debate article[66] founded with others in June 2020 the Association Science Forum Covid-19.[67] The Forum is chaired by one of the country's most distinguished virologists. Forty scholars from different faculties cooperate in a steering group, supported by circa 800 members and a group of thousands of followers on social media. The Forum educates the populace in a constructive way, often in contradiction to the eclectic and misleading information from the Agency; produces debate articles; arranges webinars, YouTube programmes and discussions; and shares the state of international knowledge in a understandable way so that people can make their own well-grounded decisions on how to respond. While official leaders have either refused to enter a dialogue or mistrusted the skilled scholars, journalists and columnists in respectable domestic and international media have monitored their view of the management of the pandemic. Experts in social and life sciences have questioned the responsible leaders' ignorance of science and lack of a truth-seeking dialogue and cooperation[68] and asked what kind of crisis communication is appearing here when the most skilled experts are excluded from decision-making. Anders Vahlne's chapter mines in detail why the alleged expert Authority did not comply with scientific standards but was only self-reliant. The Royal Swedish Academy of Sciences' commission rightly concluded in its evaluation report with a demand for the establishment of an "independent expert unit with a high level of scientific expertise in relevant areas", and also an "ethics committee with scientific expertise".[69] The lack of such a competent advising body, similar to the UK's Scientific Advisory Group for Emergencies (SAGE) and Germany's *Expertenrat*, and also its *Ethikrat*, has had fatal consequences.[70]

In spring 2021 people were still aggressively attacking any criticism of the Agency's decision whatsoever, even if many of them had grown silent after the second and third waves where the same mistakes had been repeated as before. In autumn 2021, however, with the fourth wave's acceleration, many seemed to hold on to the FHM but one could also express criticism without the former violent reactions. Public debates turned into more fair and factual discussions, even if Tegnell, Tegmark Wisell and Hallengren, with their loyal supporters, continued totally unperturbed by all other voices, and never entered any dialogue with critics. Remarkably, the FHM still does not encourage facemasks while at the same time staff at the Governmental Offices and members of the Parliament in early 2022 are instructed to use them, an embarrassing double standard (criticised by the Science Forum)[71] between self-protecting politicians and officers on the one hand and risk-bearing ordinary citizens unnerved by Tegnell's admitted reservation.[72]

Sweden's behaviour in this global crisis appears strange even in its second year. A pandemic, Krastev rightly analyses, does not "pit nations against each other"[73] but provides the most globalisation-friendly possibilities for international cooperation. This is not the case, however, for Swedish leaders where all kinds of normative comparisons with others are rejected. With regard to the population's trust in politics, such a non-cooperative attitude is fatal. In the pandemic emergency the failure or success of the political leaders decides people's image of the future. If we cannot mobilise a collective response to this crisis, how could we respond to the next one properly, for example with regard to climate change? How can someone in Sweden continue to respond to dangerous climate change with hope and trust in science and rationality if the state could not even respond adequately to the pandemic? The loss of trust is obvious, both with regard to Sweden's own citizens and with regard to the EU and the international community of nations.

Sweden's resistance to cooperating closely with other European and Nordic countries and to learning from each other has caused harm to its own interests, in politics as well as in business. The Government's blocking of common decision-making processes in the EU, such as Eurobonds for Italy,[74] a common European warning app, and an integrated European travel restriction policy offered embarrassing examples of not having understood the essence of *the Corona crisis as everybody's crisis*, where it is not the defence of one's national *Sonderweg* that is at stake but where the interdependency of all in the European project is "the most reliable source of security and prosperity".[75] Critical voices were consequently also raised in the European Council about Sweden's exceptionalist experiment undermining European solidarity.[76]

While "the whole world had gone crazy",[77] according to Tegnell, Sweden alone was supposedly applying a really rational, adequate method. In February 2021 Tegnell discounted, in a scientific journal, the massive scientific and international questioning of Sweden's and his strategy by postulating that Sweden's method was "based on the same basic principles from pandemic plans and [had] the same objectives and goals as other countries".[78] It was not. In the context of the already now quickly developing process towards one common European "health union", Sweden's merits for cooperation are not very impressive after this performance, to put it mildly. Analogously, the country's explicitly declared strategy to become "a leading life science nation"[79] is no longer very convincing either after having marginalised and excluded real science from pandemic decision-making. As if nothing has happened, however, Sweden's own national institute (SI) monitoring the international coverage of the country's pandemic handling constantly ensured for the leaders that international voices were curious rather than critical.[80] The storm of critical questioning was simply blocked off, even if the Government's highest officer for crisis management, Elisabeth Backteman, seems to have been aware of the threat of a changing international image of Sweden for the worse.[81] In internal speculations the Government even feared being discriminated against in the EU's distribution of vaccines due to the internationally critical view of the country's *Sonderweg*.[82] Nevertheless one can wonder and fear whether the Spanish saying about "playing Swedish" might become known to a wider audience because of Sweden's pandemic management where one never admits failures: *hacerse el sueco* means in Spain *playing dumb*, a skill widely practised in Sweden's pandemic emergency.[83]

Maybe the pandemic failure nevertheless also allows a hopeful seed for the long-term future, where the loss of national exceptionalism might bring something good in its wake, so that, without the burden of being best, we can grapple with the urgent challenges of our common future and earth pragmatically in cooperation with other countries. Critics might argue that my reflections and others in this book instead hinder a healthy process of reconciliation, but I am convinced that only a trustworthy confession about failures and irresponsibilities can offer a foundation for a sustainable long-term process of social healing.

According to distinguished philosopher Georg Picht, the unresolved aporias in our past will always return and challenge us.[84] History's "intrinsic power" (*Eigenmacht*) can never be subjugated and ruled by us. The irreversible und unresolved contradictions that we have produced in our past will always pursue us. One cannot simply deny them. Therefore, for the long-term coherence of the society, it is important to face them, to admit them and to learn from them. Hereby we find the hidden keys to a sustainable future. My deeper driving force in offering reflections on Sweden's shipwreck therefore should not be misunderstood as immoderate accusation, but as an attempt to search for therapeutic tools for coping with the past and efficient tools to be used in the next pandemics or national crisis.

Fear, shame and self-compassion

Another way of approaching the question of why a majority of the people has for so long supported a strategy that has put their own life and health at risk is to try out selected tools from social and cultural psychology. I am not educated in these fields and can only hope that my preliminary reflections here could inspire other scholars. In addition, I would by no means like to generalise about *the* Swedish ethnic soul and what the pandemic reveals about it. Nevertheless, my field/site studies and projects in social anthropology and contextual theology have taught me that one should never underestimate the cultural dimension and simply generalise as if all human beings everywhere and everywhen are the same. We always remain unique children of our specific social, geographical and historical context and *Zeitgeist*, at the same time as we also follow the same universal biological and cultural codes of being human in the niches of evolution in general.

In my view, Sweden's pandemic experiment has made evident that collective psychological processes of feeling fear and shame have also played a crucial role in the support for the risky management. Gustavsson has, as described earlier, explored the deeper roots of public health patriotism and also investigated these empirically.[85] Her analysis explains convincingly the overwhelming response to the Agency's strange crisis communication in the beginning. But why did this strong support endure and continue at such expense, when the first wave harvested circa 4000 lives avoidably? And why did it endure when the second and third waves accelerated due to the same mistakes as before? Why does one not, at the end of the pandemic's second year, accuse the leaders of the loss of almost 10,000–12,000 lives that could undoubtedly have been saved? Patriotism is undoubtedly at work here but can it also explain the long-term impact on the sinister cooperation of state and people? While critical voices accelerate and increase in volume in the public debates, shame creeps in slowly but surely, and suspicions gain currency as to whether one had placed one's bet on the right horse. Several of my former patriotic friends grew silent and apathetic when the second wave sped up.

How could shame studies assist us to mine this mystery more deeply? My hypothesis here is that a) the strong force of avoiding shame, at any price, explains the aggression against all kind of voices that are thematising failure, responsibility, humiliation, embarrassment and guilt,[86] and b) that the healthy potential of accepting shame and turning it into constructive learning from failure and conversion is absent after two pandemic years. Shame has both an emotional and a cognitive dimension; talking about "avoiding shame" implies both: my emotional impulse not to feel guilty, as well as the cognitive rational defence to resist others shaming me. In so far as one moves forward taking account of the past, the healthy forces of (positive) shame will grow. Shame offers an important relational skill and potential for self-criticism as it represents a crucial "social emotion" (Dan Zahavi). Favourably one can identify some seeds that might start to grow in the future. Gustavsson's question points out the direction: "What happens in a country where shame does not lead to an open national self-criticism?"[87] Continuing on this path: what could happen in a country when shame finally leads to open, constructive learning from failures?

Once people had accepted the authority of the state and the troika's (Giesecke, Carlson, Tegnell) explanations from the start in March 2020, many also turned this acceptance into a belief. I certainly do not want to blame anyone for relying with great trust on the national state to take care and to take the right action. Every citizen has a right to demand the best possible pandemic management from its Government.

However, when critical voices from highly competent scientists in harmony with international journalists and writers questioned the Government's abdication and the FHM's strange policy in April 2020, the sound high level of trust turned into an unsound belief. Was it better to defend the state policy and put one's hope to Tegnell as guardian and saviour, or should one start to collect alternative information? And why did leaders in the daily press conferences month after month not respond to the critics, but denounce them as indecent instead? The media and journalists were also following this path. Rather than investigating the powerful, they critically questioned how German ARD journalist Christian Stichler dared to ask critical questions.[88] After half a year he left the country with a peculiar film about Swedes not worrying at all, remaining in their vision of dwelling comfortably in a kind of paradisiac *Bullerby* world.[89] Science journalists suspended their duty to explore independently and turned into FHM megaphones.[90] Obviously the Agency demanded blind obedience and many preferred to practise this belief.[91]

According to polls, 84% of the people had confidence in the beginning and believed in the state's laid back method ordained top down where individual responsibility (*egenansvar*) was combined with just a few undemanding recommendations to wash hands, stay at home if sick and be careful. The majority was proud of not being exposed to *lockdowns* as in other countries but the Swedish strategy, mostly designed for the prosperous middle class, in fact *locked out* circa 20% of the population, namely citizens over 70.[92] They were advised to stay at home and to ask others for help. Such ordained exclusion from above led after a few weeks to the so-called "uproar of the elderly", where detailed questions were asked in a manifest about the consequences of ageism.[93] Such an imperative and encouragement of individual responsibility might have increased the pride of citizens in managing this crisis from below, but it also implied that the responsibility was taken from the shoulders of the state and moved to the shoulders of the individual. While my hairdresser in spring 2020 proudly answered "we do not need restrictions from above as we can fix this ourselves", she remained shamefully silent when the second wave again harvested lives avoidably due to the same errors as before.

In what scholar of legal sociology Håkan Hydén calls a "patchwork of normative fragments and regulations", often inconsistent, Sweden followed a path of combining low legality (avoiding strict regulations) and high legitimacy (aiming at high acceptance and obedience).[94] From February to November 2020 the country was convinced that this crisis could be managed even better along the path constructed by the troika. Leaders fuelled this fatal view again and again, and when the Government had nothing more to say PM Löfven assured the public in August that they had "chosen the right way" and claimed that it would have been "against the constitution"[95] not to rely on the Agency, a point of view that was sharply criticised by the Danish Parliament's commission with regard to Sweden's management where one *only* listened to the Agency.[96] In his second speech to the nation in November, Löfven encouraged individual responsibility and pointed a finger at the people: "It depends on me and you!"[97] While other national leaders, for example in Denmark, Norway and Germany, emphasised the need for social cohesion and solidarity, Löfven appealed to individualism (with a hidden shaming finger). Löfven only twice addressed his people directly in the form of a national speech.

The problem, though, was that the Agency did not inform its population correctly at all, as many thought, but provided them with dangerously false information. To this day the FHM denies or relativises aerosol transmission and presymptomatic spread, mistrusts the proven effects of facemasks and regards children as almost safe from suffering from serious Covid. The alleged experts did not in fact build on any expertise at all, but even downplayed and denied publicly the more evident insights produced by scientists all over the world and acknowledged by other nations. Their crisis communication was rather characterised by "nudging" and technocratic thinking than offering the population a clear "mental model" and map to navigate by.[98] Risk communication in Sweden produced lack of knowledge and practised a "discursive relocation of responsibility"; unfortunately it is well known in political science that this is a tendency in Swedish crisis management.[99] In short, the state, which many encountered with great trust, did not offer confidence in its citizens (to accept necessary strict restrictions) but overloaded them with individual responsibility on unreliable grounds of knowledge. The fatal virological interpretations and pandemic crisis management were combined with unprofessional and unethical crisis communication, which tried to avoid social unrest but did not provide the people with a reliable map to navigate by. Avoidable loss of almost 10,000–12,000 lives, circa 200,000 sick with Long Covid in December 2021, a "care debt" (that will take circa four years to work off (with more loss of lives and damaged health),[100] 9% unemployed, and the avoidable risk of losing trust were natural consequences.

What has all this to do with shame? My hypothesis implies that the first pandemic year in Sweden produced so many misjudgements, rationally justified failures, errors and fatal dysfunction in so many spheres of the formerly well-lubricated social fabric that staying confident in a state that immediately turned into turmoil demanded enormous mental energy to be put into convincing oneself that we are doing "pretty well",[101] a phrase which still remains Minister Hallengren's mantra in the pandemic's 19th month. The establishing of so many obvious failures in so many spheres conducted by the Agency produces shame. Not admitting any failures and displacing one's responsibility demands even more emotional, cultural and rhetorical energy. Justifying what has obviously gone wrong and denying any guilt produces one more level of shame above the level of shame due to practical failures. Such a, let us say, two-tier web of shame was spun around most of the society in the first pandemic year. Only committed actors and groups in the civil society and in some scholarly contexts were able to resist and mobilise countervailing power. One can certainly ask who has developed such a feeling and reflection; as we lack reliable studies I can here only rely on my personal experience and refer to the many thousands of people from all kinds of social spheres within the country who connected to the different activities of our Science Forum and provided us with their experiences. As I expressed once in a YouTube talk, the spiritual pain caused by the national leaders' pandemic experiment appears to be much broader and deeper than one can surmise. A natural consequence of refusing shame was to attack all these aggressively as nest befoulers and enemies of the state. Intellectuals and highly educated players – doctors, scholars, philosophers, politicians and others – were also seduced into taking their positions in this network of defending the strong state patriotically and denying all shame. Not only the Left Party[102] but also all the others betrayed their own ideology by not satisfyingly protecting the life and health of the people.

After months of constant eclectic and incomplete information mixed with disinformation, the population had become a part of this process. Therefore it should not come as a surprise that many would feel ashamed if their leaders were unmasked as incompetent.[103] Rather than exposing oneself to such shame, one could blame and stigmatise the critics of this strategy. It was obvious that Tegnell in his argument about the people's trust in the state as the key to Sweden's alleged success was speaking misleadingly. Rather the "Swedish government and citizenry had trusted each other too much",[104] and had locked each other in the so-called "corridor of opinions" where the feeling of shame at having been a part of this hindered the process of opening one's eyes. The victims themselves, the suffering and the dead, were completely lost from sight hereby.

We know very well how naturally feelings of shame turn into aggression and violence, and the feeling of being stigmatised by other countries' critical observers had to be avoided at any price. It could not be that we were doing wrong as we always do right, just wait and see, and in the end we will be proven right. In November 2021 former GD Carlson was still repeating the mantra that it is too early to evaluate anything.[105] There are no lessons to be learnt at all, not even from the "testing shipwreck".[106] Not to worry, there is nothing to be ashamed of.

From studies in shame we know well how the whole dynamic in its initial phase begins with feeling the threat of being accused of having done wrong. Shame is, as Björn Olsen rightly says, one of the worst feelings evolution has equipped us with and we do everything to avoid it.[107] Nevertheless shame can also offer an important good driving force for activating awareness and conversion. It can serve as an ethical wake-up call and increase our self-respect. The extreme stubbornness, straightforwardness and single-mindedness of Tegnell in daily press conferences on television were in this regard a heart-balm for the Swedish soul in fear of having failed. What some could see as incompetence others interpreted as an impressive steadfastness.[108] The chief epidemiologist practised in masterly fashion the arts of rhetorically turning every kind of information and question into support for his own views, comforting a majority of the epidemiologically uneducated population in a woolly state of feeling safe and rationally protected.[109] In this way, incompetence with a national mandate and nearly absolute power fuelled conformist belief that led to shame that again led to the shared belief that everything was always undoubtedly being done right. Punctum!

Expressing criticisms from below came with a social cost. Moving to the nest befoulers' camp implied in such a context serious risks of being excluded from the community, a bitter lesson that many had to experience in work places, in families and neighbourhoods, and also in universities and schools. Many sad stories about this have been shared with members of the Science Forum and other committed organisations. Analogously, many stories have been told about courageous children and families who tried to follow reliable scientific advice, for example with regard to the use of facemasks. Teachers who prioritised protection against infection lost their jobs; parents who wanted to protect family members with health risks or elderly relatives were accused by municipalities of violating the official duty of attending school; friends became un-friends; even marriages were splintered when a Tegnellian nationalist debated with a critical partner. The processes of shame, discussed earlier, obviously here also followed the well-known dynamic where one turns the danger of feeling ashamed by admitting a failure into repression and an even more aggressive defence of what one believes in. Swedes may have locked their religious beliefs deeply inside so-called private religiosity, but the ordinary cultural dynamics of developing shame over one's untruthful behaviour and belief cannot simply be pushed away.

The formerly united society was in this way threatened by a new form of disunion, where the former culture of consensus-based negotiations aimed at the good of all now became a hinderance for critical constructive thinking and acting. In synergy with the previously mentioned moral sliding, where values of individual freedom ranked highly but values of solidarity and defending the right to life for one's neighbour was weakened, this process affected the national identity substantially, and it is still much too early to prophesy about any processes of coping with the past (*Vergangenheitsbewältigung*) and reconciliation. But one might remember here a German saying among lawyers with regard to the weighing of rights to freedom vs. protecting life and health: *liberties can return, the dead cannot.*

Interestingly this dynamic is the opposite of what is recommended and practised in Christian and other religious belief.[110] The biblical stories know very well how shame can trigger violence and recommend therefore a voluntary loss of status rather than defending one's own pride and honour. Self-righteousness is regarded as a sin against God, who alone can justify as the source of justice. Compassion and self-control are virtues in Jewish-Christian faith, and it is similar in other religions. Such compassion and sensitivity to the processes of sin and shame are necessary conditions for fighting back in synergy with the Creator against the evil outcomes of shame.

Shame is in this sense connected to our handling of vulnerability and compassion. Avoiding or refusing shame implies at the same time denying one's vulnerability. To what degree Swedish decision-makers are driven by such an idolisation of power, strength and infallibility supersedes my competence. Nevertheless one can wonder what it does to a community when political leaders and leading civil servants deny their own vulnerability by refusing any criticism, responsibility, guilt and shame. Legal authorities will decide about guilt, but the lack of being able to feel shame is a personality deficit rather than a real strength if one listens to psychological theory.

Shame offers by contrast a highly constructive feeling that theologian Doris Joachim compares to a vaccine.[111] In small doses one becomes immune to the overwhelming destructive shame. The vaccine strengthens our skills in ethical thinking and acting and also our compassion. People who can wholeheartedly reveal their vulnerability can do wrong and feel ashamed. They can ask for forgiveness, forgive themselves, learn from failures and turn around and convert. Shame, however, must be distinguished from guilt. While guilt is adaptive and can lead to being held accountable by others for what I have done, shame is, according to some scholars, a feeling that threatens my well-being and can destroy it from within. According to Bréne Brown it is not helpful at all.[112] While guilt aims at what I do, shame aims at how I feel.

I do not agree at all, and would rather follow psychologists and phenomenologists who emphasise the social dimension of shame. In opposition to Brown, one should in my view not separate actions from feelings but rather interconnect them while still differentiating them. Accepting one's guilt *and* feeling ashamed about it can both, in synergy, become a force for healing. It becomes even more exciting if we regard shame as a crucial social emotion and skill. This not only makes us aware of the general anchorage of shame in interpersonal relations, but it even allows us to develop more deeply the cohesion of social (even political) life, for example in the surprising ability of so-called *vicarious shame*, a term that explains how people can experience a self-conscious emotion in reaction to the behaviour of another person.[113] Imagine what pandemic management could have been like if such a social skill together with compassion had been enhanced to flourish at its best.

Reasons for the obvious absence of such healthy self-control among the decision-makers in Sweden might be found in the country's long secularisation, but they might also be anchored in the aforementioned conformist consensus culture that obviously is especially vital among the governing Social Democrats. Many of them still cannot separate what is best for the country and what is best for the party but equate the one with the other. Might it be that here in the pandemic context we are discovering two sides of the same coin in the Swedish *Folkhem*, that is the long coherent social mobilisation towards being one of the world's leading societies with regard to welfare, coherence, equity and prosperity on the one side, and the strange dynamics of interconnected liberalism, conformism and contempt for the other on the other side?

Most probably, the marginalisation of all the Covid dead and suffering sick and the lack of commemorating them in a dignifying way, which I explored explicitly earlier,[114] also has its roots in this chord of denying failure, shame and guilt on the one hand and renewing trust and confidence on the other. Who wants to be reminded that their actions have unnecessarily led to the loss of thousands of lives? Nevertheless, not "becoming numb to the sorrow", as Joe Biden demanded,[115] and the remembrance of the suffering and dead, the arts of *Memoria passionis subversiva*, represents in my view a necessary skill for citizens in Sweden in their need to rediscover the deeper force of coherence beyond the broken trust in the disastrous SARS-CoV-2-experiment. Let us hope that this process can take place in good time before the next national crisis or pandemic appears.

For the sake of the future and the envisioned reconciling healing process, it would be interesting to see if this collective guilt and its anchorage in feeling shame that I am alleging here will offer a hinderance, in analogy to therapeutic experiences with drug-misusers, or if it can be broken by processes of admission, confession of guilt and a self-critical sound, rational evaluation with regard to failures and those to be held accountable. From Germany I know all too well that such a collective shame can be broken by open processes of sharing one's participatory guilt. My friends in post-apartheid South Africa can also tell wonderful stories about the healing power freed by the Truth Commission where stories were told by both victims and offenders. In post-Soviet Baltic states after 1989 I myself observed how senior military leaders in a shared meeting with local representatives and foreign guests asked for forgiveness, fell into tears and shared in detail how they destroyed the land and people with nuclear waste, which in the former system they had regarded as right and dutiful. They asked for forgiveness. But such healing needs a long time. It needs specific places, as well as rituals and guardians, and it might take a generation, especially for a country like Sweden "wounded by peace", as writer Elisabeth Åsbrink has thought provokingly expressed it. The term was coined by famous oncologist, writer and Auschwitz survivor Georg Klein, who used it to describe Swedes who after 200 years of peace have lost their ability to recognise evil when it appears.[116]

Bengt Lindroth speaks, in my view more aptly, about an "experience deficit" (*erfarenhetsunderskott*) that makes Sweden different from the other Nordic countries, which have experienced the painful long-term impacts of warfare in all spheres of society. According to Lindroth, "we who did not take part in the war" could not, as the other Nordic countries, draw on experiences from the Second World War and look for lessons taught to be used even now. Columnist Katrine Marçal wonders ironically if Sweden has also now implemented some kind of policy of neutrality against the virus.[117] While others fought it, we stayed cool. Emanuel Macron even declared war on the virus (French philosophers are in love with the war metaphor in a way that I as a German have serious problems with). Lacking the big crises, Swedes instead started to remember the smaller recent ones: Olof Palme's murder, the sinking of *F/S Estonia*, the tsunami in Thailand, the forest fires of 2014 and 2018 and even organised crime and all its rate of fatal shootings, which is the highest in Europe. Remembering these, however, did not offer any help but caused a decided feeling and insight that there was something wrong with the nation state and its capacity to handle a crisis adequately.[118] All crisis management was in fact characterised by serious structural, political and individual failures. So there was not much to learn.

Can something good follow then from the national pandemic crisis? Hopefully, yes, I would answer, but only if one accepts the pandemic as a crisis and self-critically analyses the Swedish experiment. Exemplarily King Carl XVI Gustaf has demonstrated how to walk into such a future by declaring the country's strategy as horribly "failed".[119] The national Corona Commission's second report characterises it as a "shipwreck" and mines in detail all that has gone wrong.[120] In February 2022 the Commission presented its final report with caustic criticism on several points (for details cf. the introductory chapter).[121] Among other things it pointed at the Government that had left all power solely to the FHM, its slowness and inefficiency and its inability to apply the precautionary principle to protect life and health. With regard to this chapter's overarching theme of learning from failure, sadly enough also the responses from Minister Hallengren, GD Tegmark Wisell and Tegnell to the Commission's criticism once more again verified the compact blocking by those responsible. Tegmark Wisell refused to accept any criticism.[122] In general she defended the whole strategy for having taken into account the "wholeness".[123] Such a view seems to place the Agency's definition of wholeness over the citizens' individual life and health und fulfils the criteria of utilitarian denial of the human dignity of every individual human being (in analogy to totalitarian regimes' placing the collective, the *Volk*, over the individual).[124] Tegnell rejects the criticism stating "that we have landed in what has been reasonable to do in every context".[125] Hallengren asserted that Sweden's picking its way was "right",[126] and repudiates any criticism. Those to be held accountable have left their positions, so that the Commission's investigation of the issue of responsibility comes to nothing. Tegnell leaves his position in March 2022; PM Löfven and GD Carlson have left earlier.

Scientists have analysed the country's pandemic response as a "disaster".[127] In the international research project investigating and comparing 17 countries in the world on the interaction of science and politics (ESCAPE), Sweden is also included. The authors highlight Tegnell's and Carlson's fatal foundational decision to go for so-called natural herd immunity and to avoid at any price a shutdown of society.[128] No other country seems to have followed such an unethical and illegal method so consistently as the Swedish FHM troika, supported by a passive Government, even if the UK, Netherlands and Denmark for a few days early on were tempted to do so.[129] The case is satisfyingly verified, so I do not need to plague the reader with further details.

Publicly the Agency downplayed the judgements from national scientists and international authorities as extreme positions, and succeeded in luring the media and political bodies to accept their policy. The authors of the ESCAPE report summarise as follows:

> The Swedish people were kept in ignorance of basic facts such as that the new coronavirus is airborne, that individuals without symptoms can be contagious and that facemasks protect. Mandatory legislation was seldom used; recommendations without any sanctions were the usual tool.[130]

In consequence they demand from the country "to start a self-critical process about its political culture and its lack of accountability of decision makers to avoid future failures as occurred with the Covid-19 pandemic".[131]

Following the public debates in winter 2021/22 I have not much hope that any of these leaders will take any responsibility for any failures, as they excel each other in rejecting any charge. But it will be interesting to follow how the majority of people, who have withdrawn their confidence in the leaders over the course of 2021, will feel and act in the year 2023. Will they confirm the responsibility of their leaders and accept that they should be shamed? Will they feel shame about having supported more or less blindly their deadly strategy? And if so, will they share their stories and feelings of shame with each other to cultivate the cultural soil for reconciliation and renewal of social coherence?

Shame can become toxic but it can also become a unique medicine and tool for healing. From drug therapy one can learn the exciting lesson about how such a constructive, healthy process of admitting, feeling and sharing shame can lead to surprisingly strong experiences of freedom and renewal. Following the experts, the most important method here is to fight the toxic shame with what modern psychotherapy has developed successfully: deepening the skill of self-compassion (*Selbstmitgefühl*).[132]

Such a self-critical self-compassion does not mean narcissistically feeling sorry for oneself but teaches the skill of an accepting, open-minded and caring mode of encountering a critical situation. The other's shaming of one's failure can in such a way be turned into an acceptance of one's imperfection and limits. Admitting a failure could in that sense cure rather than harm. "If one wants to learn from failures one must admit them",[133] as editor Sanna Rayman so aptly titled my article between the second and third waves.

Shame could then, hopefully, in post-pandemic Sweden, serve as an important compass for the protection of our human coexistence. Psychotherapy can train these skills individually but it remains open how one could imitate such a process in Sweden collectively. Maybe an alliance of doctors, psychotherapists, artists, faith communities and committed scientists can start such a process in the civil society? Maybe my suggestion to establish a National Museum of Pandemics[134] might offer such a safe place where open discussions can take place?

As an inspiration one could remind oneself of the German minister of Health, who at the beginning of the pandemic approached the public with the attitude of seeking the right way, well aware of potential failing: "We will probably need to forgive each other much in the coming months", he declared exemplarily.[135] Sadly he committed all too many failures in his hyperactivism. Economist Louise Bringselius also aptly makes us aware of the need for learning from failures, if one wants to enhance society's trust and healing after the crisis.[136] Scholar of crisis management Edward Deverell observes an obvious "risk that both inter- and intracrisis learning processes in the wake of COVID-19 are impacted negatively due to the national and international politicisation of Sweden's management of the pandemic".[137] Overcoming shame by public self-critical evaluation and individual and collective self-compassion is intimately interconnected with processes of increasing and decreasing trust and confidence. In the pandemic we learn that without such trust, in synergy with beliefs in each other and practised love towards one's neighbour, on an interpersonal small scale as well as on a large societal scale, no society can be sustained. Daring to feel ashamed and mobilising the emotional forces of self-compassion towards having done wrong seem to be central forces for learning and finding new ways of handling a pandemic.

The legal dimension

While shame represents an important skill that enhances the individual being a *zoon politicon* (political animal, Aristotle), it is also embedded in the society's morality. But society's legal dimension is also at stake. If I do something wrong that I need to be ashamed of or that others are shaming me for, I can either deny it or admit it and start the reconciling process of confession, forgiveness and healing. If a person commits what the society has defined as "crime", a similar process of investigating guilt takes place, although the state takes the other's place, representing the victim and the collective. Here also the process takes its course: investigation, assessment of guilt, sentence and fine. Sweden, sadly enough, lacks modes of holding politicians and national servants accountable. Four politicians and leading civil servants have already resigned before the Commission's final report in February 2022 and thus escaped responsibility, and Tegnell left his position in March 2022.[138] Citizens are not able to appeal directly to a Constitutional Court, and civil servants were in 1997 freed from administrative responsibility.[139] Here we also probably find a completing explanation of the persistent insensibility of the Government and the Agency. Sweden's virus politics offers a complex view of how the legal system worked and failed in the pandemic emergency. I will just briefly list some points here, as the Corona Commission has explored this in more detail and other legal investigations might take place.

1 The Agency violated its own legal instruction from the Government by not "acting on scientific grounds"[140] in its decisions, and the Government violated its duty to control the Agency and to correct it (usually by replacing the Agency's Director-General).
2 The Agency's Director-General violated the Contagious Disease Act (*Smittskyddslagen*) by reducing four times the duties of testing, registration and tracing those infected with what was classified as "socially dangerous disease".[141]
3 The Agency misinformed the populace by denying aerosol transmission and the related efficiency of facemasks, and hereby caused a considerable number of cases of the disease, with an estimated loss of 3000 lives.[142]
4 Regionally responsible Contagious Disease Doctors delayed the use of facemasks in the health care systems, including in hospitals, and on public transport.[143] The city of Halmstad even prohibited the use of protective equipment such facemasks for teachers at school by referring to the FHM in January 2021 but had to turn around later.[144]
5 The Swedish Work Environment Authority (*Arbetsmiljöverket*) did not fulfil its duty to protect employees and also pupils at schools by not recommending protective equipment and closing schools and workplaces, and the Municipalities' (private) organisation (without legal status) SKR hindered the use of protective equipment in April 2020.[145] An obvious consequence for the schools was the infection with Covid-19 of circa 35% of all children and circa 50% of all teaching staff in the country. No legal action has been taken so far to investigate this overwhelming national violation of the Labour Protection Act and the rather slack practice of controlling its application by the national Agency *Arbetsmiljöverket*. One of the most flagrant failures of this Agency was explicitly not to demand facemasks for health workers in contact with Covid patients, in spite of the demand of the law to protect one's employees.[146]
6 The Health and Social Care Inspectorate (IVO) investigated a large number of suspected cases of illegal euthanasia of the elderly but did not hand over these cases to the legal authorities.[147]
7 National codes of medical ethics were broken by both Agency leaders and individual doctors, in a way that would usually lead to withdrawing a doctor's license.[148]
8 Doctors and nursing home leaders in many places exceeded their authority in interpreting the messages from the FHM (about flattening the curve) with regard to the elderly, deciding *not* to send them to the hospital but instead offer only palliative care. The co-director of the National Board of Health and Welfare (*Socialstyrelsen*), Thomas Lindén, even published "Advice and Recommendations concerning the management of persons in care homes with Covid-19." This document was very much open to interpretation and opened the way for initiation of palliative care with depressant agents like morphine,

which are contra-indicated in Covid-19 patients and potentially lethal. It even declared that "clinical assessment of the patient does not need to be done physically". The decision to determine life and death for the patients in care homes could be performed via telephone! As a later report demonstrated, in 20% of the investigated cases no doctor had visited them. Scholar of Law Lotta Vahlne Westerhäll stated the illegality of the Board's de-prioritisation of the elderly, but its co-director Lindén refuses to accept this criticism.[149] An IVO investigation was started in late 2021 to map how many people (among the elderly and disabled) were excluded in advance from Covid-care by making a formal decision about not sending them to hospital if they showed Covid symptoms.[150]

9 The National Board of Health and Welfare (*Socialstyrelsen*) decided early in the pandemic on instructions for Covid-19 triage through its Ethical Council (SMER). One suggested applying one single criterion, biological age. This was done in a situation where people were preparing for the collapse of the health care system, and where Tegnell decided not to maximally delimit the spread but only try to keep it below the capacity of the health system. Fortunately not all doctors followed these instructions which waived the principle of everyone's equal human value in favour of the utilitarian praxis of "QALY",[151] a method that in fact assures the right of the (bodily) stronger to survive.

A pandemic puts democracy to the test. How is the division of powers working between the Legislature, Executive and the Judiciary in the situation of pandemic emergency? As my short list of legal problems in Sweden has shown, the structural division and interconnection of the powers has not worked satisfactorily at all. Sweden is not alone in having failed the test, but it would need a substantial debate and investigation of its underlying democratic structures to avoid a similar shipwreck in the next crisis, an insight already prepared by the Corona Commission's reports.

The triad of science, politics and trust

In his wide-reaching book on "Globalance", that is, the challenge to achieve global balance in the Covid and post-Covid world, Swiss ethicist and theologian Christoph Stückelberger offers constructive reflections about trust. As a central presupposition to manage a pandemic, he emphasises "the importance of scientific cooperation and a level of trust".[152] Here I would like to develop his ideas further and unfold the hypothesis that *the success or failure of pandemic management depends on how well the reciprocal interaction of science, politics and the population's trust is enacted.*

There should be no doubt about the significance of knowledge and the central importance of science and its advice for the decision-making of responsible politicians and political bodies. This is true in the context of a pandemic as well as in the context of anthropogenic climate change. From climate impact science and climate politics one can learn that listening to science saves lives. Both politicians and scientists need to trust each other, and both are urged to establish an efficient problem-solving communication. Political decisions need to be grounded in solid expert judgements that rely on the latest and most convincing states of knowledge in the relevant fields. Nevertheless the criterion of a maximum of scientific evidence might also turn into a destructive belief in over-evidence, and decision-making in a situation of an accelerating threatening crisis therefore needs to balance scientific evidence and efficient measures for protecting life and health in an urgent proactive process of a common scientific and political search for what is best for all. Waiting for all available data before taking action might be too late on the one hand, and responding too hastily might worsen a situation. As Martin Lindström aptly shows, aiming at over-evidence in a situation of pandemic urgency is risky and threatens life.[153] The Swedish method of the Agency responding, though, was constantly reactive and never proactive,[154] and mostly late rather than quick. Several evaluations in different countries have shown how efficiently quick responses have saved lives, and how slow responses have led to the loss of lives. That is why the Corona Commission clearly criticised the FHM's constant "slowness".[155]

Not only do the politicians need to listen to and rely with confidence on the most relevant and well-informed scientists but the scientists must also be able to rely on politicians who can understand and acquire their knowledge and transform advice quickly into efficient action. Politically decided actions must again then be critically monitored and evaluated by science in communication with politics. A well-functioning process in this interacting communication takes the shape of a circle: *seeing – analysing – acting – seeing anew*.

Practising this method at its best is even more important in the so-called "post-truth pandemic" and "infodemic", where a large amount of disinformation and quasi-truths are circulating, in all kinds of social and other media. Trish Greenhalgh therefore aptly requests that "scientists will have to go on the offensive" to "succeed in this new era of ideological distortion and bad faith".[156] Politics must also herein learn to handle science discerningly and carefully.

Moreover, political decision-making has to weigh different interests against each other, and in the early phase of the pandemic many weighed the protection of life and health on the one side and the protection of the society's economy on the other. Health and economy were opposed. Economists have nevertheless clearly analysed how such an opposition is counterproductive and simply false, as only a maximum of protecting life and health can support the economy in the best possible way.[157] In the same way the opposition of rights to freedom vs. restrictions to protect health also offers a dangerously misleading ethical view, as freedom always includes the other's freedom, and as rights to freedom can return while dead neighbours cannot. The state's task to prioritise life and health is obvious, both ethically and legally, even if one carefully follows the European Convention on Human Rights where every Government has to guarantee "to protect everyone's right to life and health by law".[158]

Especially in cases of deciding about adequate measures, the politicians had to act on the sometimes certain, sometimes uncertain advice in the pandemic emergency and they had to work out what kinds of restrictions could be both efficient and in acceptable proportion to delimiting the individual rights of the citizens to freedom. Democratic nations had of course a much tougher challenge here in comparison with nations governed by autocratic regimes and dictatorships, but it is impossible to discover any clear difference between the two in the efficiency of saving lives. Success instead seems to depend on the interplay of science advising politics in reciprocal confidence and on the population's trust. As the shape of reciprocal trust between people and Governments is different in democratic and autocratic contexts, I look forward to the forthcoming discussions in political science on this question.

Although politicians in Sweden traditionally involved experts, scientists and relevant scholars in policy-making, the pandemic crisis communication revealed the painful opposite. According to Sweden's distinguished economist Lars Calmfors, the interaction of science and politics has turned into a "near shipwreck" in the pandemic.[159] This stands in stark contrast to how Anthony Fauci described the attitude of president Biden in the US pandemic management:

> When he asked me to serve as his chief medical advisor he made clear to me that science must determine all that we are doing. He said, if we make a mistake, we must admit it, be responsible for it, and try to adjust it.[160]

In my view the Swedish leaders' kind of thinking and acting represents an extensive lack of trust in science, by ignoring other countries' modes of scientific-political interactions, and it also represents an embarrassing lack of respect for other countries' ethical judgements. According to Calmfors, the Agency leadership should have been replaced early on (which I in fact demanded in June 2020),[161] "due to its inability in a situation of high uncertainty not to accept that one's judgements could be wrong".[162] One might ask whether Sweden in the pandemic has put Western civilisation's cultural and ethical achievements aside by striving for natural herd immunity without the permission of the people,[163] and whether it has acted in harmony with what is described as the European Union's community of values.

The whole circle of crisis communication and the triad of trust among politics, science and the people was obviously damaged in Sweden. With fatal consequences, the Agency troika demanded and received very early in the pandemic all operative power from the Government,[164] who seemed to have abdicated from their role.[165] PM Löfven – who, in his political career as a former trade union leader, is not experienced in dialogues with scientists and lacks higher education – constantly confirmed from that time on his strong confidence in his Agency's "experts", and that he could not see any alternative than to rely solely on them.[166] The Agency did not want to bother the people with tough restrictions but rather let the contagion run reasonably through the country to achieve natural herd immunity. The promise not to overload the health system and to protect the elderly was given but never achieved, as the level of the contagion was far too high, a level that killed and infected all too many innocent. The health care system is still after 20 months not prepared to handle a pandemic.[167] Initiated voices demand the deconstruction of the Agency and the restoring of the former Infection Protection Institute (*Smittskyddsinstitutet*). Debates on the FHM's further existence will get hotter and a new Government will need to restore the broken trust by investigating what to learn from the Agency's many failures. "Trust requires transparency, not only through frequent and targeted crisis communication, but, more importantly, by engaging stakeholders and the public in risk-related decision making", the OECD states in its "first lessons" from different Governments' responses.[168] The FHM has certainly constantly informed the people around the campfire of their daily press conferences, but the Agency has not at all revealed its underlying evaluations and grounds for decision-making. Its crisis communication was characterised rather by "the opposite of the transparency and honesty that should inform communication" as the National Corona Commission states.[169]

The national Agency's strategy continuously emphasised letting the infection spread on a reasonable scale in order to protect the health care system, "flattening the curve", and achieving natural herd immunity for everyone's benefit. The fact that this was at the core of Tegnell and Carlson's policy, until a vaccine appeared on the horizon, has been proven beyond a doubt.[170] One of the most influential ethicists in Sweden, Torbjörn Tännsjö, who for decades dominated social ethics, summarised this aptly:

> It [the Agency's strategy] seems to be . . . to infect people as quickly as possible to achieve herd immunity. It sounds as if one is prepared to victimise a number of individuals – in the short run – to save more lives on the whole by saving the economy.[171]

The philosopher emphasises how such a method would be unacceptable in other countries, and concludes that "motivations are more utilitarian in Sweden than in countries that are shutting down".[172] The method, acceptable to Tännsjö, is, however, for the WHO and most ethicists unethical and illegal, and reveals a political and cultural pathology.[173] Following Tännsjö's utilitarian ethics, the National Board of Health and Welfare's instruction, prepared by Lars Sandman and the Ethical Committee, applying the controversial principle of "QALY" in the situation of triage, violates both the country's legal constitution and common European principles of human dignity and equality.[174]

Strikingly, a judicious German interdisciplinary study has clearly shown how the path of mainly relying on individual responsibility in Sweden led to a remarkable loss of lives that could have been spared if the national state had taken a similar path to other countries. The researchers show how infections and deaths could have been reduced by about 75% and 38% if the country had executed a similar lockdown to other countries.[175] In the light of the previously discussed reciprocal interplay of science, politics and trust, the passivity of politics in combination with the autocratic execution of power by the Agency, the ignorance of relevant science and the blind trust of a majority of citizens caused a dysfunctional triad where not trust but distrust, misused trust and broken trust were revealed.

The third angle in our triad, alongside science and politics, is about the people and their relation to and cooperation with their leaders and institutions, both in politics and in science. Trust and confidence in responsible leadership offers probably the most significant quality in the triad of pandemic management in a democratic society. Confucius was keenly aware of this and ranked confidence among the three essential skills: first armament, then food, but "without the people's trust nothing can stand" (XII).[176]

Sweden traditionally had a very high level of trust compared with other countries due to its long history of a consensus-based welfare society. A worrying development is, however, that this high level of trust seems to erode if one investigates the levels of local trust, especially among the younger generations in recent years. Therefore it seems even more important to emphasise how the whole population's trust can be restored after the pandemic disaster.

Other Nordic countries such as Denmark, by contrast, are characterised by a high level of trust, and this trust and preparedness of the Danish people to follow their Government's tough decisions has been analysed as a crucial factor.[177] This makes the failure in Sweden even more surprising as the country obviously, as Peter Baldwin has explained and as Gunnar Steineck's chapter in this book particularly underlines, had very good preconditions to manage the pandemic successfully. My hypothesis here is that the disaster was caused by a serious malfunction in the triad of politics, science and trust. Initiated scholars have asked if this part of Sweden's pandemic experiment implies the final end of its welfare system,[178] but I would be careful about drawing such final conclusions and instead still hope for the skill to learn from one's failures.

These violations of different laws also undermined the people's trust substantially. And it gets even worse when no one can be held ethically and legally accountable in the country since the abolishment of so-called civil servants' responsibility (*tjänstemannaansvar*) in 1987. A violation of the laws by those in whom one has great confidence causes a kind of moral and political earthquake. To admit this would imply an emotionally painful challenge that many obviously prefer to avoid. "What do we have our authorities for if we must protest against their decisions all the time?" an angry commentator wrote with regard to a reader's letter demanding a third dose of vaccine for all the elderly.[179] Citizens had to face the challenge of whether they should continue to trust blindly or start to learn lessons from the Authorities' misleading information and insecure decisions. How can one turn broken trust into trustworthy new modes of crisis communication? Will people continue to encourage blind trust and hinder the necessary process of learning from failures? Or will Sweden enter a new path of admitting failures, learning, and enhancing open, self-critical crisis communication and evaluation?

As both Baldwin and Stückelberger have pointed out, different countries have developed very diverse modes of responding to the pandemic, and sociocultural differences seem to play a central role herein, as these also impact on several dimensions such as the dynamics of trust and distrust, and the speed of decision-making together with the speed of changing behaviours. According to the so-called *Trust Barometer* from early 2020, a large number of world citizens had trust in their Government in the beginning (65%) and wanted the politicians to lead the response to the pandemic (>70%).[180] In Sweden as many as 84% of the population trusted the Agency, but they did not demand any responsibility from their Government, which nevertheless scored high percentages of support for passively supporting the Agency. As the pandemic continued to harvest innocent lives, the levels of trust lowered of course, but trust is well known for being a tenacious quality that is difficult to unsettle. In Sweden confidence remained strong and unshaken during the first wave but when people could see more clearly how the same mistakes were repeated fatally in the second wave, support for the Agency fell to circa 55% in December 2020 and to only 35% in March to June 2021.[181]

Trust cannot be measured simply in the same way as body temperature but is analysed with regard to different parameters including values and indicators such as transparency, integrity, and ethics in general, as well as innovation and reliability.[182] Forthcoming studies of trust might be able to show how and where those losses of trust have taken place and what it means for the long-term health of the society. Loss of trust usually turns into an acceleration of sociocultural and political pathologies. In the pandemic context we can also approach trust as a skill of relying on decision-makers both in science and in politics, and of preparing to follow their recommendations and measures in our ordinary daily life and work. A more general trust in the national state and in the well-functioning interaction between science and politics generates in such a model the highest possible affirmation from below and also obedience to and compliance[183] with rules from above.

Without confidence, the cooperation between science and politics can scarcely succeed in democratic societies without the use of force. This is also, by the way, the reason for the high success of vaccination in societies with high trust levels and the very worrying low rate of vaccination in low trust societies such as Russia and some Eastern European states. In countries where with good reasons people could never rely on political leaders, the vaccination rate, of for example 20% in Bulgaria, is worrying for the whole of Europe as the spread will go on and on and new mutations will take place.[184]

Another way of approaching the praxis of trust is by mining more deeply the forces of *solidarity*. The value of solidarity has been central in the Swedish ethnic soul, and issues of social justice, solidarity and equality have played an important role especially in the Social Democratic movement. Nevertheless, in Sweden too the pandemic has brought higher risks to the most vulnerable.[185] The elderly and children, but also the poorly educated with low incomes and immigrants had to carry the most demanding and often life-threatening burdens. The precariat on the neoliberal employment market was exposed to the contagion with less protection, and the troika's strategy has rightly been described as a strategy for the prosperous middle class and the rich.[186] Practising solidarity is, as Hans Diefenbacher et al. strikingly state,[187] connected to responsibility and social justice, and it provides an ethical surplus that is highly important for the quality of social life in a community. Social cooperation, love for one's neighbour and practical care instead of contempt for the weak and the other represent crucial values of social life, and one must painfully confess that this solidarity has not satisfyingly flourished in Sweden. Even the disabled have been exposed to serious risks by the FHM deciding not to offer them a booster vaccination in time.[188] While emphasising individual responsibility at its central tool in the state's response to the pandemic, solidarity among the citizens was the same time hindered by deciding on measures that did not take into account existing social inequality and injustice. One can wonder if the pandemic in Sweden as well as worldwide might teach us a lesson about the urgent need for practising trust and solidarity with and for each other:

> It remains to ask whether this surplus [of solidarity] can serve as a foundation for greater cohesion of global society and whether the term solidarity, "weak" compared to other concepts, could not reveal its strength precisely in contexts like these.[189]

An advantage was achieved by the Swedish approach as many conflicts about the proportionality of measures that were plaguing other countries could be avoided here. Corona sceptics in the German *Querdenker* movement attacked their Government violently but adored Tegnell as a hero when they demonstrated by dressing in Swedish flags and dancing in Pippi Longstocking clothes. Sweden faced such protest against the state's demands only very marginally. While other countries had to fight a movement of "knowledge resistance" among social groups of corona sceptics, in analogy to the well-known dynamics of climate sceptics, the national Agency itself developed a surprisingly strong resistance to scientific knowledge. The challenge that democratic societies usually had to face, that is to ensure a common acceptance of valid scholarly grounded general knowledge,[190] was now threatened by the state itself by its refusal to accept common scientific insights about aerosol transmission, facemasks, asymptomatic spread, children's role and the infectiousness and loss of protection among the vaccinated.

Applying my preliminary model of the triad of the reciprocal interaction of trust, science and politics, one must state that countries that were striving for a maximum of such transparent reliable and open crisis communication and decision-making were successful. Countries like Germany, New Zealand, Japan and South Korea were most successful in developing efficient and widely supported pandemic management, while countries where trust was lacking had significant problems with responding efficiently. Only China offers an exception as the dictatorship, without any concern for human rights, could apply a tough, wide-reaching zero-Covid strategy and exposed its population to the harshest possible measures. Trust or lack thereof does not play any role here. Power from above and obedience is what counts. China's virus politics also served as an instrument for global politics where they proclaimed themselves to have the best possible protection of health due to the best possible political system of communism. How convincing is the Chinese leader's claim, and is a dictatorship really the best political system for coping with a national and global crisis? China's slack line in climate politics does not really support such a view, to put it mildly.

At the other extreme from China, we find parts of Trump's USA and Bolsanaro's Brazil, where the state simply left the citizens alone to tackle the pandemic emergency. Trump nevertheless lost his election, partly due to his hyper-relaxed line, and Bolsanaro was impeached for having caused many avoidable deaths due to his passivity and denial. In addition to these, one might also mention the few nations such as Turkmenistan and Tanzania where national leaders constantly simply denied the danger of the virus, and not only left their citizens alone but also betrayed them with misleading information. Other countries successfully practised a region-wide zero-Covid strategy[191] and were able to save many lives and keep a majority healthy, even if this became much more demanding in the fourth wave when they had delayed vaccinating as many as possible and the virus variants had become more infectious. In Sweden a zero-Covid strategy was made to look ridiculous and the FHM refused it as an option, a view that was explicitly expressed by FHM GD Carlson in the Parliament's interrogation (cf. the introductory chapter). Not striving to delimit the contagion as much as possible but allowing it to run reasonably comes with a cost. Even if PM Löfven and GD Carlson assured people that they aimed at minimising the spread as well as they could, their practices did not verify their intention but revealed an avoidable loss of lives.

Personally I cannot understand why the zero-Covid vision, or its milder variant the No-Covid vision, of striving for the *lowest possible* number of new infections should not offer us the best way into a future state of endemicity.[192] On the world map of different pandemic outcomes, Sweden is located far away from the successful zero-Covid countries and those who practised a well-functioning interaction of science and politics in combination with a transparent crisis communication to ensure the people's trust.

Has everything really gone wrong in Sweden's approach? No, not at all.

Certainly Swedes have also figured out and practised wise and efficient responses that have been able to protect the population from even worse miseries. I list them briefly here:

- In the early phase the Government decided to let the national health insurance allow people with suspected symptoms to stay home from work without any considerable loss of income. A large group of employees took the opportunity, and from one day to another social mobility decreased radically, leading to a proportional decrease in the spread of Covid-19.
- The country's traditionally high level of trust in the national institutions represents a central highly valuable commodity for involving the population in taking the right preventative action. The Agency's inefficient crisis management and communication and the politicians' passivity do not negate the intrinsic value of this trust in itself. Many citizens tried to take their responsibility as seriously as possible but as they were misinformed about aerosol spread,

facemasks and children, they could only adapt their lifestyle to maximise protection in a limited way.

- Critical voices appeared on the scene early on, and they were accompanied by several professional and morally sound commissions and reports. Even if the media in general failed and acted as megaphones of power, the public discourse continued. In any case, especially from November 2020, the media offered a more open and complex source of information for the citizens, even if decision-makers deliberately did not let this have an impact on them. Supposedly half of the population from spring to autumn 2021 changed their attitude towards the reliability of the national pandemic management to a critical one.
- Sweden's former identity as a moral super power with regard to modern social welfare development has been lost. The image of Sweden was damaged, but this also offers at the same time new possibilities for reconstructing one's identity in a more realistic way beyond the time of bunker mentalities.

Nevertheless four crucial lessons taught by Sweden's experiment should become obvious after my reflections in this chapter.

1 Protecting life and health to the maximum possible degree should be undoubtedly the guiding star in a pandemic emergency, due to ethical, legal, social and even economic reasons.
2 Listening to science and transforming its insights into an efficient response saves lives, a wisdom in analogy to climate impact science's significance in ongoing dangerous climate change. The quality and form of transparent communication between politicians and scientists is crucial here. As the SARS-CoV-2-pandemic is also embedded in the processes of global environmental change and especially the interplay of animals, habitats and human societies, the lessons taught in the pandemic emergency need to be carefully integrated with science and politics in the environmental emergency of climate change. Everyone's individual health and planetary health need to be protected in an interconnected way. Ideologies that place the value of collective (public) health over the value of every individual's health are violating the equal value and dignity of human life and overriding the principles of human rights.
3 The skill of practising confidence and trust offers a crucial and complex quality of all dimensions of pandemic management. This concerns the people's trust in politics and science, as well as politicians' trust in science, and scientists' trust in apolitical decision-making. The triad of science, politics and trust implies reciprocal interrelations in a process of change. Doing harm to the best relational interaction in this triad does harm to human lives and health, and also the long-term inner peace and coherence of a society. Such damage might be caused in many ways, through obscure crisis communication, through unshakeable dogmas such as natural herd immunity, through individual rather than national responsibility (instead of both), and through scientific ignorance,

or through the lack of ethics, compassion and transparent inclusion of the people in the process of decision-making about the citizens' lives and health.

4 Learning from failures offers the most crucial skill of responding to an ongoing dangerous pandemic. Only decision-makers who can admit failures, learn from them, and adjust and change course to more efficient responses can achieve the maximum lowering of an ongoing contagion that in itself causes all the miseries in lost lives and short and long-term disease in a virus-based pandemic. Holding onto dogmatic positions and blindly applying these leads to an unacceptable avoidable loss of lives and indicates an underlying political pathology with regard to the power-sharing practice between politics, science and the trusting people to be protected. A people should not be exposed to a biopolitical "experiment" in a pandemic emergency. If a state in addition executes such an experiment following the utilitarian path against the ethics of human dignity, it will necessarily put in jeopardy and victimise its citizens' lives and health, as Lapo Lappin's chapter elucidates.

   Responding to such an emergency demands bodies and leaders in politics, science and national administration who can admit failures and therefore are able to learn and change their course in order to achieve maximal protection of their people's lives and health. In accordance with medical ethics' well-known duty-of-candour principle,[193] this should also be practised transparently in all aspects of pandemic management.

5 Individual and sociocultural processes of accepting guilt and affirming shame play a substantial role in restoring trust in each other and reciprocal trust between politicians, scientists and citizens. They can serve as central forces for healing broken trust and strengthening the coherence of a society and thereby its resilience in forthcoming crises and pandemics.

Further important lessons taught appear in the other chapters. For me it would be enough if I could throw some light on the life-enhancing potential of confessing sin, not being afraid of shame, admitting failures to learn from them and thereby strengthening individual social and political responsibility and compassion. How do we open "our eyes to the world we have been living in"?[194] How do we want to walk through the pandemic portal with such lessons learnt into a new world?

Notes

1 Cf. Anders Vahlne's chapter on the alleged experts' qualifications in the responsible Agency.

2 The term "hobby epidemiologist" was coined early in the debates to belittle and exclude critical voices against the strategy, as if the only reliable analysis could come from the FHM. Distinguished economist Lars Calmfors rebuffs the "you-aren't-an-epidemiologist-so-shut-up school" by making us aware that the pandemic covers a wide range of social spheres and demands broad interdisciplinary discussions. Calmfors, Lars. *Mellan forskning och politik: 50 år av samhällsdebatt*, Stockholm: Ekerlids Förlag, 2021: 330–334.

3 www.ndr.de/nachrichten/info/podcast4684.html .

4 The virologist was awarded the German Research Council's (DFG) "2020 Communicator Award" for outstanding communication amid the coronavirus pandemic. In March 2020 the podcast was accessed by more than 15 million people and by May the number had risen to more than 40 million, www.dfg.de/en/service/press/press_releases/2020/press_release_no_11/index.html , www.ndr.de/nachrichten/info/Podcast-mit-Drosten-und-Ciesek-Links-zu-Corona-Studien,corona2636.html .

5 https://lakartidningen.se/aktuellt/nyheter/2020/03/johan-carlson-kritiken-mot-tegnell-ar-narmast-ovardig/ , www.svd.se/kritiken-mot-tegnell-ovardigt . Carlson, in addition, declared it "indecent, when public persons simply spit out a lot of stupidities". He seems to demand blind trust in his Agency.

6 Gustavsson, Gina. *Du stolta, Du fria: Om svenskarna, Sverigebilden och folkhälsopatriotismen*, Stockholm: Kaunitz-Olsson, 2021.

7 Editors of the book celebrating my 65th birthday discussed in their introduction why I had to throw all my energy into virus politics and how this offered a natural expansion of my former research projects. Heimbrock, Hans Günter, Jörg Persch, and Filip Ivanovic (eds.). *Eco-Theology: Essays in Honor of Sigurd Bergmann*, Paderborn: Ferdinand Schöningh/Brill, 2021: XI–XII.

8 www.dn.se/debatt/folkhalsomyndigheten-har-misslyckats-nu-maste-politikerna-gripa-in/ ["The FHM has failed: Politicians must take action now"]. The 22 scholars' article (by virologists, medical scholars and doctors) opened the critical debate about Sweden's strategy. It was responded to by attacks of nest befouling, and those in power refused to respond in an objective way. A month later, the group founded the Science Forum Covid-19, one of the strongest scientific, though fully ignored, voices for an alternative pandemic management strategy in the country, https://vetcov19.se/en/ . On the Forum cf. the introductory chapter. Cf. our article on the anniversary of its publication, www.dn.se/debatt/vi-var-22-oroade-forskare-som-ville-na-de-politiskt-ansvariga/ .

9 The term was applied to the Agency by distinguished economist Lars Calmfors and the Royal Swedish Academy of Sciences' general secretary Göran K. Hansson, www.dn.se/debatt/lat-inte-prestige-hindra-en-omprovning-av-coronastrategin/ .

10 Cf. Bergmann, Sigurd. "Navigating Ethics in a Pandemic – Contempt for the Weak Versus Love of Neighbor in a Swedish Lens", *Dialog: A journal of Theology* 60:4 (2021), https://onlinelibrary.wiley.com/doi/full/10.1111/dial.12697 . On the cultural dynamics of "necrosecurity" see Lincoln who explores "the cultural idea that mass death among less grievable subjects plays an essential role in maintaining social welfare and public order". While the anthropologist's reflections characterise central right-wing dynamics in the USA the same processes seem to have been at work also in Sweden, though in a consensus society impacted by Social Democrats' ideology. Lincoln, Martha. "Necrosecurity, Immunosupremacy, and Survivorship in the Political Imagination of COVID-19", *Open Anthropological Research* 1 (2021): 46–59, www.degruyter.com/document/doi/10.1515/opan-2020-0104/pdf .

11 Commission chair Mats Melin emphasised the "shipwreck" of testing in the pandemic emergency, www.svt.se/nyheter/inrikes/mats-melin-stallt-utom-allt-tvivel-att-regionerna-var-ansvariga-for-testning .

12 www.svt.se/nyheter/inrikes/kungen-jag-anser-att-vi-har-misslyckats .

13 Historically it was not at all Oxenstierna's intention to separate the Government's and the agencies' power. The often used references to him as an argument for defending the FHM's executing of nearly autocratic power have to do with PM Löfven's inability to understand and respond to the pandemic emergency rather than to continue a historical tradition. Moreover, PM Andersson has continued since November 2021 along the same line of political abdication, even if she and Minister Hallengren pretend to be more energetic (by enacting lax and rather inefficient measures; cf. the timeline in Chapter 2).

14 www.zdf.de/gesellschaft/markus-lanz/presse-schweden-ungeschminkt-100.html .

15 *Pandemonium* means the gathering of *all demons* in one place. In John Milton's *Paradise Lost* (1667) it is the name for the Capital of Hell. The term of *Global Politosomatics* was

coined by Mika Aaltola in his investigation – in the context of the Corona pandemic – of how individuals' anxieties and fears of bodily harm interlink with the global hierarchy of spreading risk. It refers to the social political bodies interacting with individual bodies. Aaltola, Mika (ed.). *Understanding the Politics of Pandemic Scares: An Introduction to Global Politosomatics*, London: Routledge Studies in Governance and Public Policy: Routledge, 2012; Cf. Aaltola, Mika (ed.). *Understanding the Politics of Pandemic Emergencies in the Time of COVID-19: An Introduction to Global Politosomatics*, the Politics of Pandemics Vol. 1, London: Routledge, 2022.

16 That is, a high level of trust similar to other Nordic countries but different from societies with low levels of trust in Eastern Europe.

17 Leading politicians in the Government often assured people of their trust in science but in fact relied solely on the Agency, and neglected scholars at relevant academic institutions and highly creditable critics in the public debates. Anders Vahlne's chapter explains in detail why the alleged "experts", in both the FHM and the media, did not in fact represent reliable science.

18 www.kantarsifo.se/sites/default/files/reports/documents/kantar_public_sifo_allmanhetens_tillit_tankar_och_beteende_under_coronapandemin_17_december_2021.pdf .

19 Cf. note 182.

20 www.washingtonpost.com/politics/2020/05/03/risk-swedens-coronavirus-strategy-blind-patriotism/ , Gustavsson. *Du stolta, Du fria*, 132–139.

21 www.dn.se/ledare/gina-gustavsson-pandemin-hanterades-fel-men-i-stallet-for-att-ta-ansvar-marker-makthavarna-ord/ .

22 The semantic field of *trygg* is wide and includes security, safety and comfort. A newborn child can feel *trygg* carried in its mother's arms. The central Swedish value of feeling *trygg* can depend on many factors, such as belonging and making-oneself-at-home, but also on the absence of violence and threats. The discourse on *trygghet* has become central in recent public debates. Why do some feel *trygg* with regard to what others experience as *trygg*? What characterises a *trygg* place? Cf. Rönnblom, Malin, Ida Linander, and Linda Sandberg. *(O)tryggt? Texter om makt, plats och motstånd*, Stockholm: Premiss, 2021.

23 Cf. Hagevi, Magnus. "Beyond Church and State: Private Religiosity and Post-Materialist Political Opinion Among Individuals in Sweden", *Journal of Church and State* 54:4 (2012): 499–525, https://academic.oup.com/jcs/article/54/4/499/819277?login=true .

24 Cf. Moodie, John. "Sweden's Response to Covid-19 and the Limits of Individualism", www.coronatimes.net/sweden-response-covid-19-limits-individualism/ .

25 Cf. Gustavsson. *Du stolta, Du fria*, chapter four, especially 187–196. On state individualism cf. Jens Stilhoff Sörensen's chapter.

26 In a touching radio report from 1958 we can listen to an old man who has suffered seriously for years but does not want to bother the doctor unnecessarily. This might have to do with men's problems in taking care of their bodies, but after nine years of working as a pastor in Central Malmö I could tell all too many stories about loneliness and not-bothering-others that made me deeply sad.

27 www.battrestadsdel.se/asikter/kronika-besvara-inte-folkhalsomyndigheten-med-fragor-om-pandemin/ .

28 www.tidningenhalsa.se/artiklar/artiklar/20190521/bli-din-egen-lyckas-smed/ .

29 Cf. Lapo Lappin's chapter, which explores more deeply the relation of dignity and utilitarianism in Sweden's pandemic biopolitics.

30 Knausgård, Karl Ove. *Min kamp 2*, Oslo: Forlaget Oktober, 2010: 24–60. Available also as an excerpt from *My Struggle, Book Two: A Man in Love*, www.newyorker.com/books/page-turner/the-birthday-party .

31 Gustavsson. *Du stolta, Du fria*, 311–315.

32 Cf. Rosenberg, Göran. "The Crisis of Consensus in Postwar Sweden", https://static1.squarespace.com/static/56e59e9bcf80a14323cd2977/t/5780b0ca9f74568e00132634/1468051660431/consensus.pdf . One should note that "consensus" in this context is not anchored in the discourse ethics nowadays widely applied internationally,

following Jürgen Habermas' influential communicative social philosophy, a concept that was introduced in Sweden first in the 1990s. Applying discourse ethics acknowledges the most central voice to those concerned by the problem in the discourse about solutions.

33 Cf. Gustavsson. *Du stolta, Du fria*, 181–187.

34 www.dw.com/en/swedens-fm-linde-we-managed-to-flatten-the-curve/av-53846751 .

35 Baldwin, Peter. *Fighting the First Wave: Why the Coronavirus Was Tackled so Differently across the Globe*, Cambridge: Cambridge University Press, 2021: 66.

36 Cf., https://kvartal.se/artiklar/fortjanar-folkhalsomyndigheten-folkets-fortroende/ , https://kvartal.se/artiklar/paternalismen-genomsyrar-pandemikommunikationen/ , https://kvartal.se/artiklar/vetenskapligadimridaer/ .

37 www.nature.com/articles/d41586-020-01098-x .

38 Lindström, Martin. "The New Totalitarians: The Swedish COVID-19 Strategy and the Implications of Consensus Culture and Media Policy for Public Health", *SSM – Population Health* 14 (June 2021): 100788, www.sciencedirect.com/science/article/pii/S235282732100063X .

39 https://yle.fi/uutiset/3-11399713 , www.expressen.se/debatt/den-svenska-coronastrategin-tecken-pa-totalitar-utveckling/ [Ehrnrooth, Jari. "The Swedish Corona Strategy as a Sign of Totalitarian Development"], www.dagensarena.se/essa/viruspolitik-en-totalitar-demokratur/ [Bergmann. "Virus Politics in a Totalitarian Democrature"].

40 www.gp.se/kultur/kultur/coronakrisen-%C3%A4r-ett-sammanbrott-f%C3%B6r-den-svenska-modellen-1.28044594 . Rothstein thought-provokingly states that after this pandemic Sweden can no longer be regarded as a welfare state model and "the home of order, trygghet/safety, and humanitarianism on Earth".

41 Hans Magnus Enzensberger in the chapter "Swedish Autumn", in *Ach Europa!* Frankfurt am Main: Suhrkamp, 1987.

42 Sontag, Susan. "A Letter from Sweden", *Ramparts Magazine* (July 1969): 23–38, 24, www.unz.com/print/Ramparts-1969jul-00023 .

43 Schulz, Genia. *"Die Ästhetik des Widerstands" – Versionen des Indirekten in Peter Weiss' Roman*, Stuttgart: J.B. Metzler, 1986: 42.

44 www.svd.se/folkhalsonationalism-kan-forklara-svenska-coronalinjen . Cf., www.dn.se/kultur-noje/darfor-blev-svenskarna-folkhalsopatrioter/ , www.theguardian.com/world/commentisfree/2020/may/01/sweden-coronavirus-strategynationalists-britain .

45 Jerneck, Magnus (ed.). "Inledning: Konsten att bemästra en pandemi", *Statsvetenskaplig tidskrift* (*The Swedish Journal of Political Science*) 123:5 (2021).

46 Former state epidemiologist Johan Giesecke, Tegnell's and Carlson's mentor and the Agency's advisor, turned exceptionalism into arrogance and claimed that "The reason Sweden's strategy distinguishes itself internationally is because everyone else is wrong". Cf. Baldwin. *Fighting the First Wave*, 77. And Tegnell stated in his widely received radio summer talk that "the whole world had gone crazy", www.svt.se/nyheter/inrikes/tegnell-som-om-varlden-blev-galen . In his chapter on Tegnell, titled "Giesecke's boy", freelance journalist Johan Anderberg draws on his interviews with the FHM troika doctors, and describes how Giesecke is impressed with Tegnell's skill of being "a-political", that is, not influenced by others. Because of his quality of being *oberörd* (unaffected) and *orubblig* (imperturbable) Giesecke had chosen him, helped him to write his PhD and enthroned him at the Agency. As a former doctor, Tegnell tells Anderberg, he did not feel comfortable with patients who wanted a diagnosis "*inpackad i en massa fluff och medkänsla*" (packaged with lots of fluff and compassion) but preferred those who could accept a straight message. Anderberg, Johan. *Flocken: Berättelsen om hur Sverige valde väg under pandemin*, Stockholm: Bonniers, 2021: 35–38. Tegnell's personality has been described in a personal letter (8 February 2021, in the undersigned's archive) from an initiated high-ranking doctor, with special responsibility for social welfare, who has worked closely together with the troika doctors (who he experienced as "sloppy, nonchalant and unknowledgeable"). In his eyes, Tegnell suffers from what an older term diagnoses as "ixiodi", which implies "a lack of mental plasticity", and that leads to his

(well-known) "fixation on principles" and "inability to adjust misjudgements". This seems to fit well into what Giesecke shared with us about his protégé, and it fits well into my impression of Tegnell's public performance.

47 Andersson, Staffan, and Nicholas Aylott. "Sweden and Coronavirus: Unexceptional Exceptionalism", *Social Sciences* 9:12 (2020): 232, https://doi.org/10.3390/socsci9120232 .

48 Krastev, Ivan. *Is It Tomorrow Yet? Paradoxes of the Pandemic*, London: Allen Lane, 2020: 24.

49 Party leader Jimmie Åkesson demanded twice in June 2020 and March 2021 that Tegnell be dismissed, www.svt.se/nyheter/inrikes/jimmie-akesson-anders-tegnell-bor-avga , www.expressen.se/nyheter/akesson-tegnell-har-inte–forbattrats-det-har-aret-/ .

50 On the *opinion corridor* and its criticism see www.thelocal.se/20191230/swedish-word-of-the-day-asiktskorridor/ , www.svd.se/darfor-ar-iden-om-asiktskorridoren-sa-radikal .

51 www.spiegel.de/politik/ausland/corona-in-schwedens-pflegeheimen-der-eingeladene-tod-a-00000000-0002-0001–0000–000173444539 .

52 www.dn.se/insidan/svenskar-ser-ner-pa-aldre/ .

53 www.barnombudsmannen.se/globalassets/dokument-for-nedladdning/publikationer/publikationer2/barnombudsmannens-rapport–covid-19-pandemins-konsekvenser-for-barn-slutredovisning-av-regeringsuppdrag.pdf .

54 www.fub.se/nyheter/prioritera-vaccin-till-vuxna-med-downs-syndrom/ .

55 www.altinget.se/artikel/varfor-vagrar-folkhalsomyndigheten-ge-boosterspruta-till-uppenbara-riskgrupper , www.arbetarbladet.se/2021-11-14/om-smittan-okar-varfor-vantar-anders-tegnell , www.arbetarbladet.se/2021-10-31/glomde-ni-pa-riktigt-de-funktionsnedsatta-igen .

56 www.dagensmedia.se/medier/digitalt/fhm-forsvarar-sig-har-ar-mejlvaxlingen-mellan-presschefen-och-jan-scherman/ . For a differentiated analysis of the public discourse in the professional media, the authorities, sciences, critics and the social media's strong voices and groups see Kajsa Klein's enlightening chapter.

57 www.dn.se/ledare/gina-gustavsson-det-ar-inte-bara-trollen-som-harjar-i-den-svenska-coronadebatten/ .

58 https://sverigesradio.se/artikel/dold-facebookgrupp-forsoker-paverka-svenska-intressen-utomlands , www.dn.se/ledare/gina-gustavsson-allt-som-stor-sverigebilden-ar-inte-informationspaverkan/ .

59 www.dagensmedia.se/medier/digitalt/fhm-forsvarar-sig-har-ar-mejlvaxlingen-mellan-presschefen-och-jan-scherman/ , www.dagensmedia.se/medier/dagspress/fhm-chefens-hyllning-det-ar-tack-vare-medierna-som-vi-natt-vara-mal/ . FHM Press office leader Christer Jansson confirms that his Agency has to actively deal with "suspicious political influence [*informationspåverkan*]", a central term used in psychological warfare, a discipline that Jansson is educated in as officer in the Swedish Defence. Scholars at the Swedish Defence University, however, investigated how Russia treated the story about the coronavirus as a battlefield in Sweden by sharing damaging narratives against Swedish interests in the pandemic, www.fhs.se/forskning/forskningsprojekt/informationspaverkan–sarbarheter-och-effekter.html .

60 Scholar of strategic communication James Pamment stated on the radio program that the Facebook group which he had hacked, where scientists and citizens critically discussed Sweden's strategy, represented what military defence denotes as dangerous impact. He withdrew his postulate later on Twitter and disappeared from the debates for a long while. Nevertheless he later published an essay on "The Role of Nonstate Actors in Counter-branding the Swedish Covid-19 Response" the Swedish response in a dubious online journal, www.koreascience.or.kr/article/JAKO202121061509446.page , where he describes the Facebook group as a "quite typical mixture of legitimate and illegitimate communication techniques used by activist groups" and attacks the critics' communication with others and the media. One might wonder how Sweden can rightly complain about the oppression of the media and free opinion in illiberal and autocratic countries while at the same time applying similar methods in its own country by threatening and

denouncing critical voices about the country's pandemic management. The question will not fade away with the pandemic because strong forces, where National Television and Radio are also involved, have recently gotten the Government to establish a new Agency for Psychological Defence. Who will investigate and "counter-brand" what such an Agency will practise further on?

61 https://kvartal.se/artiklar/nar-fri-asiktsbildning-blev-ett-hot/ .

62 https://eu.usatoday.com/story/opinion/2020/07/21/coronavirus-swedish-herd-immunity-drove-up-death-toll-column/5472100002/ .

63 Gustavsson. *Du stolta, Du fria*, 97–159.

64 Brecht, Bertolt. *Das Leben des Galilei (1939–55)*, vol. 14, Frankfurt am Main: Suhrkamp, 1998.

65 https://tt.omni.se/forskare-i-upprop-till-regeringen/a/RRdG2d .

66 See note 8.

67 https://vetcov19.se/en/ , www.youtube.com/channel/UCarSBJ6PFC8_6oFJ9pwvqvQ .

68 Bringselius, Louise. "Coronapandemin, förvaltningen och tilliten: En forskningsagenda", in Jerneck. *Statsvetenskaplig tidskrift*, 179–188, 186; Nylén, Lars. "Påbud och efterlevnad: En fråga om effektiv kriskommunikation", in Jerneck. *Statsvetenskaplig tidskrift*, 223–240, 234; Calmfors. *Mellan forskning och politik*, 331–336.

69 *What Can We Learn from the Pandemic? Research Syntheses and Recommendations for the Future – the Royal Swedish Academy of Sciences' Expert Group on COVID-19*, Stockholm, 2021, https://s3.eu-de.cloud-object-storage.appdomain.cloud/kva-image-pdf/2021/11/covidrapport_slutrapport_sammanfattning_211130_eng.pdf .

70 www.gov.uk/government/organisations/scientific-advisory-group-for-emergencies/about , https://de.wikipedia.org/wiki/Corona-Expertenrat_der_Bundesregierung , www.ethikrat.org/en/?cookieLevel=not-set&cHash=4cedc8fcdda0b368d4409bb0febbe036 .

71 www.dn.se/debatt/dubbelmoral-fran-politiker-om-behovet-av-munskydd/ .

72 www.dn.se/sverige/tegnell-svart-att-andra-attityden-till-munskydd/ .

73 Krastev. *Is It Tomorrow Yet?* 8.

74 Diefenbacher, Hans, Johannes J. Frühbauer, Benjamin Held, Frederike van Oorschot, Dorothee Rodenhäuser, and Hannes Vetter. "Die Idee der Solidarität in der Corona-Pandemie", in Held, Benjamin, Thomas Kirchhoff, Frederike van Oorschot, Philipp Stoellger, and Ines-Jacqueline Werkner (eds.). *Corona als Riss: Perspektiven für Kirche, Politik und Ökonomie*, Universitätsbibliothek Heidelberg, 2020: 149–184, https://books.ub.uni-heidelberg.de/heibooks , 165.

75 Krastev. *Is It Tomorrow Yet?* 18.

76 https://ecfr.eu/article/commentarysweden_goes_it_alone_the_eus_coronavirus_exception/ .

77 See note 46.

78 https://onlinelibrary.wiley.com/doi/full/10.1111/apm.13112 .

79 www.regeringen.se/artiklar/2021/11/nationell-samverkan-for-en-ledande-life-science-nation/ .

80 In April 2020 the Institute reported many critical articles on Sweden's corona strategy but claimed that a majority of these were merely curious. The Institute noted that foreign media are discussing whether one could rely on the Swedes' high degree of trust and on the country's crisis management, https://si.se/corona-strategin-bekraftar-sverigebilden/ .

81 Elisabeth Backteman mentions nothing in the Government's extensive internal crisis planning document in summer and autumn 2020 about citizens' life, health and the struggling health workers, but points at national threats from the risk of social unrest (p. 62) and a damaged image of Sweden abroad (p. 48). Regeringskansliet, Justitiedepartementet, *Hösten 2020 Planeringsunderlag*, 2020–09–01.

82 This is an odd piece of information that appears in the documents handed over to the Corona Commission, www.svd.se/regeringen-hade-okanda-moten-med-fhm-kritiker .

83 "Hacerse el sueco" means *to play Swedish*. It is not meant to be any kind of insult to the Swedish people. The saying might have derived from the Latin word "soccus", "log". It

means not understanding or not hearing something – just like how we "play dumb" so we do not have to be responsible for or aware of something. *Soccus* turned to *suecos* and the expression became popular when Swedish sailors docked in Spanish ports. To avoid certain inconvenient obligations and affairs, they *kept their distance* by using the *lack of Spanish language skills* as an excuse to basically get out of doing something, www.citylifebarcelona.com/odd-spanish-expressions-hacerse-el-sueco/ . Playing Swedish then means burying one's head in the sand and getting out of doing something without taking responsibility.

84 Picht, Georg. *Der Begriff der Natur und seine Geschichte*, Stuttgart: Klett Cotta, 1989: 9. Cf. also Koselleck, Reinhard. *Vergangene Zukunft: Zur Semantik geschichtlicher Zeiten*, Frankfurt am Main: Suhrkamp, 1988: 61, on how the intrinsic power of history grows in analogy to its doability in modernity.

85 www.di.se/debatt/patriotism-forklarar-stodet-for-svenska-coronastrategin/ .

86 For the analytic differentiation of shame, guilt, humiliation and embarrassment see Dan Zahavi in his enlightening lecture at the rich "Respect and Shame in Healthcare and Bioethics Workshop" at the Wellcome Centre, 22 December 2021, www.youtube.com/watch?v=cu-YzabbS5o .

87 Gustavsson. *Du stolta, Du fria*, 122.

88 www.dn.se/nyheter/sverige/vem-ar-tysken-som-staller-tegnell-mot-vaggen/ .

89 "Bullerby" is the name of a Swedish village and the title of Astrid Lindgren's famous children's book series. Germans talk about *Bullerby-syndrome*, that is, the stereotypical idealisation of paradisiac Sweden in German-speaking countries, www.daserste.de/information/politik-weltgeschehen/weltspiegel/reportage/sendung/schweden-corona-und-der-traum-von-bullerbue-104.html . Cf. also Stichler's (depressing but striking) essay on "Sweden's *Sonderweg* into self-isolation", where Swedes have simply become used to corona, stay relaxed and move to their summer cottage, www.zeit.de/politik/ausland/2020-07/covid-19-schweden-quarantaene-konjunktur-corona-krise/komplettansicht .

90 www.svd.se/einhorn-journalister-ska-inte-agna-sig-at-pr .

91 On the hinderances and difficulties for people in achieving and judging, and also applying, correct information from reliable sources see Kajsa Klein's chapter.

92 www.folkhalsomyndigheten.se/nyheter-och-press/nyhetsarkiv/2020/mars/personer-over-70-bor-begransa-sociala-kontakter-tills-vidare/ .

93 www.mittskifte.org/petitions/aldreupproret .

94 Hydén, Håkan. "Corona – en rättspolitisk utmaning!" *Statsvetenskaplig tidskrift* (*The Swedish Journal of Political Science*) 123:5 (2021): 315–342, 333–335.

95 www.dn.se/nyheter/sverige/lofven-coronakrisen-har-skapat-stora-revor-i-valfarden/ , www.svd.se/stefan-lofven-sitter-over-valet-om-partiet-vill-ha-mig .

96 www.ft.dk/-/media/sites/ft/pdf/publikationer/haandtering-af-covid19-foraar-2020.ashx , pp. 397, 414.

97 www.regeringen.se/tal/2020/11/statsminister-stefan-lofvens-tal-till-nationen-den-22-november-2020/ .

98 Wallin, Annika. "Okunskap och riskkommunikation: Att knuffa eller ge en karta", *Statsvetenskaplig tidskrift* (*The Swedish Journal of Political Science*) 123:5 (2021): 213–222. On the deficits of Sweden's official crisis communication cf. also Nylén. "Påbud och efterlevnad", 223–240.

99 Jerneck. *Statsvetenskaplig tidskrift*, 17.

100 The term *vårdskuld* refers to the number of postponed treatments and surgeries. While national statistics show the actual number of Covid-deaths, it is more difficult to calculate the number of Covid-related deaths due to the accumulated *vårdskuld*, which it is estimated will take circa four years to work off in Sweden.

101 www.dn.se/sverige/hallengren-sverige-har-kommit-val-ut-ur-detta/ .

102 https://kvartal.se/artiklar/vansternsprinciper/ .

103 Cf. Jens Stilhoff Sörensen's chapter.

104 Baldwin. *Fighting the First Wave*, 80.
105 www.dagensmedicin.se/specialistomraden/infektion/johan-carlson-om-kritiken-for-tidigt-att-saga/ .
106 www.dn.se/ledare/gunnar-jonsson-lofven-och-tegnell-borde-inte-blunda-for-testha veriet/ .
107 www.youtube.com/watch?v=dASRSkXh3ds&t=5s .
108 According to Anderberg. *Flocken*, 38, Tegnell had been chosen by Giesecke for the position as chief epidemiologist because of his capacity for being *orörd* (untouched) and *orubblig* (imperturbable).
109 For a discussion of Tegnell's confusing rhetoric see Lena Einhorn, www.dn.se/kultur-noje/lena-einhorn-sa-surrade-sverige-fast-sig-vid-masten-i-hanteringen-av-pandemin/ , and an analysis of the Government's and Agency's fatal *folie à deux*, www.dn.se/kultur/lena-einhorn-sa-forvandlades-strategin-mot-pandemin-till-en-massans-dardans/ .
110 Cf. Huizing, Klaas. "Shame on you! Scham als Grundbegriff einer protestantischen Ethik", *Zeitschrift Für Evangelische Ethik* 57:2 (2013): 89–101.
111 www.kirche-im-hr.de/sendungen/21-ueber-scham-verletzlichkeit-und-staerke/ .
112 https://fs.blog/brene-brown-guilt-shame/ .
113 Cf. Welten, Stephanie, Marcel Zeelenberg, and Seger Breugelmans. "Vicarious Shame", *Cognition & Emotion* 26 (2012): 836–846.
114 Bergmann, Sigurd. "Memoria Passionis Subversiva: The Moral Power of Remembrance in the Pandemic – in a Swedish Lens", in Erbele-Küster, Dorothea, and Volker Küster (eds.). *Between Pandemonium and Pandemethics: Responses to Covid-19 in Theology and Religions*, Leipzig: EVA, 2022.
115 23 February 2021, www.independent.co.uk/news/world/americas/us-politics/biden-memorialcoronavirus-b1805906.html .
116 Klein, Georg. *Skapelsens fullkomlighet och livets tragik: Essäer*, Stockholm: Bonniers, 2005.
117 www.dn.se/nyheter/varlden/katrine-marcal-britterna-lever-i-ett-undantagstillstand/ .
118 Lindroth, Bengt. *Vi som inte var med i kriget: Om Sverige, Norden, Europa & coronan*, Stockholm: Carlssons, 2021: 256–257.
119 www.dn.se/sverige/kungen-om-pandemin-vi-har-misslyckats/ .
120 https://coronakommissionen.com/ . For a summary see https://coronakommissionen.com/wp-content/uploads/2021/10/summary-sweden-in-the-pandemic.pdf .
121 https://coronakommissionen.com/publikationer/slutbetankande-sou-2022-10/ .
122 https://tt.omni.se/fhm-s-generaldirektor-ratt-vara-forsiktiga/a/V92Kzp .
123 https://sverigesradio.se/artikel/tegmark-wisell-forsvarar-coronastrategin-avgorande-att-vi-tittat-pa-helheten .
124 Cf. Jens Stilhoff Sörensen's chapter.
125 www.gp.se/nyheter/sverige/anders-tegnell-l%C3%A4mnar-folkh%C3%A4lsomyndig heten-1.67484714 .
126 https://tt.omni.se/hallengren-om-kritiken-det-var-ratt-vagval/a/Or2w11 .
127 https://time.com/5899432/sweden-coronovirus-disaster/ .
128 Cf. Emil J. Bergholtz's chapter.
129 https://medium.com/@barbara_c/how-the-mitigation-strategy-tempted-northern-europe-and-convinced-only-sweden-f6fb9197d49a .
130 Brusselaers, Nele, David Steadson, Kelly Bjorklund, Sofia Breland, Jens Stilhoff Sörensen, Andrew Ewing, Sigurd Bergmann, and Gunnar Steineck. "Evaluation of Science Advice During the COVID-19 Pandemic in Sweden", *Humanities and Social Sciences Communications* 9, Article number: 91 (2022), www.nature.com/articles/s41 599-022-01097-5 .
131 *Ibid*.
132 Schöps, Corinna. "Du darfst Dich schämen", *DIE ZEIT, Doctor*, 2 Mai 2020, 6–13. Cf. on the method of MFC (Mindful Self Compassion), www.aerzteblatt.de/archiv/174949/Achtsames-Selbstmitgefuehl-Moege-ich-freundlich-zu-mir-sein .

133 www.altinget.se/artikel/debatt-att-lara-av-misslyckanden-kraver-att-man-erkanner-dem .
134 www.dagensarena.se/essa/om-doendets-konst/ .
135 "Wir werden in ein paar Monaten wahrscheinlich viel einander verzeihen müssen." The message was in my view exemplary but the minister had to admit all too many failures later on, with the result that it lost its salty impact, www.tagesspiegel.de/politik/wir-werden-einander-verzeihen-muessen-warum-jens-spahn-mit-diesen-ungewoehnlichen-worten-richtig-liegt/25772260.html .
136 Bringselius, Louise. "Coronapandemin, förvaltningen och tilliten: En forskningsagenda", *Statsvetenskaplig tidskrift* (*The Swedish Journal of Political Science*) 123:5 (2021): 179–188, 180.
137 Deverell, Edward. "Att lära av pandemin: Interkrislärande, intrakrislärande och reformer i krisens efterspel", *Statsvetenskaplig tidskrift* (*The Swedish Journal of Political Science*) 123:5 (2021): 361–378, 361.
138 PM Stefan Löfven, FHM GD Johan Carlson, Leader of the Governmental Crisis Group Elisabeth Backteman, and PM secretary Nils Vikmång. Cf., www.dn.se/sverige/forra-krishanteraren-har-lamnat-regeringskansliet/ , www.gp.se/nyheter/sverige/anders-tegnell-l%C3%A4mnar-folkh%C3%A4lsomyndigheten-1.67484714 .
139 Sweden abandoned civil servants' responsibility (*tjänstemannaansvar*) in 1975. In 2018 the Parliament decided to re-establish it but the Government delayed this. A new proposal was rejected in the Parliament in 2020, www.riksdagen.se/sv/dokument-lagar/dokument/motion/_H8023152 .
140 www.riksdagen.se/sv/dokument-lagar/dokument/svensk-forfattningssamling/forordning-20131020-med-instruktion-for_sfs-2013-1020 .
141 www.altinget.se/artikel/experter-sveriges-smittskyddslag-har-inte-efterfoljts .
142 www.gp.se/debatt/obegripligt-att-munskyddskrav-inte-inf%C3%B6rs-mot-omikron-1.63685437 .
143 https://lakartidningen.se/aktuellt/nyheter/2021/01/aven-skane-infor-munskydd-for-alla-i-vardlokaler/ . Carl Johan Sonesson, political chair of Region Skåne, decided (contrary to FHM decisions) to use facemasks in health care work as early as 26 October 2020 (Facebook *Moderaterna i Skåne* 26 October 2020). Regarding the use of facemasks on public transport, Sonesson tried to initiate this but encountered resistance from contagious disease doctor Eva Melander questioning its evidence (Twitter, Eva Melander 5 November 2020). For a detailed description of his commitment and controversies see *Sonesson, Carl Johan. Skånes kamp mot coronan: En personlig berättelse*, Lund: Samizdat, 2021.
144 www.svt.se/nyheter/lokalt/halland/halmstad-forbjuder-munskydd-i-skolans-lokaler .
145 www.dn.se/debatt/aterinfor-smittskyddsinstitutet-som-fristaende-myndighet/ , https://ka.se/2020/04/27/arbetsgivarna-lag-bakom-att-tona-ner-krav-pa-munskydd/ .
146 Cf. Bringselius. "Coronapandemin, förvaltningen och tilliten", 182.
147 www.ivo.se/publicerat-material/nyheter/2020/ingen-region-har-tagit-fullt-ansvar-for-individuell-vard/ .
148 https://ledarsidorna.se/plus/foljer-folkhalsomyndighetens-ledning-lakarnas-etiska-regelverk/ .
149 www.dagensarena.se/innehall/professorn-att-prioritera-bort-aldre-strider-mot-lagen/ .
150 www.sydsvenskan.se/2021-11-17/efter-skandalen-i-skane-ivo-ska-granska-fler-aldreboenden .
151 The quality-adjusted life year or quality-adjusted life-year (QALY) is a generic measure of disease burden, including both the quality and the quantity of life lived.
152 Stückelberger, Christoph. *Globalance: Ethics Handbook for a Balanced World Post-Covid* (Globethics.net, 2020), www.globethics.net/globalance , 39.
153 Lindström, Martin. "Covid-19-pandemin och den svenska strategin: Epidemiologi, postmodernism och svensk exceptionalism", *Statsvetenskaplig tidskrift* (*The Swedish Journal of Political Science*) 123:5 (2021): 93–124.

154 Former state epidemiologist Annika Linde in her interview, www.washingtonpost.com/world/2020/11/18/sweden-coronavirus-surge-policy/ .
155 www.svd.se/undermaligt-senfardigt-haveri–har-ar-kritiken .
156 www.project-syndicate.org/onpoint/science-in-the-post-truth-age-by-trish-greenhalgh-2021–01 .
157 www.ifo.de/publikationen/2020/article-journal/das-gemeinsame-interesse-von-gesundheit-und-wirtschaft , www.hhs.se/en/research/sweden-through-the-crisis/saving-lives-or-saving-the-economy/ , www.washingtonpost.com/outlook/2020/10/20/sweden-economy-pandemic-strategy/#comments-wrapper .
158 www.echr.coe.int/documents/convention_eng.pdf .
159 www.su.se/nyheter/forskaren-som-vill-bidra-till-b%C3%A4ttre-politik-1.581815; cf. Calmfors. *Mellan forskning och politik*, 331–336.
160 www.zeit.de/2021/45/anthony-fauci-immonologe-usa-corona-pandemie-zukunft-donald-trump/komplettansicht .
161 www.dn.se/insandare/byt-ut-ledningen-for-folkhalsomyndigheten/ .
162 Calmfors. *Mellan forskning och politik*, 328.
163 www.n-tv.de/panorama/Drosten-lehnt-Durchinfektion-bei-Juengeren-ab-article21665735.html .
164 www.altinget.se/artikel/fhm-onskade-och-fick-avgorande-inflytande-over-regeringens-beslut .
165 https://kvartal.se/artiklar/regeringen-har-abdikerat/ .
166 www.svd.se/stefan-lofven-sitter-over-valet-om-partiet-vill-ha-mig .
167 https://tt.omni.se/varden-inte-redo-for-en-ny-pandemi/a/28okvG .
168 www.oecd.org/coronavirus/policy-responses/first-lessons-from-government-evaluations-of-covid-19-responses-a-synthesis-483507d6/#back-endnotea0z3 .
169 https://coronakommissionen.com/wp-content/uploads/2022/02/summary_20220225.pdf .
170 www.svd.se/fhms-tidiga-strategi-var-flockimmunitet , https://emanuelkarlsten.se/tegnell-mejlen-sa-fick-flockimmuniteten-faste-hos-folkhalsomyndigheten/ .
171 Tännsjö, Torbjörn. "Är den svenska strategin utlitaristisk?" [Is the Swedish strategy utilitarian?], in Gafvelin, Åke, and Lapo Lappin (eds.). *Filosofi och pandemi*, Skellefteå: Norma, 2021: 32.
172 *Ibid.*, 33.
173 www.abc.net.au/religion/the-ethics-of-swedens-herd-immunity-strategy/12764868 .
174 Cf. Lapo Lappin's chapter and Bergmann. "Navigating Ethics in a Pandemic".
175 https://papers.ssrn.com/sol3/papers.cfm?abstract_id=3603976 .
176 *Analects*, here quoted from Chinese Literature comprising *The Analects of Confucius, the Sayings of Mencius, the Shi King, the Travels of Fa-Hien and the Sorrows of Han*, Hamburg: Tradition Classics, no year.
177 www.tandfonline.com/doi/full/10.1080/01402382.2021.1909964 , https://sverigesradio.se/artikel/higher-vaccination-rate-in-denmark-where-people-trust-authorities-more .
178 www.dn.se/debatt/bristerna-i-aldreomsorgen-kan-sanka-valfardspolitiken/ .
179 "Vad har vi våra myndigheter till om vi ska protestera mot beslut hela tiden", www.dn.se/insandare/ge-alla-over-60-ar-en-tredje-dos-vaccin/ .
180 Edelman Trust Barometer Special Report Spring 2020, 5 May 2020. CSt 46.
181 While in April 2020 one could see support of 73% for the FHM and 63% for the Government's pandemic management, https://novus.se/coronastatus-0420-2/ , one finds in February 2021 57% support for the Agency and 38% for the Government (according to MSB, www.msb.se/siteassets/dokument/aktuellt/pagaende-handelser-och-insats/coronaviruset , Figure 1, p. 4). In January 2022 the confidence in Tegnell and the FHM again decreased to circa 50%, and surprisingly trust in health care has also dropped from 64 to 49%. Cf., www.gu.se/sites/default/files/2020-10/6.%20Stort%20f%C3%B6rtroende%20f%C3%B6r%20Folkh%C3%A4lsomyndigheten%20och%20

1177%20under%20coronapandemin%20final.pdf, https://novus.se/nyheter/2021/01/fortroendet-kring-corona-for-myndigheter-och-regeringen-rasar/ , www.dn.se/sverige/dn-ipsos-sjunkande-fortroende-for-sjukvarden/ . In general, by following the regular studies from the Swedish Trust Barometer, one can observe a negative trend with decreasing *trygghet* and worsened neighbourhood trust in the local society, www.aftonkuriren.se/?p=134345 . Corona's impacts on these trends still need to be analysed.

182 Edelman Trust Barometer, Special Report Spring 2020, 5 May 2020, CSt 166.

183 Peter Baldwin suggests that compliance works as a better term than trust, but due to the wide range of scientific reflections on trust I prefer the term and will use terms like compliance and obedience as terms of practical outworkings of trust. Baldwin. *Fighting the First Wave*, 281.

184 www.politico.eu/article/covid-vaccination-eastern-europe-trust-fourth-wave-vaccine/ .

185 Elderly children, immigrants, and less educated groups with lower incomes have been exposed to higher risks. Corona revealed the existing class society, www.dagensarena.se/essa/sa-synliggjorde-coronan-klassamhallet/ .

186 www.dn.se/ledare/elsa-kugelberg-den-svenska-coronastrategin-ar-till-for-medelklassen/ .

187 Diefenbacher et al. "Die Idee der Solidarität in der Corona-Pandemie", 179f.

188 www.altinget.se/artikel/varfor-vagrar-folkhalsomyndigheten-ge-boosterspruta-till-uppenbara-riskgrupper .

189 Diefenbacher et al. "Die Idee der Solidarität in der Corona-Pandemie", 179: "Zu fragen bleibt, inwiefern dieser Überschuss als Grundlage für einen verstärkten Zusammenhalt der Weltgesellschaft dienen kann und ob der im Vergleich zu anderen Konzepten »weiche« Begriff der Solidarität nicht gerade in diesen Zusammenhängen seine Stärke zeigt".

190 https://iai.tv/articles/asa-wikforss-why-do-we-resist-knowledge-auid-1245 .

191 https://zerocovidalliance.org/; cf. our call for Sweden to join the pan-European zero-Covid movement, www.altinget.se/artikel/11-forskare-sverige-bor-ansluta-sig-till-ett-paneuropeiskt-nollcovid-upprop .

192 www.bruegel.org/2021/02/aiming-for-zero-covid-19-europe-needs-to-take-action/ , www.thelancet.com/journals/lancet/article/PIIS0140-6736(21)00186-0/fulltext .

193 In medicine doctors and health workers sign up to the basic "duty of candour", owed to all patients, whereby one admits mistakes made, apologises, and does one's best to make amends. Cf. www.theguardian.com/society/2021/dec/20/omicron-is-terrifying-so-why-wont-we-learn-from-past-mistakes .

194 Krastev. *Is It Tomorrow Yet?* 2.

7

EPIDEMIOLOGY AND COVID-19

Why numbers are important and can be misleading

Nele Brusselaers

A personal note

When Wuhan in China was affected by this new Covid-19 virus in December 2019, many people (including professionals) were thinking that this was something "far far away". As a clinical epidemiologist and medical doctor with further education in hospital hygiene and infection control, I was following all media reports from the start. Although I had never worked with epidemics or massive outbreaks (few epidemiologists had!), infectious diseases and epidemics had always intrigued me. Even during medical education, we learned little about outbreaks and epidemics and just some basic hospital infection control measures. Yes, chronic infections and some acute infections were covered, and the importance of vaccinations for those pathogens with an epidemic-potential. Who would have thought that every medical professional, every person, would be confronted with this pandemic from 2020 and onwards?

In my early days as fulltime researcher, I conducted several projects on hospital-acquired infections, and I started working on the human microbiome around 2016 – or how bacteria and viruses influence our long-term health. Many medical professionals have considerably less professional experience and training considering epidemics or any "communicable" infectious disease, and for sure less experience with epidemiology. Yet different voices can bring in useful insights into this multifaceted issue affecting us all (e.g., healthcare organisation, treatment, diagnostics). Without doubt, this pandemic revealed itself to be complex on many different levels, from global/national/regional infection control to healthcare and society (including economy, legal aspects, and others).

As a Belgian living in Sweden for many years (including most of 2020), I closely followed the developments in both countries and elsewhere. I quickly and clearly noticed a dis-concordance in Sweden between the scientific community and the

DOI: 10.4324/9781003289364-8

communication of the Swedish authorities, as we described in detail in the report of our contribution to the *Escape* project.[1]

In this chapter I aim to give an overview of some relevant basic concepts and pitfalls of epidemiology using examples of how the Swedish Covid-19 pandemic was handled or could have been handled, while not going into depth on the more advanced infectious disease epidemiology. I do not aim to evaluate or compare the overall Swedish management of the pandemic with other countries. I do not want to give a judgement on the chosen path or underlying reasons. Yet, as a professor in epidemiology, I want to highlight some questionable decisions and communications made in a country known for its long history of infectious disease epidemiology and reputable nationwide health registers and data collection.

What is epidemiology, and why is this scientific discipline important?

Before Covid-19, the scientific discipline of epidemiology was barely known to the general public, and not even recognised as an important research discipline in many countries around the world. Yet epidemiological data have been collected and used for centuries. How can you know the burden of a disease in your country/region/hospital, if you do not know how many individuals get this disease every year, and how many people become chronically ill? How can you plan how many hospital beds and healthcare personnel you need, if you do not know how many patients need surgery, intensive care, dialyses, rehabilitation, and other treatment? How can you evaluate if a smoking cessation campaign or mass vaccination works? How do you know which individuals are at highest risk to develop a disease or have a more rapid deterioration?

These are just a handful of examples of when epidemiology has shown its use and importance. Although you need statistics to analyse the collected data, the biggest challenge is how you collect and interpret the necessary data. How do you design the studies and data collection process? How do you obtain a representative sample of the population of interest, and prevent errors in design and interpretation?

Critical thinking, looking at "*the bigger picture*" and at the methodological details at every step, is essential for the epidemiologist. Even the best statistician cannot repair a poor study design or suboptimal data collection.

Why we need timely and accurate data

Nobody, including professionals in healthcare, epidemiology, and policymaking, can entirely trust one's gut feeling or expert opinion when it comes to epidemics. How epidemics evolve depend on the causal pathogen and how individuals and society respond to the emerging threat. When the situation in Italy was getting out of hand, most European countries were slow to react (and are still slow to react with each new wave of infections). The whole handling of this global pandemic showed that there is quite a big divergence between theory and practice, and that there are clearly other factors at play besides science and history.

Even if you do not yet have data for your country, there is data from other countries and from previous epidemics and outbreaks nationally and internationally. Efforts could have been taken to be prepared (as advised by the World Health Organization early on) – but who would have guessed a tiny virus could have disrupted our lives to this extent in this advanced era of human development?

In Sweden, it was communicated (unsupported by any data) that Covid-19 would not spread in Sweden, that the numbers were decreasing (while daily numbers were still going up), that there would not be a second, third, and fourth wave.[2] One of the first "signals" that something weird was going on in Sweden was when Anders Tegnell, the State Epidemiologist at FHM, proclaimed that the number of Covid-19 infections in Sweden were going down, that Sweden had had the worst of it already in early March 2020,[3] while the reported numbers were still increasing daily. This message was in sharp contrast to what was happening in other European countries and elsewhere, all struggling to get prepared for a drastic increase in demand for healthcare. Sweden had been slow from the start to recommend strict infection control measures.[4] Yet, FHM also clearly argued against international recommendations from the World Health Organization, European Centre for Disease Control, and others.[5] The standard answer from FHM seemed to be that there was insufficient evidence, that there were not enough data.[6] Nevertheless, *absence of evidence is not evidence of absence*, and the amount of reports and studies on Covid-19 have increased rapidly from the start of the pandemic. FHM and other officials communicated regularly that the effect of any measurements and the consequences of the pandemic can only be evaluated 1–2 years later,[7] apparently disregarding all previously accumulated experience in epidemics and infection control, and the importance of infectious disease modelling.[8]

Sweden is recognised globally as one of the countries with the most comprehensive health data collection, with various high quality nationwide registries which can be linked using the personal identification number. Sweden has also been described as a "paradise for epidemiologists" because of the impressive and unique amount of available healthcare data in a format usable and extremely valuable for scientific research.[9] Therefore, it would be presumed data collection on Covid-19 should be easy to implement within the existing data collection framework. Yet there have been major issues with delays of multiple days and even weeks (reporting of daily cases and deaths), pauses in reporting, restricted testing, inconsistencies between numbers between the different official sources (FHM, National Board of Health and Welfare, Statistics Sweden), multiple changes in case definitions[10] (Figure 7.1).

Some municipalities did not declare their mortality figures in elderly care; and reporting of death rates on regional level were not transparent.[11] The delays in reporting were of concern, especially during the peaks of infection[12] – since this was constantly denied or minimalised by FHM. When you looked at the daily numbers, the actual number of cases was underreported making it seem like the

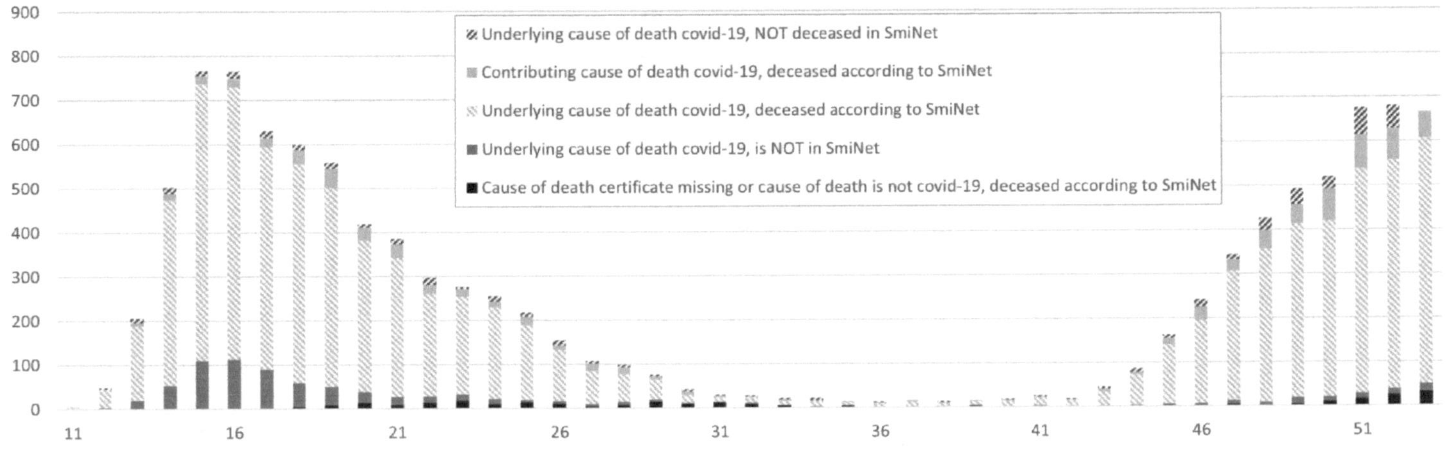

FIGURE 7.1 Covid-19 as cause of death in Sweden: discrepancies between the different official databases FHM presents the number of deaths of the infected calculated on the basis of laboratory-confirmed Covid-19 cases from individuals who died within 30 days of a positive test result. The National Board of Health and Welfare's statistics are based on the cause of death certificate. SmiNet is an electronic monitoring system for reporting in accordance with the Swedish Communicable Diseases Act.

Source: www.socialstyrelsen.se/statistik-och-data/statistik/statistik-om-covid-19/statistik-over-antal-avlidna-i-covid-19/datakallor-for-avlidna-i-covid-19/ https://twitter.com/CovidXIX/status/1485236623960952834/photo/1

Graph by the author.

number of daily deaths were going down (Figure 7.2); and barely anyone seemed to die during the weekend.[13] Consequently, the numbers of Covid-19 deaths on a given day could keep increasing for days or even weeks after the actual day. In Belgium in contrast, a nationwide Covid-19 reporting system was initiated in January 2020, weeks before community spread was reported.[14] Through this mandatory Belgian reporting system, all new hospitalisations and deaths were reported daily every morning by each hospital and elderly care facility – with no major re-adjustments later on.[15]

Data presentation and visualisation

Different Covid-19 statistics have been reported including number of cases, hospitalisations, deaths, and excess mortality. It is never good practice to cherry-pick a single number and disregard the other available data. All data collection systems have specific flaws and challenges as also described in more detail later in the chapter. Data visualisation and communication to the public have often been misleading in Sweden (and elsewhere) when reporting numbers from Sweden and other countries (cf. Edvinsson's and Höög's chapters).[16] There were also concerns about data-manipulations, in particular of Covid cases and paediatric cases and deaths in Sweden, especially in the light of the restricted testing policy in children (cf. Höög's and Bergholtz's chapters).[17] Different scaling (i.e., Y-axes) were also used by FHM or Public Media to present graphs and numbers, which always seemed to imply the situation in "the other country" was worse than Sweden. FHM, and especially Anders Tegnell, often made incorrect or misleading statements related to Covid-19 in the media (e.g., on travel patterns, or proportion of immigrants, that children are not infectious, that there is no pre-symptomatic spread of the virus, and others).[18] For these statements, sources were not communicated, results were misrepresented or misinterpreted, and findings or studies were cherry-picked.[19]

How do you design a good epidemiological study?

We were unable to identify any peer-reviewed and published scientific original papers describing studies with an epidemiological study design on Covid-19 in Sweden written by the apparent key persons behind the Swedish strategy at FHM (Tegnell, Carlson, Giesecke),[20] published in 2020–2021. There was one study on the mortality of patients with Covid-19 admitted to the intensive care unit during the first wave of the pandemic in Spring 2020 with Tegnell among the co-authors – which is mentioned later when describing selection bias.[21] Although multiple statements have been made by FHM based on apparent epidemiological data, the sources, methodology and limitations were usually difficult or even impossible to assess, and clearly insufficiently communicated to the public. The apparent Swedish data underlying many of these statements would not have survived the usual scrutiny occurring during the scientific peer-review process. In addition, Tegnell and colleagues cherry-picked findings from (properly conducted) epidemiological

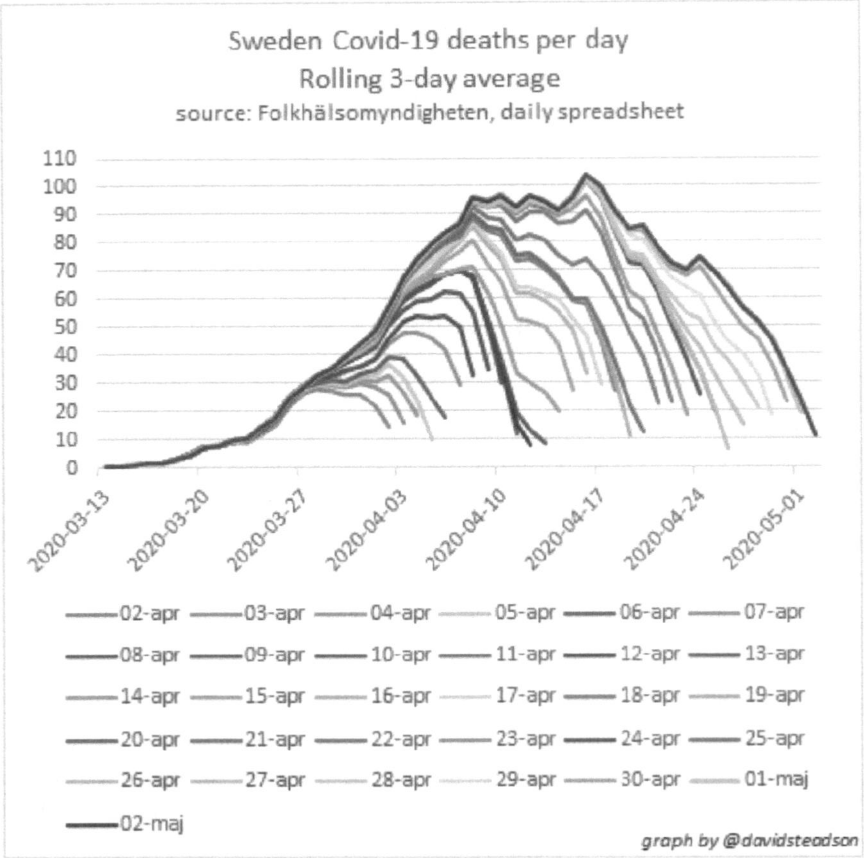

FIGURE 7.2 Number of deaths per day as reported by FHM with the different colours representing the retrospectively updated daily numbers

Source: Reproduced with permission from David Steadson @davidsteadson; *https*://twitter.com/DavidSteadson/status/1256709606950256640?s=20.

studies, mispresenting them, or not putting these findings in an appropriate and comprehensive context (cf. Vahlne's chapter). Many of the statements by FHM/ Tegnell have been debunked in debate articles by scientists (including those from *Vetenskapsforum*) in debate articles, peer-reviewed scientific papers (including letters, editorials), traditional and social media (cf. Vahlne's chapter).[22]

The design stage of an epidemiological study is the most important stage, since you determine how you will enrol study participants, collect data (which data you ideally should collect and can collect), and which problems are likely to occur. First of all, you need a good research question and a clear aim/objective since you are always limited in the amount of data you can collect. Different study designs have been used to monitor and assess the Covid-19 outbreak, which can mainly be categorised in *intervention studies* (e.g., efficiency of Covid-19 vaccines or treatments) and *observational studies* in which no active intervention is applied as part of the study. Observational studies can be grouped in descriptive studies[23] and analytical studies,[24] and if we go outside clinical research, there are also *correlation* or *ecological studies*.

Descriptive studies on Covid-19 include monitoring cases, number of hospitalisations, and deaths in which trends are monitored over time and in different places. "Descriptive" implies that these studies are only useful to describe the situation, yet not analyse the situation as in analytical studies. In other words, descriptive data are insufficient to compare the Covid-19 situation in different countries.[25] Case-reports and case-series are also descriptive, yet yield very low scientific value because of the remaining uncertainty (e.g., former US President Trump who developed Covid-19 and used a certain treatment combination).[26]

In *analytical studies*, the association between one or multiple factors (exposures) and one or multiple outcomes is evaluated (e.g., what are the risk factors for hospitalisation with Covid-19?). Analytical studies can be categorised in cohort studies, case-control studies, or cross-sectional studies, depending on when and how you collect all information, and especially which study participants will be enrolled.

In *cohort studies*, you start with a group of individuals, part with a risk factor (e.g., older age, obesity) and part without – and you assess who developed the outcome (e.g., death by Covid-19).

In *case-control studies* you select individuals based on presence or absence of the outcome, and you will look at potential predictors (e.g., deceased individuals with Covid-19 are more likely to be older than those who did not die from Covid-19).

In *cross-sectional studies*, you will collect information on potential risk factors and the outcome at the same time, making it difficult to determine which came first. For example, if you assess the weight of individuals as a risk factor for Covid-19 based on the seroprevalence (i.e., prior infection), since some people may have gained or lost weight because of the infection.

In *ecological studies*, you do not have information on the exposures or outcomes of individuals but only of groups of individuals (aggregated data). An example would be if you would compare the seroprevalence of Covid-19 in different countries, and compare it to the proportion of children wearing bicycle helmets. It could well be that a correlation exists, yet it is unlikely in this example that it would be causal. Yet, ecological studies on Covid-19 can also gain useful insights if *biologically plausible* associations are investigated.[27]

An example of a statement based on an ecological design would be FHM claiming that the mortality numbers during the first year in Norway are better because they have a lower proportion of immigrants than in Sweden.[28] According to Tegnell, Sweden was also doing better than Belgium – a very densely populated country centrally located in Europe with 375 inhabitants/km^2 compared to the 25/km^2 in Sweden, with a slightly larger population size of 11.6 million vs. 10.4 million – stating that Sweden has a similar proportion of individuals with a migration background.[29]

Problematic here is that you do not know, on an individual level, if those who die have a migrant background; and Tegnell and his team apparently did not check the proportions of individuals with a migration status in these regions – since these claims were simply incorrect.[30] What we do know is that people with a migrant status and socio-economically vulnerable groups were indeed over-represented among those who were infected and died in Sweden (based on cross-sectional individual-level data).[31] This seems an obvious consequence of the Swedish strategy and narrative as communicated by Tegnell/FHM, "It's only the others becoming sick/who die", as we described in our *Escape* project.[32]

Some basics of infectious disease epidemiology

If an (infectious) disease is usually present in a community, this is referred to an *endemic* situation – which may still be higher than the desired level (e.g., presence of malaria in some regions, while eliminated in other regions).[33] If the observed number of cases is markedly above the expected number, this is called an *epidemic*, or *outbreak* if occurring in a more limited geographic area.[34] If there are several cases of a disease, but it is not entirely clear if they are caused by the same cause (e.g., pathogen, toxin, chemical), this is called a *cluster*.[35]

The World Health Organization took notice of a *cluster* of cases of atypical "pneumonia of unknown cause" in Wuhan on December 31st, 2019.[36] From around January 9th, 2020, the World Health Organization talked about an *outbreak*, on January 30th a Public Health Emergency of International Concern (PHEIC, not a typical epidemiological term) and from March 11th, a pandemic.[37]

Figure 7.3 is a visual representation of the timeline for infection by Covid-19. When an individual can transmit an infection (infectious period) depends on the pathogen. This does not necessarily coincide with the symptomatic period, which can also vary in severity depending on patient characteristics and the amount of

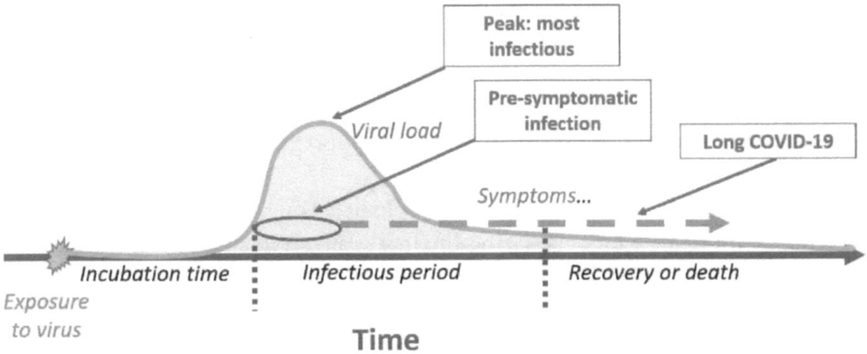

FIGURE 7.3 Timeline of incubation, infectiousness, and recovery for Covid-19

Source: Graph by the author.

the pathogen transmitted (viral dose). For Covid-19 it was established early that pre-symptomatic transmission is possible, meaning that individuals who did not develop any symptoms yet may already have transmitted the disease to others.[38] For Covid-19, there has been discussion about the extent of potential asymptomatic spread from early in the pandemic, and it is established that people with very minor symptoms can be infectious.[39] In Sweden asymptomatic and pre-symptomatic spread were denied repeatedly by FHM, as also seen by the recommendations for quarantine (only those symptomatic) and selection for testing.[40] It was also insinuated repeatedly to the public that children could not become ill or transmit the disease.[41]

Common errors in epidemiology

One of the dogmas in epidemiology is "*correlation is not causation*". It is not because you find an association between chocolate consumption and math test results, that chocolate makes you smarter.[42] If you would assess this in a setting where only the rich can afford chocolate and education, it is no surprise you find a correlation. There could be a biological mechanism as well, but with one single study showing an association, mass-chocolate consumption cannot be recommended to the entire world population. In other words, epidemiologists look at the bigger picture, considering prior (clinical, societal, and other) knowledge and especially previously published research – expanding the body of scientific knowledge with each study.

Common errors for epidemiological studies are shown in Figure 7.4 and can occur in any study design. Especially lack of *power* (*random error*) is common if the

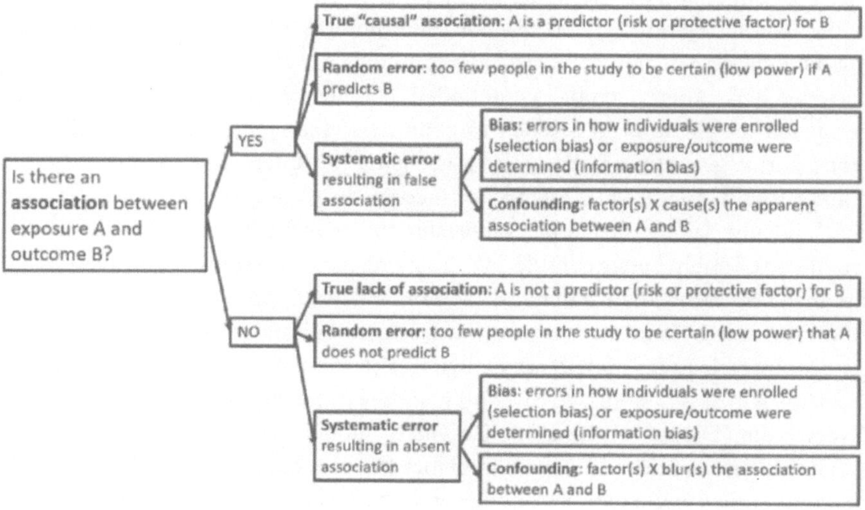

FIGURE 7.4 How to interpret epidemiological studies on potential associations

Source: Graph by the author.

study size is too small. *Biases* and *confounding* may be more difficult to detect or anticipate, since they need reasoning and some prior knowledge of the studied potential predictors (exposures) and outcomes, or similar situations – and how individuals will be recruited or enrolled. It is often difficult to motivate potential study participants to participate in a study, especially if a considerable effort is requested (extensive or unpleasant data collection including taking samples) or a long follow-up is required.

Which type of bias may occur also depends on the study design. In particular if you start your study from selecting those with/without the exposure (cohort) or with/without the outcome (case-control). *Selection bias* occurs if those selected individuals with a certain exposure or outcome are not representative for all individuals in a certain setting (e.g., only deaths from Covid-19 occurring in the hospital are counted, only adults are tested, only the most severely ill are followed-up while individuals with mild symptoms drop out of a study). In Sweden there were early studies to test for prior Covid-19 infections among blood donors and pregnant women.[43] From one side it is good to use existing resources and study data for urgent research questions such as surveillance purposes,[44] but on the other side it is also clear that these study participants represent a healthier section of the Swedish society.[45]

Information bias appears when there are errors in the determination of an exposure or of outcome, and can happen if, for example, the diagnostic procedure of Covid-19 is suboptimal resulting in over- or underreporting of the disease (respectively false positives and false negatives).

Confounding occurs when there is at least one other factor blurring the potential association between an exposure and an outcome. An example would be claiming that a certain country is managing the pandemic better than others by just looking at the exposure (country) and the outcome (number of deaths) while disregarding differences in demographics, socio-economic factors, population density, travel patterns, and other potential confounders.[46] FHM repeatedly and consistently compared the situation in Sweden to countries which were fairing considerably worse at that given time point without nuancing the different risk profiles of these countries and confounding factors, or incorrectly presenting the data.[47] Sweden was suddenly claimed not to be comparable to the other Nordic countries which faired considerably better considering the number of infections and deaths during the first 1.5 year of the pandemic.[48] The other Nordic countries (Denmark, Finland, Norway, Iceland) have a long mutual socio-cultural history, strong political ties, comparable population density and travel patterns, similar lifestyle, and speak a language which is as similar to Swedish that they can communicate with few issues (Norwegian, Danish, Icelandic).[49] Countries should also be compared by their baseline characteristics (i.e., situation before the pandemic), and not based on the outcome (for example number of cases or deaths/million) which will be evaluated.

If confounding and systematic errors are present, this hampers the *internal validity* of a study, meaning that we cannot trust the presented findings. Even if the study has an acceptable internal validity, it does not mean *external validity* will also be good. It is not because something is found in a certain setting that this will be the same everywhere. For example, if a study found no association between obesity and the risk of Covid-19 in a group of fit elite athletes, this does not mean there is no association in other populations. The results of this selected group (selection bias) of very healthy individuals are therefore not generalisable to the general public. Results from studies in adults should also not be generalised to paediatric populations.

Case ascertainment

The use of a common case definition allows for standardisation of the cases of interest both within an ongoing outbreak investigation and possibly between outbreak investigations that differ over time or geographic location, as described in the textbook of *Field Epidemiology*.[50] Case definitions include criteria for person, place, time, and clinical features and should be specific to the outbreak under investigation.

For Covid-19, there are several case definitions used: the (suspected) infected individual, the hospitalised individual (in intensive care or elsewhere), and the individual who died because of Covid-19; and those who have prolonged symptoms of Covid-19 (so-called long-Covid).

As you see, the case definition per se does not include a diagnostic test, especially early in an outbreak when the causal pathogen is not yet identified. The *clinical presentation* of individuals with Covid-19 has evolved over the two years of the pandemic, with new variants of the virus presenting with slightly different dominating symptoms. Even with the same variant, symptoms may vary – and for Covid-19, many individuals were asymptomatic or only had mild symptoms.[51] In Sweden, individuals who were not (yet) symptomatic were disregarded as potential cases, as shown by the ineligibility for testing and absent need for quarantine after high-risk exposure as in other countries.[52] Although studies on self-reported symptoms may include individuals who did not have Covid-19 (false positives), they are still useful for surveillance purposes – and to estimate the true extent of the problem.[53]

Considering diagnostic tests, we know that it is unrealistic and unaffordable to have 100% accurate tests which can be used on a large scale. Clinical diagnoses are also imperfect because of varying symptoms, severity, and possible other pathologies with similar symptoms. For every diagnostic test, there is a trade-off between *sensitivity* and *specificity*. An optimal sensitivity implies that everyone with the disease is detected as such; and optimal specificity implies that those who test positive are all truly positive and nobody is diagnosed with the disease while being healthy. For tests requiring high sensitivity it is better to identify too many people who may have the disease (resulting in some false positives) since the consequences of not detecting cases are severe (e.g., timely detection of cancer improves survival). With highly sensitive tests, further examinations could be performed to confirm the diagnosis (e.g., cancer screening). With high specificity it is important that nobody is diagnosed incorrectly as having the disease. A high specificity of a test is important if a positive test result will result in major consequences for the individual (e.g., the therapeutic decision to start chemotherapy or operate).

When individuals are incorrectly classified based on their disease status, we talk about *misclassification*. In *non-differential misclassification* this can go both ways, with false positives and false negatives being as likely to the same extent. In *differential misclassification*, either false positives or false negatives are more likely to occur. Both main categories of misclassification, non-differential and differential misclassification, can be due to lower sensitivity (more false negatives) and/or lower specificity (more false positives). The difference between non-differential misclassification and differential misclassification is rather that non-differential misclassification will only dilute (decrease) the strength of the associations studied, that is, decrease the size of the effect measures (any effect measure), while differential misclassification can either increase or decrease the strengths of the associations studied, that is, either increase or decrease the size of the effect measures (any effect measure).

If you want to detect a dangerous infectious disease such as HIV, you want to miss as few cases as possible (i.e., low number of false negatives) – and aim for maximum *sensitivity*. For Covid-19, missed cases may not go into isolation and continue the chain of infection. If you have a more sensitive case definition you may also be better able to predict the burden and near future of the spread of the infection in the society. In general, it could be considered better to over-estimate the upcoming need for healthcare capacity increase than to underestimate this, since it does take time to reorganise hospitals and create more beds and recruit/reorganise more personnel.

Yet, in Sweden, large-scale testing was not prioritised, and access to testing was restricted or complicated by long waiting times.[54] Compared to countries like China or New Zealand, Sweden was never able to (and never intended to) detect close to all active infections, symptomatic and (yet) asymptomatic. This was also shown by discrepancy between the number of reported infections, the number of deaths, and the reported acquired immunity (as discussed in Edvinsson's chapter) and the relatively high case-fatality in Sweden.[55] Although some infections may have not been detectable anymore when the individuals were finally tested, the proportion of people testing positive was clearly higher than in countries following the WHO-promoted test-and-trace strategy. On January 8th, 2021, it is for example very clear that more than 20–30% of the administered tests were positive, compared to less than 1% in Australia and less than 3% in the other Nordic countries (Figure 7.5).

Even while community spread was reported in several European countries, and there was accumulating evidence for asymptomatic infection, only symptomatic individuals coming from Covid-19 hotspots could receive testing during the early phase of the pandemic in Sweden.[56] Wider spread testing for active infections was only available from June 2020 and onwards, again for symptomatic individuals only.[57] Self-testing (without professional help) was commonplace and recommended by FHM based on a small pilot study with both self-testing and

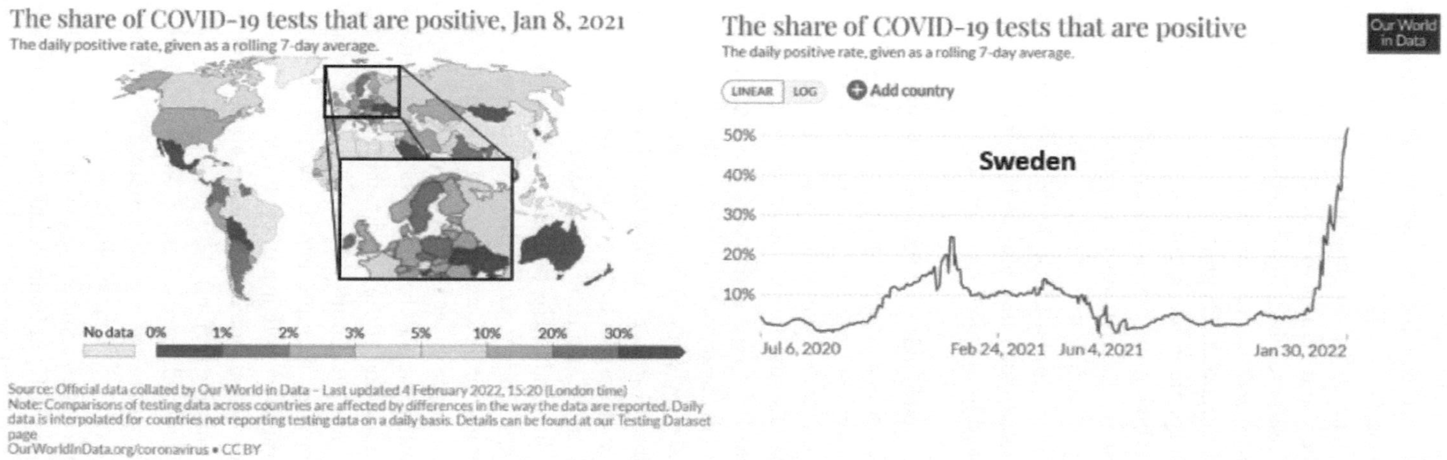

FIGURE 7.5 The proportion of Covid-19 tests with a positive result on January 8th, 2021 (globally) and between July 2020 and January 2022 (Sweden)

Source: Adapted from *Our World in Data*. Hannah Ritchie, Edouard Mathieu, Lucas Rodés-Guirao, Cameron Appel, Charlie Giattino, Esteban Ortiz-Ospina, Joe Hasell, Bobbie Macdonald, Diana Beltekian and Max Roser (2020) – "Coronavirus Pandemic (COVID-19)". *Published online at OurWorldInData.org*. Retrieved from: https://ourworldindata.org/coronavirus [Online Resource].

professional testing,[58] with the risk of getting poor quality samples and false negative results – again examples of selection bias, and ascertainment most likely resulting in an underreporting of cases.

During 2020, FHM was repeatedly claiming infection was reasonably under control (despite rising numbers and restrictive testing), while at the same time claiming herd immunity was almost reached, ignoring the number of deaths which would accompany such high infection levels based on international case-fatality estimates (cf. Edvinsson's and Bergholtz's chapters).

During the summer of 2020, there was a controversy in Sweden about tests giving false positive results – which is the downside of highly sensitive tests.[59] Why would a few more positive cases (and consequent isolation) be more problematic than unaware cases who keep spreading the infection? The higher numbers? Is it better to misdiagnose active cases, leading to an underreporting of the numbers, than having a few false positives which may also include individuals who would test positive a few days later and just made the cut-off for positivity at the time of the test?

Access to testing has been restricted. Children and elderly were often denied access to testing or down-prioritised; and if waiting times for testing increased, several individuals would already test negative (yet potentially keep spreading the infection when waiting for the test).[60] These are textbook examples of *selection bias*, that is, who is selected for a study; and *ascertainment or diagnostic bias*, since the diagnostic method is suboptimal. This resulted in *underreporting* of cases, as it seems more likely to be classified as false negative than false positive.

The number of hospitalised individuals is based on a combination of the number of severe cases, the available healthcare capacity, and the admission criteria. Sweden has among the lowest number of hospital beds and intensive care unit (ICU) beds in Europe.[61] Already early on in the pandemic, there were signs and official documents circulated in the hospitals indicating that, for example, obese and elderly individuals should not receive ICU.[62] Access to hospitalisation or even outpatient clinics was also restricted because of waiting times and limitations for transferral. Officials denied that triage has happened at the level of hospitalisation or ICU, yet the distribution of age and other patient characteristics suggests otherwise.[63] This was especially apparent when looking at the age distribution at the ICU, with an underrepresentation of the eldest age groups.[64] Many elderly individuals in retirement homes or living at home in multiple regions of Sweden did not receive potentially life-saving healthcare and were just offered morphine without physical examination by a medical doctor, informed consent, or notification of the family (as officially documented in multiple regions).[65]

Denying access to healthcare will have an effect on the number of reported hospitalisations, again an example of *selection bias* resulting in differential misclassification and underreporting of cases. One example of the consequences was the reportedly high survival of individuals admitted with Covid-19 to the ICU.[66] If you do selectively deny access to the ICU, and only admit those with the highest probability of survival, your results will consequently be biased towards a higher survival and findings cannot be generalised to ICU populations in other countries.[67] Comparisons of the representativeness of the Swedish and other Covid-19 hospitalised and ICU populations[68] should also take into account the time-dependent strain on the healthcare (during the peaks of the different waves) and improvement of treatment over time because of accumulating international evidence on treatment possibilities and efficacy.

The case definition of Covid-19 deaths has also been discussed and criticised in Sweden. While in some countries suspected cases were included particularly at the early phase of the pandemic (often because of limited test capacity, especially post-mortem), a less sensitive definition was used in Sweden. One argument used was that not everyone who died with Covid actually died of Covid, and that "old" or "sick" people would have died anyway (as if everyone in a retirement home has a life expectancy of maximally one year).[69] It was argued that those who died were "*dry tinder*", yet it has been shown that this argument cannot explain the excess mortality in Sweden during the pandemic (cf. Edvinsson's and Bergmann's chapters).[70]

If someone tested positive for Covid and was hospitalised because of the severe symptoms, it was not impossible that he or she died many weeks later. These individuals were not considered Covid deaths by FHM if the death occurred more than 30 days after the diagnosis (in contrast to the National Board of Healthcare data).[71] Although 30-day mortality is a common measure of occurrence in epidemiology, this is an estimate based on the numbers occurring within a set timeframe. Using this measure does not change the cause of death, the "eligible" deaths just occur within the timeframe and not later. When counting the actual number of deaths without a time restriction, this approach would again have resulted in *misclassification* in the direction of lower numbers of cases.

Conclusion

In this non-comprehensive overview of the Covid-19 pandemic in Sweden from an epidemiology perspective, it is quite clear that FHM has made questionable decisions and communications to the public. In this chapter I tried to highlight that many common mistakes are made against the basic principles of epidemiology – and not even going into complex infectious-disease modelling. In the beginning of the pandemic, I thought it was incompetence, yet I do suspect a more deliberate communication strategy and idiosyncratic motives, at least to some extent. The three key persons from FHM are all trained physicians who should have sufficient knowledge about infectious diseases and infection control.[72] Tegnell, as State Epidemiologist, obtained master training in epidemiology from the same school where I studied (London School of Hygiene and Tropical Medicine), a global authority in epidemiology and in infectious diseases. Giesecke has been seen as an authority in Infectious Disease Epidemiology, as Professor at Karolinska Institutet, author of a handbook on the topic, and WHO and ECDC expert.[73] Combined with what we learned through our efforts on the *Escape* project and the other chapters of this book, it seems clear that FHM went deliberately against scientific evidence, scientific integrity, and basic knowledge of epidemiology and infection control. I can only conclude that all this fits within a deliberate herd-immunity strategy. Changing strategy was no option despite accumulating evidence on economic, human, and personal costs. This strategy was not to be questioned by people within FHM, nationally and internationally, and certainly not adjusted or abandoned. Yes, it has been the first time that every currently living adult has been exposed to such a global and rapidly evolving infectious threat to humankind, affecting everyone's daily life. Yes, things could have gone better in every country, and hopefully every country will learn from their mistakes. We can only hope that this will result in a better response and outcome when the next pandemic will hit our globe. Yet, we cannot improve a response to any ongoing or new threat if optimisation based on acquired and accumulating scientific evidence is not allowed, and discussions are shunned. The word "science" comes from the Latin "scientia" which means knowledge. Science should consequently be based on demonstrable and reproducible data – aiming for measurable, generalisable, and reproducible results through testing and analysis, a process known as the scientific method. Science should be based on facts and evidence, not on opinions, religion, beliefs, ideology, or personal preferences.

Notes

1 Brusselaers, Nele, David Steadson, Kelly Bjorklund, Sofia Breland, Jens Stilhoff Sörensen, Andrew Ewing, Sigurd Bergmann, and Gunnar Steineck. "Evaluation of Science Advice During the COVID-19 Pandemic in Sweden", *Humanities and Social Sciences Communications* 9, Article number: 91 (2022), www.nature.com/articles/s41599-022-01097-5 .

2 Brusselaers, N., S.C.L. Kamerlin, and P. Wittung-Stafshede. "Swedish Scientists Call for Evidence-Based Policy on COVID-19", in Schneider, L. (ed.). *For Better Science – By Leonid Schneider, on Research Integrity, Biomedical Ethics and Academic Publishing*, 2020, https://forbetterscience.com/; Vogel, G. "'It's Been So, So Surreal.' Critics of Sweden's Lax Pandemic Policies Face Fierce Backlash", *Science Magazine*, October 2020; Bjorklund, K., and A. Ewing. "The Swedish COVID-19 Response Is a Disaster. It Shouldn't Be a Model for the Rest of the World", *Time*, 14 October 2020; Dawod, N., and H.O. Berg. "'Tror inte på ett stort utbrott i Sverige' – Folkhälsomyndigheten och Socialstyrelsen om coronaviruset" ["I do not believe in a major outbreak in Sweden" – The Swedish Public Health Agency and the National Board of Health and Welfare About the Coronavirus], *Aftonbladet*, 26 February 2020. Folkhälsomyndigheten. "Ingen spridning av det nya coronaviruset i Sverige" [No spread of the new coronavirus in Sweden] 13 February 2020, www.folkhalsomyndigheten.se/nyheter-och-press/nyhetsarkiv/2020/februari/ingen-spridning-av-coronavirus-i-sverige/ .

3 Andersson, M. "Tegnell om virusfallen: Jag tror att det värsta nu är över" [Tegnell About the Virus Cases: I Think the Worst Is Over Now] *Omni*, 5 March, 2020, https://omni.se/tegnell-om-virusfallen-jag-tror-att-det-varsta-nu-ar-over/a/zG1Aq9; Karlsten, E. "Sant och falskt om citat från Folkhälsomyndigheten och Anders Tegnell", 19 March 2020, https://emanuelkarlsten.se/sant-och-falskt-om-vad-statsepidemiolog-anders-tegnell-sagt/ .

4 Brusselaers et al. "Evaluation of Science Advice in the COVID-19 Pandemic in Sweden".

5 *Ibid.*

6 *Ibid.*; Bjurwald, L., E. Schönholzer, and A. Andén. "Maktens granskare eller maktens megafoner? Svensk journalistik under coronapandemin" [Investigators of Power or Megaphones of Power? Swedish Journalism During the Corona Pandemic]. (Näringslivets medieinstitut [Business media institute], 2021).
7 Sayers, F. "Swedish Covid-19 Chief Anders Tegnell: Judge Me in a Year/Why We Aren't Wearing Masks in Sweden", *Unherd*, 24 July 2020, https://unherd.com/2020/07/swedens-anders-tegnell-judge-me-in-a-year/ .
8 Sjödin, H., A.F. Johansson, A. Brännström, Z. Farooq, H.K. Kriit, A. Wilder-Smith, C. Åström, J. Thunberg, M. Söderquist, and J. Rocklöv. "COVID-19 Healthcare Demand and Mortality in Sweden in Response to Non-Pharmaceutical Mitigation and Suppression Scenarios", *International Journal of Epidemiology* 49:5 (2020): 1443–1453; Kamerlin, S.C.L., and P.M. Kasson. "Managing COVID-19 Spread with Voluntary Public-Health Measures: Sweden as a Case Study for Pandemic Control", *Clinical Infectious Diseases* 71:12 (2020): 3174–3181.
9 Adami, H.-O. "Sweden: A Paradise for Epidemiologists?" *The Lancet* 347:9001 (1996): 588. Cf. also Steineck's chapter in this volume.
10 Villani, L., M. McKee, F. Cascini, W. Ricciardi, and S. Boccia. "Comparison of Deaths Rates for COVID-19 Across Europe During the First Wave of the COVID-19 Pandemic", *Frontiers in Public Health* 8 (2020), www.frontiersin.org/article/10.3389/fpubh.2020.620416 . The infection fatality rate of COVID-19 in Stockholm – Technical Report (20094–2), F.P.H. Agency), Editor. 2020: Sweden. Assessment of COVID-19 surveillance case definitions and data reporting in the European Union. Briefing: Requested by the ENVI committee, E. Parliament, Editor. 2020; Gummesson, J. "Tegnell pausar svensk insamling av coronadata" [Tegnell pauses Swedish collection of corona data], *Svenska Dagbladet*, 27 April 2020.
11 Brusselaers et al. "Evaluation of Science Advice in the COVID-19 Pandemic in Sweden"; Sörensen, J. "Terror in Utopia: Crisis (mis-) Management During the Covid-19 Pandemic in Sweden", *Sociološki pregled* 54:3 (2020): 961–1007.
12 "Why Do COVID-19 Deaths in Sweden's Official Data Always Appear to Decrease?" 13 November 2020, https://ourworldindata.org/covid-sweden-death-reporting .
13 "Understanding How Sweden Reports Its Coronavirus Figures", *The Local, Sweden*, 14 April 2020, www.thelocal.se/20200414/understanding-swedens-figures-on-the-coronavirus/ .
14 For details see, www.sciensano.be/en/health-topics/coronavirus .
15 *Ibid.*
16 Funck, M.A. "Åtta av tio coronapatienter överlever intensivvård" [Eight out of ten corona patients survive intensive care], *Sveriges Radio*, 12 April 2020, https://sverigesradio.se/artikel/7450992; Kostsehub, N. "Stopping COVID-19 with Misleading Graphs", *Towards Data Science*, 19 June 2020, https://towardsdatascience.com/stopping-covid-19-with-misleading-graphs-6812a61a57c9 .
17 Bjorklund and Ewing. "The Swedish COVID-19 Response Is a Disaster"; Vogel, G. "COVID-19 Data in Paper About Swedish Schoolchildren Come Under Fire", *Science* 371:6533 (2021): 973–974.
18 Karlsten. "Sant och falskt om citat från Folkhälsomyndigheten och Anders Tegnell"; Capar, R.-I. "Tegnell: Larger Immigrant Population Led to Faster Corona Spread in Stockholm", *Norway Today*, 20 October 2020, https://norwaytoday.info/news/tegnell-larger-immigrant-population-led-to-faster-corona-spread-in-stockholm/; Steineck, G., A. Ewing, J. Lötvall, J. Sörensen, and A. Vahlne. "Tegnell kvalificerar sig inte ens som hobbyepidemiolog" [Tegnell Does Not Even Qualify as a Hobby Epidemiologist], *Göteborgs-Posten*, 1 January 2021.
19 Steineck et al. "Tegnell kvalificerar sig inte ens som hobbyepidemiolog".
20 Brusselaers et al. "Evaluation of Science Advice in the COVID-19 Pandemic in Sweden". Edwards, C. "Who Are the People Behind Sweden's Coronavirus Strategy?" *The Local, Sweden*, 1 June 2020, www.thelocal.se/20200601/whos-who-in-swedens-coronavirus-debate/ .

21 Chew, M.S., P.J. Blixt, R. Åhman, L. Engerström, H. Andersson, R.K. Berggren, A. Tegnell, and S. McIntyre. "National Outcomes and Characteristics of Patients Admitted to Swedish Intensive Care Units for COVID-19: A Registry-Based Cohort Study", *European Journal of* Anaesthesiology 38:4 (2021): 335–343.
22 Brusselaers et al. "Evaluation of Science Advice in the COVID-19 Pandemic in Sweden".
23 Grimes, D.A., and K.F. Schulz. "Descriptive Studies: What They Can and Cannot Do", *The Lancet* 359:9301 (2002): 145–149.
24 Grimes, D.A., and K.F. Schulz. "An Overview of Clinical Research: The Lay of the Land", *The Lancet* 359:9300 (2002): 57–61.
25 Iacobucci, G. "Covid-19: Comparing Sweden's Response with the UK's Is 'Misleading,' Experts Argue", *BMJ* 370 (2020): m3765.
26 Gallagher, J. "Dexamethasone, Remdesivir, Regeneron: Trump's Covid Treatment Explained", *BBC*, 9 October 2020, www.bbc.com/news/health-54418464 .
27 Pana, T.A., S. Bhattacharya, D.T. Gamble, Z. Pasdar, W.A. Szlachetka, J.A. Perdomo-Lampignano, K.D. Ewers, D.J. McLernon, and P.K. Myint. "Country-Level Determinants of the Severity of the First Global Wave of the COVID-19 Pandemic: An Ecological Study", *BMJ Open* 11:2 (2021); Khorram-Manesh, A., E. Carlström, A.J. Hertelendy, K. Goniewicz, C.B. Casady, and F.M. Burkle. "Does the Prosperity of a Country Play a Role in COVID-19 Outcomes?" *Disaster Medicine and Public Health Preparedness* (12 August 2020): 1–10, https://pubmed.ncbi.nlm.nih.gov/32782059/ .
28 Capar. "Tegnell: Larger Immigrant Population Led to Faster Corona Spread in Stockholm".
29 *Ibid.*
30 *Ibid.*
31 Hansson, E., M. Albin, M. Rasmussen, and K. Jakobsson. "Large Differences in Excess Mortality in March-May 2020 by Country of Birth in Sweden" (In Swedish), *Läkartidningen* (29 June 2020): 117, https://pubmed.ncbi.nlm.nih.gov/32619245/; Rostila, M., A. Cederström, M. Wallace, M. Brandén, B. Malmberg, and G. Andersson. "Disparities in COVID-19 Deaths by Country of Birth in Stockholm, Sweden: A Total Population Based Cohort Study", *American Journal of Epidemiology* 190:8 (2021): 1510–1518; Strang, P., P. Fürst, and T. Schultz. "Excess Deaths from COVID-19 Correlate with Age and Socio-Economic Status. A Database Study in the Stockholm Region", *Upsala Journal of Medical Sciences* 125:4 (2020): 297–304; Calderón-Larrañaga, A., S. Dekhtyar, D.L. Vetrano, T. Bellander, and L. Fratiglioni. "COVID-19: Risk Accumulation Among Biologically and Socially Vulnerable Older Populations", *Ageing Research Reviews* 63 (2020): 101149.
32 Brusselaers et al. "Evaluation of Science Advice in the COVID-19 Pandemic in Sweden".
33 Hickey, M., J. Elliott, and S.L. Davison. "Hormone Replacement Therapy", *BMJ* 344 (2012): e763.
34 *Ibid.*
35 *Ibid.*
36 *Timeline: WHO's COVID-19 Response*, 2021, 13 July 2021, www.who.int/emergencies/diseases/novel-coronavirus-2019/interactive-timeline .
37 *Ibid.*
38 Bai, Y., L. Yao, T. Wei, F. Tian, D.Y. Jin, L. Chen, and M. Wang. "Presumed Asymptomatic Carrier Transmission of COVID-19", *JAMA* 323:14 (2020): 1406–1407; You, Y., X. Yang, D. Hung, Q. Yang, T. Wu, and M. Deng. "Asymptomatic COVID-19 Infection: Diagnosis, Transmission, Population Characteristics", *BMJ Supportive & Palliative Care*, 30 July 2021; Li, C., Y. Zhu, C. Qi, L. Liu, D. Zhang, X. Wang, K. She, Y. Jia, T. Liu, D. He, M. Xiong, and X. Li. "Estimating the Prevalence of Asymptomatic COVID-19 Cases and Their Contribution in Transmission – Using Henan Province, China, as an Example", *Frontiers of Medicine* 8 (2021): 591372; Subramanian, R., Q. He, and M. Pascual. "Quantifying Asymptomatic Infection and Transmission of COVID-19

in New York City Using Observed Cases, Serology, and Testing Capacity", *Proceedings of the National Academy of Sciences of the United States of America* 118:9 (2021): e2019716118; Peirlinck, M., K. Linka, F. Sahli Costabal, J. Bhattacharya, E. Bendavid, J.P.A. Ioannidis, and E. Kuhl. "Visualizing the Invisible: The Effect of Asymptomatic Transmission on the Outbreak Dynamics of COVID-19", *Computer Methods in Applied Mechanics and Engineering* 372 (2020): 113410; Gandhi, M., D.S. Yokoe, and D.V. Havlir. "Asymptomatic Transmission, the Achilles' Heel of Current Strategies to Control Covid-19", *NEJM* 382:22 (2020): 2158–2160.

39 Bai et al. "Presumed Asymptomatic Carrier Transmission of COVID-19"; You et al. "Asymptomatic COVID-19 Infection"; Li et al. "Estimating the Prevalence of Asymptomatic COVID-19 Cases and Their Contribution in Transmission"; Subramanian et al. "Quantifying Asymptomatic Infection and Transmission of COVID-19 in New York City"; Peirlinck et al. "Visualizing the Invisible"; Gandhi et al. "Asymptomatic Transmission".

40 Brusselaers et al. "Evaluation of Science Advice in the COVID-19 Pandemic in Sweden".

41 *Ibid.*; Steineck et al. "Tegnell kvalificerar sig inte ens som hobbyepidemiolog".

42 Cf. Vigen, T. "Spurious Correlations", December 2021, www.tylervigen.com/spurious-correlations .

43 Castro Dopico, X., S. Muschiol, M. Christian, L. Hanke, D.J. Sheward, N.F. Grinberg, J. Rorbach, G. Bogdanovic, G.M. McInerney, T. Allander, C. Wallace, B. Murrell, J. Albert, and G.B. Karlsson Hedestam. "Seropositivity in Blood Donors and Pregnant Women During the First Year of SARS-CoV-2 Transmission in Stockholm, Sweden", *Journal of Internal Medicine* 290:3 (2021): 666–676.

44 Lindahl, J.F., T. Hoffman, M. Esmaeilzadeh, B. Olsen, R. Winter, S. Amer, C. Molnár, A. Svalberg, and Å. Lundkvist. "High Seroprevalence of SARS-CoV-2 in Elderly Care Employees in Sweden", *Infection Ecology & Epidemiology* 10:1 (2020): 1789036.

45 Castro Dopico et al. "Seropositivity in Blood Donors and Pregnant Women".

46 Kashnitsky, I., and J.M. Aburto. "COVID-19 in Unequally Ageing European Regions", *World Development* (136 December 2020): 105170; Drefahl, S., M. Wallace, E. Mussino, S., Aradhya, M. Kolk, M. Brandén, B. Malmberg, and G. Andersson. "A Population-Based Cohort Study of Socio-Demographic Risk Factors for COVID-19 Deaths in Sweden", *Nature Communications* 11:1 (2020): 5097.

47 Karlsten. "Sant och falskt"; Capar. "Tegnell"; Steineck et al. "Tegnell kvalificerar sig inte ens som hobbyepidemiolog"; Iacobucci. "Covid-19".

48 Amiri, A. "Role of Social Distancing in Tackling COVID-19 During the First Wave of Pandemic in Nordic Region: Evidence from Daily Deaths, Infections and Needed Hospital Resources", *International Journal of Nursing* Sciences 8:2 (2021): 145–151. Nanda, M., Aashima, and R. Sharma. "COVID-19: A Comprehensive Review of Epidemiology and Public Health System Response in Nordic Region", *International Journal of Health Services* 51:3 (2021): 287–299; Ahrenfeldt, L.J., M. Otavova, K. Christensen, and R. Lindahl-Jacobsen. "Sex and Age Differences in COVID-19 Mortality in Europe", *Wiener klinische Wochenschrift* 133:7–8 (2021): 393–398; Yarmol-Matusiak, E.A., L.E. Cipriano, and S. Stranges. "A Comparison of COVID-19 Epidemiological Indicators in Sweden, Norway, Denmark, and Finland", *Scandinavian Journal of Public Health* 49:1 (2021): 69–78.

49 Mens, H., A. Koch, M. Chaine, and A. Bengaard Andersen. "The Hammer vs Mitigation – A Comparative Retrospective Register Study of the Swedish and Danish National Responses to the COVID-19 Pandemic in 2020", *APMIS* 129:7 (2021): 384–392.

50 Gregg, M.B. *Field Epidemiology*, New York: Oxford University Press, 2002.

51 Bai et al. "Presumed Asymptomatic Carrier Transmission of COVID-19"; You et al. "Asymptomatic COVID-19 Infection"; Li et al. "Estimating the Prevalence of Asymptomatic COVID-19 Cases"; Subramanian et al. "Quantifying Asymptomatic Infection and Transmission of COVID-19 in New York City"; Peirlinck et al. "Visualizing the Invisible"; Gandhi et al. "Asymptomatic Transmission".

52 Brusselaers et al. "Evaluation of Science Advice in the COVID-19 Pandemic in Sweden".
53 Ekström, S., N. Andersson, A. Lövquist, A. Lauber, A. Georgelis, I. Kull, E. Melén, and A. Bergström. "COVID-19 Among Young Adults in Sweden: Self-Reported Long-Term Symptoms and Associated Factors", *Scandinavian Journal of Public Health*, 2021: 14034948211025425; Sudre, C.H., K.A. Lee, M.N. Lochlainn, T. Varsavsky, B. Murray, M.S. Graham, C. Menni, M. Modat, R.C.E. Bowyer, L.H. Nguyen, D.A. Drew, A.D. Joshi, W. Ma, C.G. Guo, C.H., Lo, S. Ganesh, A. Buwe, J.C. Pujol, J.L. du Cadet, A. Visconti, M.B. Freidin, J.S. El-Sayed Moustafa, M. Falchi, R. Davies, M.F. Gomez, T. Fall, M.J. Cardoso, J. Wolf, P.W. Franks, A.T. Chan, T.D. Spector, C.J. Steves, and S. Ourselin. "Symptom Clusters in COVID-19: A Potential Clinical Prediction Tool from the COVID Skymptom Study App", *Science Advances* 7:12 (2021).
54 Brusselaers et al. "Evaluation of Science Advice in the COVID-19 Pandemic in Sweden".
55 Karadag, E. "Increase in COVID-19 Cases and Case-Fatality and Case-Recovery Rates in Europe: A Cross-Temporal Meta-Analysis", *Journal of Medical Virology* 92:9 (2020): 1511–1517.
56 Brusselaers et al. "Evaluation of Science Advice in the COVID-19 Pandemic in Sweden"; *Timeline of ECDC's Response to COVID-19*, 13 July 2021, www.ecdc.europa.eu/en/covid-19/timeline-ecdc-response .
57 Bjorklund, K. "The Inside Story of How Sweden Botched Its Coronavirus Response", *Foreign Policy*, 22 December 2020.
58 Brusselaers et al. "Evaluation of Science Advice in the COVID-19 Pandemic in Sweden". Folkhälsomyndigheten (Public Health Agency). "Egenprovtagning covid-19 för personal inom hälso- och sjukvård samt omsorg" [Self-sampling covid-19 for staff in health and medical care and care], 29 May 2020, www.folkhalsomyndigheten.se/publicerat-material/publikationsarkiv/e/egenprovtagning-covid-19-for-personal-inom-halso–och-sjukvard-samt-omsorg/; Nyström, M., and T. Mossige-Norheim. "Sveriges nya coronastrategi: Fler ska testas" [Sweden's new corona strategy: 'More to be tested'], *Expressen*, 30 April 2020; Folkhälsomyndigheten (The Public Health Agency). "Utvärdering av egenprovtagning som metod för påvisning av SARS-COV-2 – Ett pilotprojekt" [Evaluation of Self-Sampling as a Method of Detection of SARS-COV-2 – A Pilot Study] (01369–2020), www.folkhalsomyndigheten.se/smittskydd-beredskap/utbrott/aktuella-utbrott/covid-19/information-till-varden/personal-inom-halso–och-sjukvard/stod-infor-etablering-av-rutiner-for-egenprovtagning-for-covid-19/; Folkhälsomyndigheten (The Public Health Agency). "Stöd inför etablering av rutiner för egenprovtagning för covid-19" [Support for the establishment of routines for self-sampling for covid-19], www.folkhalsomyndigheten.se/smittskydd-beredskap/utbrott/aktuella-utbrott/covid-19/information-till-varden/personal-inom-halso–och-sjukvard/stod-infor-etablering-av-rutiner-for-egenprovtagning-for-covid-19/ , www.folkhalsomyndigheten.se/smittskydd-beredskap/utbrott/aktuella-utbrott/covid-19/information-till-varden/personal-inom-halso–och-sjukvard/stod-infor-etablering-av-rutiner-for-egenprovtagning-for-covid-19/ .
59 "False Positive Test Cases", *Pantasniaga*, 4 September 2020, www.pantasniaga.com/false-positive-test-cases/ .
60 Brusselaers et al. "Evaluation of Science Advice in the COVID-19 Pandemic in Sweden".
61 Bauer, J., D. Bruggmann, D. Klingelhofer, W. Maier, L. Schwettmann, D.J. Weiss, and D.A. Groneberg. "Access to Intensive Care in 14 European Countries: A Spatial Analysis of Intensive Care Need and Capacity in the Light of COVID-19", *Intensive Care Medicine* 46:11 (2020): 2026–2034, https://ec.europa.eu/eurostat/statistics-explained/index.php?title=Healthcare_resource_statistics_-_beds; Hospitals in Europe Healthcare data. European Hospital and Healthcare Federation. 2018, www.hope.be/

wp-content/uploads/2018/07/2018_Hospitals-in-EU-28-Synthesis-final-for-publication-002.pdf .

62 Brusselaers et al. "Evaluation of Science Advice in the COVID-19 Pandemic in Sweden"; Wiken, J. "Larm om att patienter prioriteras bort – IVO gör tillsyn på Karolinska" [Alarm That Patients Are Not Given Priority – IVO Investigates Karolinska], *SVT Nyheter*, 1 May 2020, www.svt.se/nyheter/inrikes/larm-om-att-patienter-prioriteras-bort-ivo-gor-tillsyn-pa-karolinska .

63 Kamerlin et al. "Managing COVID-19 Spread with Voluntary Public-Health Measures"; Chew et al. "National Outcomes and Characteristics"; Bergman, J., M. Ballin, A. Nordström, and P. Nordström. "Risk Factors for COVID-19 Diagnosis, Hospitalization, and Subsequent All-Cause Mortality in Sweden: A Nationwide Study", *European Journal of Epidemiology* 36:3 (2021): 287–298.

64 Kamerlin et al. "Managing COVID-19 Spread with Voluntary Public-Health Measures"; Chew et al. "National Outcomes and Characteristics"; Bergman et al. "Risk Factors for COVID-19 Diagnosis"; Larsson, E., O. Brattström, C. Agvald-Öhman, J. Grip, F. Campoccia Jalde, K. Strålin, P. Nauclér, A. Oldner, D. Konrad, B.P. Persson, L.I. Eriksson, and J. Mårtensson. "Characteristics and Outcomes of Patients with COVID-19 Admitted to ICU in a Tertiary Hospital in Stockholm, Sweden", *Acta Anaesthesiologica Scandinavica* 65:1 (2020): 76–81.

65 Brusselaers et al. "Evaluation of Science Advice in the COVID-19 Pandemic in Sweden"; The Swedish Health and Care Inspectorate (IVO): Ingen region har tagit sitt fulla ansvar för individuell vård och behandling. (No region has taken full responsibility for individual care and treatment.) 24 November 2020, www.ivo.se/publicerat-material/nyheter/2020/ingen-region-har-tagit-fullt-ansvar-for-individuell-vard/ . Socialdepartementet, Regeringen: Regeringskanseliet: Granskning av äldreboenden presenterad. (Government Offices: Examination of nursing homes presented) 7 July 2020. Sweden, www.regeringen.se/artiklar/2020/07/granskning-av-aldreboenden-presenterad/?TSPD_101_R0=082953afa5ab20004ba88ffa4ab39ed8e5201bca4ded40bcf66de5ab4fc8797d623713cfa9a34325086554df241430005f7972f2e294ff885c146e4d669226d5f5e79e937e21b93bad917c74e957011ab2c3129313857e560b6795356dbfaac0; Ballin, M., J. Bergman, M. Kivipelto, A. Nordström, and P. Nordström. "Excess Mortality After COVID-19 in Swedish Long-Term Care Facilities", *Journal of the American Medical Directors Association* 22:8 (2021): 1574–1580.

66 Funck. "Åtta av tio coronapatienter överlever intensivvård"; Kostsehub. "Stopping COVID-19 with Misleading Graphs"; Strålin, K., E. Wahlström, S. Walther, A.M. Bennet-Bark, M. Heurgren, T. Lindén, J. Holm, and H. Hanberger. "Mortality Trends Among Hospitalised COVID-19 Patients in Sweden: A Nationwide Observational Cohort Study", *The Lancet Regional Health – Europe* 4 (2021), www.thelancet.com/journals/lanepe/article/PIIS2666-7762(21)00031-4/fulltext .

67 Chew et al. "National Outcomes and Characteristics"; Nanda et al. "COVID-19"; Larsson et al. "Characteristics and Outcomes".

68 Ahlström, B., R. Frithiof, M. Hultström, I.M. Larsson, G. Strandberg, and M. Lipcsey. "The Swedish Covid-19 Intensive Care Cohort: Risk Factors of ICU Admission and ICU Mortality", *Acta Anaesthesiologica Scandinavica* 65:4 (2021): 525–533.

69 Brusselaers et al. "Evaluation of Science Advice in the COVID-19 Pandemic in Sweden".

70 Rizzi, S., J. Søgaard, and J.W. Vaupel. "High Excess Deaths in Sweden During the First Wave of COVID-19: Policy Deficiencies or 'Dry Tinder'?" *Scandinavian Journal* of *Public Health* 50:1 (2022): 33–37.

71 Brusselaers et al. "Evaluation of Science Advice in the COVID-19 Pandemic in Sweden"; Villani et al. "Comparison of Deaths Rates for COVID-19". The infection fatality rate of COVID-19 in Stockholm – Technical Report (20094–2), F.P.H. Agency), Editor. 2020: Sweden, www.folkhalsomyndigheten.se/contentassets/53c0dc391be54

f5d959ead9131edb771/infection-fatality-rate-covid-19-stockholm-technical-report.pdf . Assessment of COVID-19 surveillance case definitions and data reporting in the European Union. Briefing: Requested by the ENVI committee, E. Parliament, Editor. 2020, www.europarl.europa.eu/RegData/etudes/BRIE/2020/652725/IPOL_BRI(2020)652725_EN.pdf .

72 Edwards. "Who Are the People Behind Sweden's Coronavirus Strategy?"

73 Giesecke, J. *Modern Infectious Disease Epidemiology*, 3rd ed., London: CRC Press, 2017.

8

THE POLITICAL ECONOMY OF ESTIMATING IMMUNITY LEVELS

Rodney Edvinsson

Background

During the spring and summer of 2020, the Public Health Agency of Sweden (*Folkhälsomyndigheten*, FHM) and leading scientists advising the agency were assuming that Sweden, or at least Stockholm, was soon to reach herd immunity. This was a vital assumption to legitimize the herd immunity strategy that de facto was practiced (i.e. a strategy to let the healthy part of the population, especially children, as discussed by Johanna Höög in this book, be infected at a pace that would not overburden health services, while at the same time isolating the so-called risk groups).

This chapter begins by discussing evidence on the infection fatality rate, IFR, presented during spring and summer 2020, internationally and from Sweden. This evidence pointed towards a very high IFR for high-income countries, at around 1 per cent, which would entail 50–100,000 deaths in Sweden or 0.5–1 per cent of the population of 10.3 million. This evidence is next contrasted with the assessments of representatives and some collaborators of FHM, showing how they downplayed the empirical evidence selectively to argue that Sweden, or at least Stockholm, soon was to reach herd immunity. What is remarkable is that representatives of and advisers to FHM claimed that there was a very low IFR as late as in the summer and autumn of 2020, despite wide empirical evidence to the contrary. These claims entailed that Sweden would have to have a much greater spread of infection than the Western European countries, and a much lower IFR. A more tentative discussion follows at the end of how this discrepancy can be analyzed from political-economic, sociological and historical perspectives.

International empirical evidence on IFR

Table 8.1 summarizes the international empirical evidence on IFR and implied IFR for Sweden, which can be compared to Table 8.2 on Swedish evidence, and

DOI: 10.4324/9781003289364-9

TABLE 8.1 Comparison of empirical evidence internationally, the implied IFR for the population of Sweden and implied Covid-19 deaths for Sweden if 70 per cent of all age groups are infected, at different points in time before the second wave.

Date published	*Based on the following evidence or reasoning*	*Further assumptions*	*Claimed or implied IFR*	*Implied IFR of Sweden, adjusted for difference in CDR in 2019*	*Implied Covid-19 deaths in Sweden if 70% infected*
14/4-2020	14th passenger of Diamond Princess died. 712 infected in total.[1]	Adjusted for difference in demographics of infected on Diamond Princess and Sweden.	2.0	1.0	75,000
8/5-2020	6% tested positive for antibodies in Belgium in mid-April.[2]	6,826 Covid-19 deaths in Belgium up to 22/4. Reported deaths assumed to be actual deaths.	1.0	0.9	65,000
13/5-2020	5% of Spanish population had antibodies 27/4–11/5.[3]	Excess mortality, 893 in one million by 3/5.[4] No further adjustment for specificity and sensitivity.	1.8	1.8	130,000
5/6-2020	6.9% tested positive for antibodies in Belgium in mid-May.[5]	9,158 Covid-19 deaths in Belgium up to 22/5. Reported deaths assumed to be actual deaths.	1.2	1.1	75,000
13/8-2020	6% prevalence in England 20/6–13/7. IFR estimated to 0.9% based on reported deaths, but 1.58% based on excess mortality.[6]		1.6	1.6	115,000
1/9-2020	Study shows IFR in Iceland 0.3%, IFR among aged 70–79: 2.4%.[7]	Adjustment based on age composition and relative difference in age IFR	0.3	0.9	55,000

TABLE 8.2 Comparison of empirical evidence on Sweden.

Date, 2020	*Based on the following evidence or reasoning*	*Further assumptions*	*Claimed or implied IFR*	*Implied IFR for demographic of Sweden*	*Implied Covid-19 deaths in Sweden if 70% infected*
9/4	2.5% active infection in Stockholm 27/3–3/4 (i.e. around 60,000 persons).[15]	56 Covid-19 deaths per day 30/3–19/4, on average. 10 net days viral shedding.	0.9	1.3	90,000
12/5	0.9% active infection in Sweden 21/4–24/4.[16]	81 Covid-19 deaths per day 27/4–10/5 on average. 10 net days viral shedding.	0.9	0.9	65,000
20/5	In Stockholm 7.3% of visitors to health centres had antibodies 3/5–9/5.[17]	2191 Covid-19 deaths in Stockholm 9/3–13/5. No adjustment for sensitivity and specificity.	1.3	1.7	120,000
18/6	5% had antibodies among blood donors in 9 regions 25/5–31/5.[18]	5460 Covid-19 deaths in Sweden 9/3–4/6. No adjustment for sensitivity and specificity or age distribution. *Bias* = 1.	1.0	1.0	75,000
18/6	0.3% active infection in Sweden 25/5–28/5.[19]	34 Covid-19 deaths per day 1/6–14/6 on average. 10 net days viral shedding.	1.1	1.1	80,000
4/9	18.7% had antibodies in Rinkeby-Kista 22/6–24/6.[20]	167 per 100,000 inhabitants in Rinkeby-Kista died. CDR in the area 4.8 per 1000. Excess deaths not used. No adjustment for sensitivity and specificity.	0.9	1.6	120,000

Assumptions: Covid deaths in a week was the maximum of reported deaths and excess deaths.[21] IFR was assumed to be 33 per cent higher in Sweden than in Stockholm, which is the ratio for mortality rates before the pandemic. Deaths occur, on average, three weeks after infection, and immunity is detected, on average, two weeks after infection.

Table 8.3 on the estimates and speculations by representatives and collaborators of FHM. The implied IFR for Sweden in Tables 8.1, 8.2 and 8.3 is adjusted for the difference in crude death rate (CDR) of various populations. The last column presents the level of Covid-19 pandemic deaths in Sweden if 70 per cent of the population in Sweden would be infected, given that herd immunity was assumed to be reached at 60–80 per cent infection (today we know it is above that level with new mutations). The number is rounded off to the closest 5,000 (closest 1,000 in Table 8.3 for values below 20,000). All calculations are kept as simple as possible, to facilitate transparency in the comparison.

As discussed in Martin Lindström's chapter, the extent of the threat posed by Covid-19 in winter and early spring 2020 was unknown, but during the spring and summer 2020 more and more empirical evidence became available. Despite claims by adherents of the herd immunity strategy, most data, if interpreted and adjusted in a manner that is not biased (for example to demographics), quite early the pandemic pointed towards a high IFR. Most importantly, on the cruise ship Diamond Princess, 2 per cent of the infected died, 14 of 714 that tested positive. Twelve of these patients had died by the end of March, so by then, it should have been clear that the IFR was very high. The last patient died on the 14th of April. For a country with the Swedish age distribution, this would give an IFR of 1 per cent or above. For herd immunity, at 70 per cent of the population infected, it would require around 75,000 deaths in Sweden. This does not take into account that older passengers on the cruise ship probably had better health than the average person of the same age and that reaching herd immunity through natural infection would put an additional burden on health care.

For some countries, the case fatality rate was quite low in spring 2020, but this was largely due to a younger population being affected in the early stages of the pandemic. Iceland was early to test a majority of those infected. Admittedly, a study for Iceland estimates IFR at 0.3 per cent.[8] According to this study, however, only 1 per cent of the infected Icelanders were over 80 years old. Thirty per cent of the deceased were under 70 years of age. As many as 2.4 per cent of those infected in the age group 70–79 died. With the same age-related IFR as in Iceland, the IFR in Sweden would be about 0.9 per cent at an even spread of infection. In Singapore, only 0.05 per cent of PCR-positive persons died, but young guest workers made up 96 per cent of those infected, whereas only 0.3 per cent were persons over the age of 70.[9] Australia and New Zealand had a case fatality rate in spring 2020 substantially below other countries, but was still above 1 per cent if adjustments are made to the lag between infection and death.[10]

Antibody studies provided early important clues on the spread of the pandemic, but no tests are perfect. First, it takes time to develop antibodies, and then different tests may show different results. Sensitivity is the share of true positives that test positive with the test (i.e. with a high sensitivity few real positives are missed). Specificity is the share of positively tested that are not false positive. If the specificity

TABLE 8.3 Comparison of claims by researchers associated with FHM, the implied IFR for the population of Sweden and implied Covid-19 deaths for Sweden under various assumptions, at different points in time before the second wave.

Source/ claimant	*Date, 2020*	*Based on the following evidence or reasoning*	*Further assumptions in this study*	*Claimed or implied IFR*	*Implied IFR for demographic of Sweden*	*Implied Covid-19 deaths in Sweden if 40% infected*	*Implied Covid-19 deaths in Sweden if 70% infected*
Giesecke[31]	17/4	Only 0.1% will die from the pandemic		0.1	0.1	4,000	7,000
FHM[32]	21/4	Model shows that 17% infected in Stockholm by 11/4, based on 2.5% active infection 27/3–3/4 and 5 days viral shedding	1,850 Covid-19 deaths in Stockholm 9/3–1/5	(0.5)	(0.6)	25,000	45,000
Giesecke[33]	1/5	20–25% of Stockholm had the infection up to 29/4	2,252 Covid-19 deaths in Stockholm 9/3–20/5	(0.4)	(0.6)	24,000	41,000
Giesecke[34]	8/5	IFR is 0.1–0.2%, slightly higher than for influenza		0.1–0.2	(0.1–0.2)	4,000–8,000	7,000–14,000
Britton[35]	10/5	IFR is 0.39% based on 2.5% on-going infection in Stockholm March/April and 5 days window of testing positive		0.39	0.39	16,000	28,000
Tegnell[36]	20/5	Claim that 20% in Stockholm have immunity, not 7% as shown by antibody study of FHM	2,252 Covid-19 deaths in Stockholm 9/3–17/5	(0.5)	(0.6)	26,000	45,000
Analysis unit of FHM[37]	16/6	Models show 0.6% IFR in Stockholm, based on 2.5% active infection 27/3–3/4, official death rates, and 10 net days viral shedding	FHM admits that actual IFR is 28% higher if excess mortality is used	0.8	(1.0)	40,000	75,000

TABLE 8.3 (Continued)

Source/ claimant	*Date, 2020*	*Based on the following evidence or reasoning*	*Further assumptions in this study*	*Claimed or implied IFR*	*Implied IFR for demographic of Sweden*	*Implied Covid-19 deaths in Sweden if 40% infected*	*Implied Covid-19 deaths in Sweden if 70% infected*
Tegnell[38]	16/6	14% had antibodies among all tested in Stockholm [despite positive bias], entailing above 20% infected by 16/6	2,691 Covid-19 deaths in Stockholm 9/3–7/7	(0.6)	(0.8)	30,000	55,000
Tegnell[39]	19/6	The 5% that had antibodies among blood donors in 9 regions 25/5–31/5 are not representative; the true number is over 20%	5,992 Covid-19 deaths in Sweden 9/3–5/7	(<0.3)	(<0.3)	<12,000	<21,000
Carlson, press conference	16/7	35–40% immune in Stockholm, double the share with antibodies among those chosen to take antibody test [unrepresentative], due to t-immunity	2,708 Covid-19 deaths in Stockholm 9/3–23/7	(0.3)	(0.3)	13,000	22,000
Tegnell[40]	27/8	At least 20% immune in Sweden	6,458 Covid-19 deaths in Sweden 9/3–17/9	(0.3)	(0.4)	17,000	30,000

Note: The same assumptions apply as in Table 8.2. Numbers in parenthesis: calculations based on the sources, but not explicitly claimed by those.

and the sensitivity are known, it is possible to find out how many have had the infection based on antibody studies, applying the following formula:[11]

$$\text{adjusted prevalence} = \frac{\text{crude prevalence} + \text{specificity} - 1}{\text{sensitivity} + \text{specificity} - 1} \tag{1}$$

Dividing the mortality rate, the ratio of deaths from Covid-19 (reported or excess deaths) to the population, with the adjusted prevalence yields an estimate of the IFR of the invested population. When estimating IFR further adjustments may be made to estimate the probable IFR for the target population, for example Sweden as a whole with its specific age composition, which may deviate from the investigated population:

$$\text{IFR}_{\text{target population}} = \frac{\text{IFR}_{\text{investigated population}}}{\text{bias of the investigated population}} \tag{2}$$

For example, assume that the crude prevalence of the investigated population in a study is 6 per cent, specificity 98 per cent, sensitivity 90 per cent, mortality rate 40 deaths per 100,000 and the bias 0.8 (i.e. the IFR is expected to be 20 per cent lower in the investigated population due to, for example, a larger share of young people). Then, the adjusted prevalence of the investigated population is $(0.05 + 0.98 - 1)/(0.9 + 0.97) = 4.5$ per cent. The IFR of the target population is $0.0004/0.045/0.8 = 1.1$ per cent. Further adjustments have to be made if, for example, reported deaths are used and excess deaths are substantially higher.

Some antibody studies indicated a low IFR. However, interpreting those can be difficult. That antibody tests give an upper limit for IFR in Covid-19 is not true if the proportion with antibodies is low or the sample is non-representative. For example, if the specificity is 98 per cent and sensitivity 100 per cent, then testing a population with no positives will, on average, yield a result of 2 per cent positively tested, and therefore not provide any clue at all of the actual IFR.

With antibody tests performed on larger populations, there was growing evidence of a high IFR. Antibody studies from Belgium, Spain and UK – the countries that were among those hit hardest during spring 2020 – all indicated that the share of the population with antibodies was in the range of 5–7 per cent.[12] It would entail an IFR at around 1 per cent for Belgium, but above 1.5 per cent for England and Spain if excess mortality is used. The high IFR and England and Spain may be indications of substantial stress on the health services.

According to *The Economist*, as of February 2022, the excess deaths of several countries with low vaccination levels were approaching 1 per cent of the population.[13] For example, the excess mortality of Bulgaria 20th of April 2020 to 6th of February 2022 was 0.948 per cent of the population, which in Sweden would entail around 100,000 deaths.

Evidence from Sweden on IFR

Actual empirical evidence from Sweden, presented in Table 8.2, including that collected by FHM, indicated a high IFR in accordance with the international studies. Although data from FHM on Covid-19 deaths correspond quite well to excess mortality in the latter part of 2020, early in the pandemic official Covid-19 deaths were underestimated, especially in Stockholm. For the present study, the maximum of excess deaths and official deaths in one week is used as a proxy for the actual number of people that died from the infection in that week. It is important to estimate unreported deaths for countries where actual deaths are much higher than the reported deaths, but also early during the pandemic when testing was at a very low level. For example, *The Economist* estimates that up to 27th of February 2022 there were 20 million global excess deaths, while there were 6 million official global Covid-19 deaths.[14] When excess deaths are higher than the reported deaths, it can be assumed that the difference between excess deaths and reported deaths is a suitable indicator of unreported deaths. However, unreported deaths cannot be negative, and excess deaths should not be used as an indicator of actual deaths if the number is below reported deaths. An assumption is also made that, on average, deaths occurred three weeks after infection, and immunity was developed after two weeks.

The FHM has conducted surveys of how many have been tested positive for on-going infection. 9th of April a study from Stockholm was presented showing that 2.5 per cent had an active infection March 27–April 3. There is uncertainty on how long an infected is tested positively, and sensitivity is not 100 per cent. Median estimates of mild cases range from nine to over 20 days.[22] According to a meta-study the probability of a false-negative result in an infected person reaches its lowest point of 20 per cent on day 8.[23] Making the same assumption as FHM[24] of a ten net days window for testing positive would entail an IFR of 0.9 per cent. However, Stockholm has a younger population than the rest of the country, and pre-pandemic mortality (in 2019) was 33 per cent higher for Sweden than for Stockholm. The Stockholm study would therefore entail an IFR as high as 1.3 per cent for Sweden. Two studies showed that an estimated 0.9 per cent of the population had an on-going infection on April 21–24 and 0.3 per cent May 25–28, which would entail an IFR of around 1 per cent as well.

The first antibody study was presented by FHM 20th of May, showing that in Stockholm 7.3 per cent of visitors to health centres had antibodies May 3–May 9.[25] This would entail an IFR of 1.1 per cent in Stockholm if visitors to health centres were representative of the population, but even higher in Sweden, at 1.5 per cent, adjusting for differences in CDR in Sweden compared to Stockholm. This was at a similar level as indicated by the test of on-going infection in Stockholm. Stockholm was probably hit very hard at the beginning of the pandemic, not unlike the situation in Spain and England. Here no adjustments are made to sensitivity and specificity due to the uncertainty of these values. Assuming a sensitivity of 99.4

per cent and a specificity of 98.9 per cent in accordance with the claims of FHM would yield an adjusted prevalence of 6.3 per cent, while assuming a sensitivity of only 80 per cent would entail an adjusted prevalence of 7.9 per cent. In both cases the estimated IFR for Sweden would be substantially above 1 per cent. The representativity can also be questioned, but there are no strong reasons to suspect a bias in any direction. The antibody study also indicated that the older age group had lower prevalence of antibodies, and making adjustment for the age difference would yield an even higher estimated IFR.

According to a study of FHM from 18th June 2020, 5.0 per cent of blood donors tested in late May were seropositive in nine regions within outpatient care.[26] Unadjusted for sensitivity and specificity, and assuming no bias, it would yield an IFR of 1.1 per cent.

A random study of antibodies from Rinkeby-Kista,[27] which can be considered representative, indicated an IFR around 1 per cent or above.

The point of Tables 8.1 and 8.2 is not the exact numbers, but to show that empirical evidence both internationally and from Sweden indicated, as early as in spring 2020, that reaching herd immunity in Sweden through natural infection would have required mortalities at a much higher level than was experienced, in the range of 50,000–100,000, as compared to 15,000 actual deaths in Sweden before the population was vaccinated in autumn 2021. This empirical evidence is largely in line with a study of different scenarios presented by Henrik Sjödin et al. (with Joacim Rocklöv as the corresponding author) on 7th April 2020.[28] Under no changes in behaviour and policy, this study predicted 50,695 deaths assuming all critical care demands were satisfied, but an additional 47,507 deaths from critical care shortage (totalling 98,202 deaths). However, with 50 per cent reduction in contacts in ages 0–59 years and 90 per cent reduction in ages 60+ years the number of deaths could be kept down to 5,117 according to the study, while even harsher restrictions would have reduced the number of deaths to just 166. The empirical evidence presented in this chapter entails that even if Sweden failed to keep down deaths compared to Nordic countries, the restrictions that were implemented may have saved as much as 50,000 lives, while an additional 10,000 lives may have been saved if the same strategy would had been followed as in, for example, Norway. The main reason why 50,000–100,000 lives were not lost in Sweden is that Sweden had to abandon the herd immunity strategy.

In autumn 2020 some countries, especially in central Europe that previously had kept deaths rates low, became even less stringent than Sweden, with dire consequences during the second wave. Figure 8.1 demonstrates that the stringency index (ranging from 0 to 100 per cent) in Europe weighed by population came in line with Sweden from June 2020.[29] The "Swedish experiment" became international. Sweden was used internationally as an example to abandon restrictions. Europe dismantled its restrictions too fast. While reported deaths per million of inhabitants due to Covid-19 was twice as large in Sweden compared to Europe in the first half of 2020, afterwards Europe had more reported deaths per inhabitant

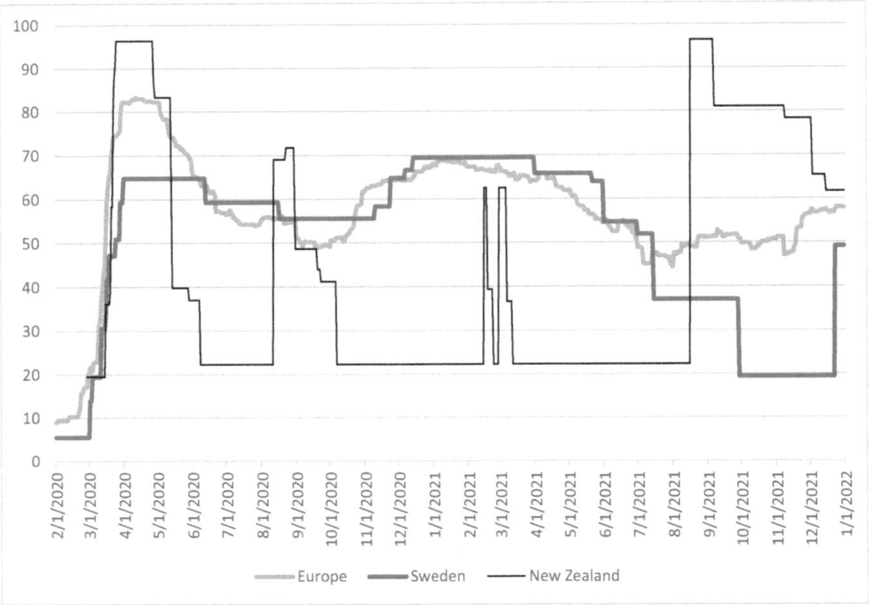

FIGURE 8.1 The stringency index in Sweden, Europe (weighed by population) and New Zealand in 2020–2021

Source: Our World in Data. Hannah Ritchie, Edouard Mathieu, Lucas Rodés-Guirao, Cameron Appel, Charlie Giattino, Esteban Ortiz-Ospina, Joe Hasell, Bobbie Macdonald, Diana Beltekian and Max Roser (2020) – "Coronavirus Pandemic (COVID-19)". *Published online at OurWorldInData.org.* Retrieved from: https://ourworldindata.org/coronavirus [Online Resource]

than Sweden. As pointed out in Emil J. Bergholtz's chapter, when the spread of the virus is at a low level, restrictions do not have to be so harsh. For example, New Zealand has successfully followed a zero-Covid strategy, but during most of the pandemic its stringency index has been below that in both Europe and Sweden (see Figure 8.1).

Claims of immunity levels and IFR by researchers supporting the Swedish strategy

Table 8.3 summarizes claims of immunity levels by various researchers linked to FHM: Anders Tegnell, state epidemiologist, Johan Carlson, the Director-General of the agency, Johan Giesecke, the architect behind the Swedish strategy, and Tom Britton, who helped the agency to get the mathematics right. It was Giesecke who recruited Carlson and Tegnell to FHM, and has called them "my boys".[30] The table shows that there was a systematic bias, in that these researchers put IFR lower or much lower than what was indicated by empirical evidence in Tables 8.1 and 8.2, but their estimates differed considerably compared to each other.

Discussion on the tests of on-going infection

On the 21st of April 2020, the FHM[41] presented a model that 17 per cent had been infected by the 11th of April in Stockholm, and a prognosis this would increase to 26 per cent on the 1st of May. It was strongly argued that herd immunity was within reach. The first version of their model had to be withdrawn since according to one of the scenarios the number of infected people in Stockholm exceeded the number of inhabitants.[42] The whole model was based on the incorrect assumption that a person tested positive only for five days. The starting point was the empirical observation that 2.5 per cent of Stockholm's population had tested positive for Covid-19 from March 27 to April 3 (see Table 8.2). It was estimated that 17 per cent had had the virus on April 11. How could one leap from 2.5 per cent to 17 per cent? The model assumed that you can only test positive for the virus for five days, and then you become immune. Let's say then that 2.5 per cent fall ill every five days. It will be 0.5 per cent per day. After 34 days, you get 17 per cent. Simplified, with a sickness rate of 0.5 per cent per day during March and the beginning of April for 34 days, you would get the figure that FHM's model gets for April 11. At the same rate, you get 27 per cent on May 1, which was exactly what FHM's model said. But in reality, infected persons test positive for significantly longer than five days, not infrequently even after they have recovered.

Tom Britton constructed a mathematical model showing that 40 per cent infection rate could be sufficient to reach herd immunity,[43] instead of 60–80 per cent as generally assumed. Britton further used the study by FHM to predict that deaths from corona would not be higher than 12,000 after herd immunity had been reached:[44]

> More than 3,000 Swedes have so far died from the coronavirus, but according to a recent estimate by Tom Britton, professor of mathematical statistics at Stockholm University, the pandemic will probably have claimed between 8,000 and 20,000 Swedes' lives in the end.
>
> The starting point in the calculations was an estimate from the FHM on how many people in Stockholm County had been infected by the virus up to and including 6 April, which was 15 per cent. By dividing the number of deaths up to and including April 30 (1,406 people), as it takes about three weeks from the time of infection to death, with the number of estimated infections, Tom Britton estimated a fatality rate of 0.39 per cent.
>
> But I think the fatality rate will decrease somewhat in the future, because we will probably be better at treating the sick and protecting the elderly. So, my best guess is that there will be about 12,000 dead, says Tom Britton to TT.

A qualified guess is here that Britton's number of 8,000 rests on an IFR of 0.2 per cent and herd immunity reached at 40 per cent infection rate, 12,000 on an IFR of 0.3 per cent and herd immunity at 40 per cent, and 20,000 on an IFR of 0.4 per cent and herd immunity 50 per cent.

Besides the problem of the assumption of five days viral shedding, most deaths occurred in the estimation sample during a period when the excess mortality was at its highest compared to the reported mortality (due to the low rate of testing in the early phases of the pandemic). Another problem was to use a study of Stockholm, with a much younger population, to estimate the death rates for the rest of the country.

In a later study from June, the analysis unit of FHM dropped the assumption of five days viral shedding.[45] As stated in the report:

> We surveyed the literature of the PCR testing window (also known as the duration of viral shedding) in order to come up with a valid parameterization for our purposes. Our chosen value of ten days is based largely on Hu et al. (2020).
>
> We also considered the following studies that included and presented results separately for patients with milder infections. Zheng et al. (2020) report a median testing window of 14 days in a subset of 22 hospitalized patients with mild disease in China, which is shorter compared to the median of 21 days reported for 74 patients with severe disease. Yongchen et al. (2020) find a median testing window of 10 days among 11 nonsevere hospitalized patients in China, and a median of 18 days among 5 asymptomatic cases. Other studies surveyed included both a mix of mild, moderate and severe hospitalized cases, but did not report results by group. There is considerable variation in the estimates, but such studies typically reported median values of 12–20 days.

The analysis unit of FHM estimated the IFR to 0.6 per cent, in Stockholm based on the same data, but with the assumption of ten days window for testing positive (in the lower band of estimates of the duration of viral shedding, although the net value should also adjust for sensitivity), while an assumption of five days would only entail an IFR of 0.3–0.4 per cent. The report also admitted that the estimate of 0.6 per cent could be an underestimation as well, due to higher excess mortality than reported mortality:

> During weeks 13–17, when 97% of the deaths in our estimation sample occurred, the ratio of excess mortality to confirmed deaths in Stockholm was 1.24. When we weight this ratio by the weekly shares of deaths in the estimation sample, we get a factor of 1.28. Taken at face value, our IFR estimate should be adjusted upward with the same factor. We can't incorporate the excess mortality numbers formally into our current estimation framework, however, since we cannot link the deaths to any cases and hence not to any onset dates. In light of this, we're therefore inclined to view our original IFR estimates as conservative, rather than presenting adjusted numbers.

Furthermore, the report does not consider that the crude death rate in Sweden is 33 per cent higher than in Stockholm. Multiplying 0.6 by 1.28 and by 1.33 yields an IFR of 1.0 per cent, in accordance with international studies. No calculation on the IFR was made using the national surveys by FHM, available 8th of May, which would have shown an IFR closer to 1 per cent as well (see Table 8.2).

Hence, using the same empirical evidence, 2.5 per cent with on-going infection in March/April, while assuming a 0.3 per cent IFR and 40 per cent infection rate yields 12,000 deaths under herd immunity, assuming a 1.0 per cent IFR and 70 per cent infection rate yields 75,000 deaths under herd immunity. The various unrealistic assumptions of, for example, Tom Britton added up to decreasing actual levels of estimated deaths under a state of herd immunity reached by natural infection by as much as 75–90 per cent!

The discussion on antibodies in April and May 2020

Before FHM presented its antibody study in 20th May, there were several other antibody studies studying Swedish conditions, but not all of them were representative of the population at large.

In a *Lancet* article Giesecke argued:[46]

> PCR testing and some straightforward assumptions indicate that, as of April 29, 2020, more than half a million people in Stockholm county, Sweden, which is about 20–25% of the population, have been infected (Hansson D, FHM, personal communication). 98–99% of these people are probably unaware or uncertain of having had the infection; they either had symptoms that were severe, but not severe enough for them to go to a hospital and get tested, or no symptoms at all. Serology testing is now supporting these assumptions.

The serology testing that Giesecke referred to, was a study conducted of employees at one hospital in Stockholm (Danderyds sjukhus). Despite that it is well known that health workers were much more exposed to the virus than the rest of the population, Giesecke still assumed that hospital staff was representative of the surrounding population. His claim of 20–25 per cent immunity in Stockholm would still entail an IFR of 0.4 per cent in Stockholm (not taking into account higher CDR in Sweden), which contradicted his earlier claim of 0.1 per cent[47] and later of 0.1–0.2 per cent.[48]

A press release from the Karolinska hospital 18th of May claimed that:[49]

> About 15 per cent of healthy people in Stockholm have undergone or are now infected with the virus that causes Covid-19. It shows results from the research study conducted at Karolinska University Hospital. . . .
>
> We have sampled a large number of employees with different tasks, both close to patients and not close to patients, and have thus gained an idea of the spread of the infection in Stockholm's working population. Our data then

> indicate that about 15 per cent have or have had SARS-CoV-2 coronavirus infection, says Joakim Dillner, professor of infection epidemiology and responsible for the Covid-19 study.

At a press conference the same day, Tegnell purported that the study from Karolinska[50] was in line with the models of FHM. The problem was that the study also showed that 7 per cent of the hospital staff had an on-going infection, which could be compared to between 0.9–2.5 per cent of Stockholm's population according to studies of FHM that had been published by then, which indicate that infection rate of the hospital staff was at least three times larger than for the population. Using the formula (1), and assuming $bias = 7/2.5$, would yield that only 5 per cent of inhabitants of Stockholm had been infected.

When the first antibody studies by FHM were presented in 20th May, showing that only 7.3 per cent of visitors to health centres in Stockholm had antibodies, Anders Tegnell commented:[51]

> "It is not 7 per cent now. We are somewhere at 20 per cent plus in Stockholm," Anders Tegnell about the figures.

Commenting on the result of FHM, Tom Britton argued:[52]

> One explanation is that FHM's previous forecast was seriously wrong, and also mine. FHM reported that there was a lot of uncertainty about their previous forecast and no one believed it was exact. But this is a large deviation. I'm hesitant.
>
> The second possibility is that the previous forecast showed how many would have been infected. The new prognosis is instead based on how many people have antibodies. Thus, not everyone infected may receive antibodies, at least not at a level that can be detected by the tests, says Britton.

The discussion in summer 2020

Despite that decisive empirical evidence from Sweden and internationally in April, May and early June indicated that IFR of Covid-19 was at the level of 1 per cent if the infection spreads smoothly in the population of a high-income country, and that herd immunity through natural infection would entail at least 50,000 deaths in Sweden, supporters of the Swedish strategy continued to argue for a position that herd immunity was not far away. After the 20th of May, the narrative shifted in various ways. The share of those tested for antibodies voluntarily was used instead, which had a positive bias, given that those wanting to test themselves did so because they suspected having had the infection. It was claimed that immunity was much higher than those having antibodies, which contradicted the claims by FHM of very high sensitivity.

In the Polish newspaper *Gazeta Wyborcza*,[53] Giesecke claimed on June 13 that Stockholm would reach herd immunity in mid-June (although the level that is needed for herd immunity deviated from Britton):

AGNIESZKA LICHNEROWICZ: When will you reach herd immunity in Stockholm?

JOHAN GIESECKE: Soon. In mid-June.

AGNIESZKA LICHNEROWICZ: Does it mean that 60 or 70 per cent of the residents will be immune to the virus?

JOHAN GIESECKE: We can only say that 60 per cent of residents will get Covid-19 by then. We do not know if they are resistant, although everything indicates this. Other coronaviruses circulate among us that lead to the building of herd immunity. It is therefore unlikely that this would be different.

On the 16th of June, *Dagens Nyheter* published an article that 14 per cent of those tested in Stockholm had antibodies.[54] Despite a strong positive bias for those testing themselves voluntarily, Tegnell used it to argue for an even higher immunity level in Stockholm:[55]

> According to state epidemiologist Anders Tegnell, this means that the figures reflect the situation about a month ago:
>
> It takes a couple of weeks to develop antibodies from the time you get sick, so the number is actually significantly higher today. We are working on this and considering that we have a doubling time of the number of cases of about ten days, it should be a little over 20 per cent. But we have to count on it properly, says Tegnell.

Tegnell's claim of the doubling of cases every ten days was contradicted by the number of deaths and hospitalizations decreasing in May and June. Karin Tegmark Wisell, who later in 2021 replaced Johan Carlson as the head of FHM, stated:[56]

> 50,000 tested provides a good statistical basis for the whole group and the figures agree quite well with how we see that the incidence has been and they feel reasonable even compared to other surveys, says Karin Tegmark Wisell, head of department at the Public Health Agency of Sweden.

Commenting on a study by FHM three days later, Tegnell argued:[57]

> In another study, 400 blood donors per week in the nine regions were tested for antibodies. There, the proportion with antibodies increased from 1.6 per cent in week 17 to 5.0 per cent in week 22.
>
> Both groups on the different occasions have relatively low values, probably because they are people who have remained isolated, says Anders Tegnell.

> We have other surveys in society that show significantly higher values, so I do not think you should focus so much on individual values, but look at the trends. Then we gradually put together several surveys into a common result.
>
> We have been saying that we could be up to a little over 20 per cent in May. It seems that we are there, but it is not certain.

Assumption of 20 per cent immunity in late May would entail an IFR of below 0.3 per cent, while using the actual empirical data would quadruple the estimate. The claims of a high level of immunity continued during the summer.

At the Public Health Agency's press conference on 16 July 2020 the Agency's Director-General Johan Carlson estimated that 35–40 per cent in Stockholm have had the infection, that is, close to the assumed herd immunity of a 40 per cent infection rate. This meant an IFR of just about 0.3 per cent. The main argument was to point out that the share of positive tests for antibodies in Stockholm (not representative of the population) was around 20 per cent and to double it due to possible t-cell-immunity. His guesses were dubious given the lack of representativity of those choosing to test themselves for antibodies and claims of FHM that their antibody test had 99.4 per cent sensitivity. These discrepancies of what was said by different parts of FHM was never explained or questioned in the general debate. The view that actual immunity was twice as large as the number having antibodies continued to be held, and as late as the FHM's press conference 27 August 2020, Tegnell estimated that at least 20 per cent had immunity in Sweden.

The political economy of herd immunity

This chapter shows that while both international and Swedish studies indicated a very high IFR, at around 1 per cent or even above, and that herd immunity through natural infection would entail that 50,000–100,000 would die in Sweden, researchers linked to FHM continued to claim that herd immunity was immanent during spring and summer 2020. They also directly contradicted the empirical evidence published by the FHM itself. Their claims were sometimes based on empirical evidence, but those were distorted in various ways, pushing the interpretation to reach a low IFR:

- Studies that included participants that were more prone to have been infected, or had lower mortality, than the Swedish population were taken as representative for Sweden as a whole.
- It was claimed that the infected were a much larger group than persons developing antibodies, contradicting empirical evidence on high sensitivity of antibody tests.
- It was argued that the immunity level to reach herd immunity was much lower than previously thought.
- Reported deaths were used instead of excess death in the early phase of the pandemic when there was a large discrepancy.

- It was implicitly assumed that the IFR could be substantially held down by isolating the risk groups, while at the same time pointing out that it was not possible to shelter communities from the pandemic.

The statements in Table 8.3 were not consistent with each other, which may indicate the FHM and researchers collaborating with the agency did not have a common view. Britton had a quite consistent idea of the IFR and showed how he changed his guesstimates. Anders Tegnell's statements were often seemingly contradictory, for example, in claiming on June 16 that the immunity level was over 20 per cent in Stockholm, and then on June 19 that it was over 20 per cent in Sweden, despite that it being known that Stockholm had a much wider penetration of the virus. Giesecke most blatantly ignored the empirical evidence, claiming as late as May 8 that Covid-19 was not much more serious than influenza (although admitting later, in April 2021, that he got some things wrong).[58] The only sound analysis in Table 8.3 based on empirical evidence concerning assumptions that were made and transparency was the estimation of 0.6 per cent IFR in Stockholm, which was, as admitted, a "conservative" estimate given the excess mortality was not taken into account. This study was largely marginalized by the leading representatives of FHM who continued to push for the view that herd immunity was being approached in summer 2020, at least in Stockholm. Studies based on more realistic assumptions, such as Henrik Sjödin et al. warning early in the pandemic of up to 100,000 deaths if the herd immunity strategy would be fully implemented,[59] were ignored or ridiculed.

Science is not about always being right, especially when there is no empirical evidence or the latter point in different directions, but a scientific method cannot entail that empirical evidence is disregarded or twisted selectively to suit specific policies. A scientific method entails an openness for empirical evidence to falsify one's hypotheses. Unfortunately, actual research practices do not always conform to such ideals. Thomas Kuhn has shown that researchers often stick to the paradigm they learned, even when empirical evidence contradicts those, and anomalies are ignored and downplayed.[60] Paradigmatic change is not a smooth process and often occurs when the empirical evidence becomes overwhelming, which pushes the old paradigm to the fringes (as happened internationally with the herd immunity strategy in 2021).

Alvesson and Spicer argue against the one-sided hypothesis that organizations mobilize cognitive capabilities.[61] Functional stupidity entails that stupidity and ignorance can play a functional role in organizations, for example by marginalizing doubt and blocking communicative acts, with positive outcomes such as the strengthening of cohesion of the organization. Functional stupidity is often dominant in a context where image and symbolic manipulation is important. This would, for example, entail that if health authorities prioritize pleasing politicians and the public opinion over saving lives, such organizations would be prone to practicing functional stupidity. Historically, good crisis management is rather the exception. Incompetent crisis management is the most common response to chocks, which is underpinned by various vested interests.

Government politicians and the Swedish press tended to assume that expert authorities represented science could not be wrong, and always acted in the public interest. A relaxed and incompetent attitude in the face of large crises has some historical roots in Sweden.[62] The passivity of FHM and other Swedish agencies has similarities to the inaction of *Medicinalstyrelsen*, which had the overall responsibility for health care, during the Spanish flu 1918–1920.[63] The physician Arnold Josefson proposed active measures, such as prolonged school vacations, suspended military training (800 young conscripts later died because the training was not suspended) and a ban on meetings of various kinds, which his opponents called meaningless. An argument against restrictions was also that it was better to attain immunity as fast as possible, given that the disease course is milder early in an epidemic than later.[64]

Sweden's model of state agencies is unique internationally,[65] which as discussed by Sigurd Bergmann in this book was established by Chancellor Axel Oxenstierna in the 17th century. No representative of the Government may decide how a subordinate state agency shall apply the law or decide an individual case. This kind of feudal vestige gives the agencies a lot of power over their activities. Civil servant liability was abolished in 1974, which entails that unelected civil servants displaying grave negligence, incompetence and favouritism can continue being employed without consequences as long as they retain their loyalty to the power structure. Although Sweden had a left-wing Government during the pandemic, and the pandemic mostly hurt social layers voting for the Social Democrats (immigrants, workers and elders), those formulating the Swedish strategy were heavily influenced by views that were also held by the international right. Criticism of state agencies has historically been viewed as negative in Sweden, as undermining their authority. For example, when the physician Arnold Josefson criticized *Medicinalstyrelsen* for their "nihilistic" attitude to the Spanish flu, he was blasted for venting his suggestions in public.[66] Similar arguments were directed against critiques of the handling FHM during the Covid-19 pandemic.

The field of political economy emphasizes that the state is not a neutral agent that is completely free from interest groups or cognitive biases. Public choice theory and applications of game theory on politics explain how political decisions can result in outcomes that are not preferred by the general public. The interest of a vocal minority with much to lose is often satisfied to the detriment of a majority that is not vocal. Marxism[67] points out that the state ultimately serves the dominant social class, and there is a connection between civil servants and the bourgeois class, through family and other connections, shaping their ideological and moral outlook, although not in a deterministic manner.

If the policy is to be based on science, and respect for human lives, the starting point should be to recognize that science is a process where established expert knowledge must be questioned. Balance of power is an important institutional principle for both scientific endeavour and government. A lesson is that other, independent, researchers also need to make their reviews and estimates during an on-going crisis, and the political leadership, the media and the public should just accept that analyses from authorities, experts and researchers could differ. Another lesson is that scientific practice needs to be based on ethics, and never to be used to hurt people either directly or indirectly – but how to at least approach such an ideal is a major challenge for social sciences to answer in the future.

Notes

1 *Our World in Data*, https://ourworldindata.org/; Russel, Timothy et al. "Estimating the Infection and Case Fatality Ratio for Covid-19 Using Age-Adjusted Data from the Outbreak on the Diamond Princess Cruise Ship", https://cmmid.github.io/topics/Covid19/diamond_cruise_cfr_estimates.html (2020).
2 VRT. "Just 6% of Belgians Have Antibodies Against Covid-19", 8 May 2020, www.vrt.be/vrtnws/en/2020/05/08/just-6-of-belgians-have-antibodies-against-Covid-19/ .
3 Carreño, Belén. "Spanish Antibody Study Suggests 5% of Population Affected by Coronavirus", *Reuters*, 13 May 2020, www.reuters.com/article/us-health-coronavirus-spain-idUSKBN22P1IK; Pollán, Marina et al. "Prevalence of SARS-CoV-2 in Spain (ENE-Covid): A Nationwide, Population-Based Seroepidemiological Study", *Lancet* 396:10250 (2020): 535–544.
4 *Our World in Data.*
5 VRT. "6.9% of Blood Samples Contain Novel Coronavirus Anti-Bodies", 5 June 2020, www.vrt.be/vrtnws/en/2020/06/05/6-9-of-blood-samples-contain-novel-coronavirus-anti-bodies/ .
6 Ward, Helen et al. "Antibody Prevalence for SARS-CoV-2 in England Following First Peak of the Pandemic: REACT2 Study in 100,000 Adults", *medRxiv*, 2020.
7 Gudbjartsson, Daniel et al. "Humoral Immune Response to SARS-CoV-2 in Iceland", *The New England Journal of Medicine* 383 (2020): 1724–1734.
8 *Ibid.*
9 Tan, Trevor et al. "Coronavirus Disease 2019 (Covid-19): The Singapore Experience. A Review of the First Eight Months", *Annales Academy of Medicine Singapore* 49 (2020): 764–778.
10 *Our World in Data.*
11 Based on Sempos, Christopher, and Lu Tian. "Adjusting Coronavirus Prevalence Estimates for Laboratory Test Kit Error", *American Journal of Epidemiology* 190:1 (2021): 109–115.
12 VRT. "Just 6% of Belgians"; VRT. "6.9% of blood samples"; Ward et al. "Antibody Prevalence for SARS-CoV-2 in England"; Carreño. "Spanish Antibody Study"; Pollán. "Prevalence of SARS-CoV-2 in Spain".
13 *The Economist.* "Tracking Covid-19 Excess Deaths Across Countries", 21 February 2022, www.economist.com/graphic-detail/coronavirus-excess-deaths-tracker .
14 *The Economist.* "The pandemic's true death toll: Our daily estimate of excess deaths around the world", 27 February 2022, www.economist.com/graphic-detail/coronavirus-excess-deaths-estimates .
15 FHM. "Resultat från undersökning av förekomsten av Covid-19 i region Stockholm", 2020, www.folkhalsomyndigheten.se/nyheter-och-press/nyhetsarkiv/2020/april/resultat-fran-undersokning-av-forekomsten-av-Covid-19-i-region-stockholm .
16 FHM. "Nya resultat från undersökning av förekomsten av Covid-19 i Sverige", 2020, www.folkhalsomyndigheten.se/nyheter-och-press/nyhetsarkiv/2020/maj/nya-resultat-fran-undersokning-av-forekomsten-av-Covid-19-i-sverige/ .
17 FHM. "Första resultaten från pågående undersökning av antikroppar för Covid-19-virus", 2020, www.folkhalsomyndigheten.se/nyheter-och-press/nyhetsarkiv/2020/maj/forsta-resultaten-fran-pagaende-undersokning-av-antikroppar-for-Covid-19-virus/ .
18 FHM. "Första resultaten om antikroppar efter genomgången Covid-19 hos blodgivare", 2020, www.folkhalsomyndigheten.se/nyheter-och-press/nyhetsarkiv/2020/juni/forsta-resultaten-om-antikroppar-efter-genomgangen-Covid-19-hos-blodgivare/ .

19 FHM. "Nya resultat om förekomst av Covid-19 i Sverige", 2020, www.folkhalsomyndigheten.se/nyheter-och-press/nyhetsarkiv/2020/juni/nya-resultat-om-forekomst-av-Covid-19-i-sverige/ .
20 FHM. "Förekomsten av antikroppar mot SARS-CoV-2 i stadsdelsområdet Rinkeby-Kista, Stockholm, 22–24 juni 2020", 2020, www.folkhalsomyndigheten.se/contentassets/2cf102cd299c4382b9a0447dc0626356/forekomsten-antikroppar-rinkeby-kista.pdf .
21 www.folkhalsomyndigheten.se and www.scb.se .
22 Kucirka, Lauren, Stephen A. Lauer, Oliver Laeyendecker, Denali Boon, and Justin Lessler. "Variation in False-Negative Rate of Reverse Transcriptase Polymerase Chain Reaction – Based SARS-CoV-2 Tests by Time Since Exposure", *Annals of Internal Medicine*, M20–1495 (13 May 2020); Wikramaratna, Paul et al. "Estimating False-Negative Detection Rate of SARS-CoV-2 by RT-PCR", *medRxiv*, 2020.
23 Kucirka et al. "Variation in False-Negative Rate".
24 FHM. "Estimates of the Number of Infected Individuals During the Covid-19 Outbreak in the Dalarna Region, Skåne Region, Stockholm Region, and Västra Götaland Region, Sweden", 2020, www.folkhalsomyndigheten.se/publicerat-material/publikationsarkiv/e/estimates-of-the-number-of-infected-individuals-during-the-Covid-19-outbreak/ .
25 FHM. "Första resultaten från pågående undersökning av antikroppar för Covid-19-virus".
26 FHM. "Första resultaten om antikroppar efter genomgången Covid-19 hos blodgivare".
27 FHM. "Förekomsten av antikroppar mot SARS-CoV-2 i stadsdelsområdet Rinkeby-Kista".
28 Sjödin, Henrik et al. "Covid-19 Health Care Demand and Mortality in Sweden in Response to Non-Pharmaceutical (NPIs) Mitigation and Suppression Scenarios", 2020, www.medrxiv.org/content/10.1101/2020.03.20.20039594v2.full.pdf .
29 Based on *Our World in Data*.
30 Karlsten, Emanuel. "Tegnell-mejlen: Berättelsen om Johan Giesecke och Folkhälsomyndigheten", 2020, https://emanuelkarlsten.se/tegnell-mejlen-berattelsen-om-johan-giesecke-och-folkhalsomyndigheten/ .
31 "Johan Giesecke One Year on: Did Sweden Succeed?" *UnHerd*, 16 April 2021, www.youtube.com/watch?v=0017zNe7obo .
32 FHM. "Skattning av peakdag och antal infekterade i Covid-19-utbrottet i Stockholms län februari-april 2020", 2020, www.folkhalsomyndigheten.se/contentassets/2da059f90b90458d8454a04955d1697f/skattning-peakdag-antal-infekterade-Covid-19-utbrottet-stockholms-lan-februari-april-2020.pdf .
33 Giesecke, Johan. "The Invisible Pandemic", *The Lancet* 395:10238 (2020): E98.
34 Svahn, Clas. "Giesecke: Om ett år är övriga Norden i kapp Sveriges dödstal", *Dagens Nyheter*, 8 May 2020, www.dn.se/nyheter/sverige/giesecke-om-ett-ar-ar-ovriga-norden-i-kapp-sveriges-dodstal/ .
35 Nilsson, Johan. "Tiondelarna som avgör tusentals svenskars öde", *Svenska Dagbladet*, 10 May 2020, www.svd.se/tiondelarna-som-avgor-tusentals-svenskars-ode .
36 *SVT*. "FHM:s antikroppstester avviker från prognoserna – matematikern 'ser två förklaringar'", 20 May 2020, www.svt.se/nyheter/inrikes/antikroppstester .
37 FHM. "The Infection Fatality Rate of Covid-19 in Stockholm – Technical Report", 2020, www.folkhalsomyndigheten.se/contentassets/53c0dc391be54f5d959ead9131edb771/infection-fatality-rate-Covid-19-stockholm-technical-report.pdf .
38 Svahn, Clas, and Mia Holmgren. "Antikroppar hos en av sju testade i Stockholm", *Dagens Nyheter*, 16 June 2020, www.dn.se/nyheter/sverige/var-sjunde-stockholmare-har-utvecklat-antikroppar/ .
39 *SVT*. "FHM:s antikroppstester".
40 FHM Press Conference, 27 August 2020.
41 FHM. "Skattning av peakdag".
42 See Emil J. Bergholtz's chapter.
43 Majlard, Jan. "Ny kalkyl: Stockholm kan nå flockimmunitet i juni", *Svenska Dagbladet*, 9 May 2020, www.svd.se/ny-berakning-stockholm-kan-na-immunitet-i-juni .

44 Nilsson. "Tiondelarna som avgör tusentals svenskars öde". Author's translation from Swedish.
45 FHM. "The Infection Fatality Rate of Covid-19 in Stockholm".
46 Giesecke. "The Invisible Pandemic".
47 *Newsvoice*. "Prof Johan Giesecke: Dödligheten för Covid-19 endast 0,1% – 'Lockdown är fel coronastrategi'", 18 April 2020, https://newsvoice.se/2020/04/prof-johan-giesecke-dodligheten-for-Covid-19-endast-01-lockdown-ar-fel-coronastrategi/ .
48 Svahn. "Giesecke".
49 Sjölund, Kim. "Stor studie kartlägger coronasmitta i Stockholm", 2020, https://news.cision.com/se/karolinska-universitetssjukhuset/r/stor-studie-kartlagger-coronasmitta-i-stockholm,c3114898 . Author's translation from Swedish.
50 Pramsten, Sara. "Studie: 15 procent på Karolinska har haft viruset", *Läkartidningen*, 18 May 2020, https://lakartidningen.se/aktuellt/nyheter/2020/05/studie-15-procent-pa-karolinska-har-haft-viruset/ .
51 *SVT*. "FHM:s antikroppstester". Author's translation from Swedish.
52 *Ibid.*
53 Lichnerowicz, Agnieszka. "Szwedzki zakaźnik: Lockdown nie ratuje nikogo. W Polsce odsuwacie zgony na później", *Gazeta Wyborcza*, 13 June 2020, https://wyborcza.pl/magazyn/7,124059,26026860,szwedzki-zakaznik-lockdown-nie-ratuje-nikogo-w-polsce.html?disableRedirects=true . Author's translation from Polish.
54 Svahn and Holmbren. "Antikroppar hos en av sju testade i Stockholm".
55 Author's translation from Swedish.
56 Svahn and Holmbren. "Antikroppar hos en av sju testade i Stockholm". Author's translation from Swedish.
57 *SVT*. "Långsam ökning av andelen personer med antikroppar", 19 June 2020, www.svt.se/nyheter/inrikes/6-1-har-antikroppar-enligt-undersokning-fran-fhm . Author's translation from Swedish.
58 *UnHerd*. "Johan Giesecke One Year on".
59 Sjödin et al. "Covid-19 Health Care Demand and Mortality in Sweden".
60 Kuhn, Thomas. *The Structure of Scientific Revolutions*, Chicago: University of Chicago Press, 1962.
61 Alvesson, Mats, and André Spicer. "A Stupidity-Based Theory of Organizations", *Journal of Management Studies* 48:7 (2012): 1194–1220.
62 See also Anders Vahlne's and Jens Stilhoff Sörensen's chapters.
63 Åman, Margareta, *Spanska sjukan: den svenska epidemin 1918–1920 och dess internationella bakgrund*, Uppsala: Uppsala universitet, 1990.
64 *Ibid.*, 166.
65 Peterson, Olof, *Den offentliga makten*, Lund: Studentlitteratur, 2017.
66 Åman. *Spanska sjukan.*
67 Miliband, Ralph. *The State in Capitalist Society*, London: Weidenfeld and Nicolson, 1969.

9

CHILDREN AT THE FRONT LINE OF THE COVID-19 PANDEMIC

Johanna Höög

Introduction

Children are left to our mercy, which is why they are supposed to be a country's most protected citizens. One could consider this a pillar of a civilized society. Unfortunately, this is far from true in practice. In recent Swedish modern history, there have been two catastrophes that severely shook the entire population – the sinking of the cruise liner *Estonia* in 1994 and the tsunami in Southeast Asia on Christmas Day 2004. 852 persons succumbed in the *Estonia* shipwreck. Of the 137 survivors, no one was under 12 years of age. Unfortunately, there was also little to be done to protect children during the tsunami catastrophe, and 543 Swedes died, of which 120 were children below 16 years of age.[1] However, during these kinds of disasters one can argue that children might just not survive as easily in those suddenly dangerous situations.

When this catastrophe came, we had time to prepare, and children could have been protected. Sweden, a country known for a high quality of life and family-friendly lifestyle, decided to keep schools open with minor protective measures in place. At the same time, children with symptoms were not tested during large parts of the pandemic, making the spread of Covid-19 amongst children uncontrolled. This chapter will describe and discuss how Swedish children were treated under the biggest medical and scientific crisis the country has experienced in a century.

When the Covid-19 pandemic spread over the world, most countries reacted by closing schools and universities for in-person teaching. It was logical to protect children until it was known what kind of disease this new virus caused and how it affected children specifically.

In Sweden, most schools were not only kept open, but they also went on like normal (Figure 9.1). The precautions communicated by the Public Health Agency of Sweden (FHM) was that pupils should wash their hands, stay at home if sick and

DOI: 10.4324/9781003289364-10

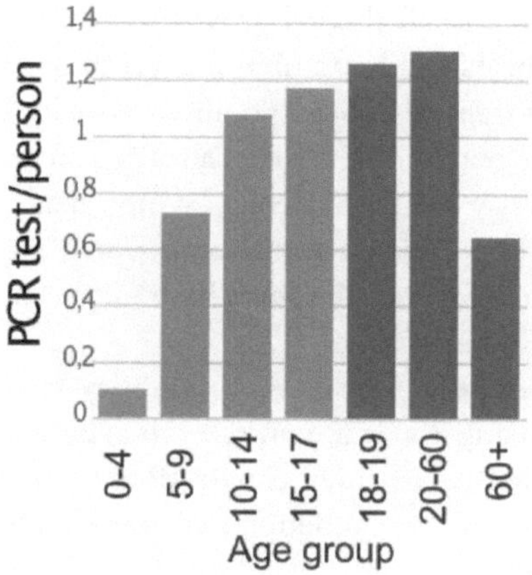

FIGURE 9.1 Children in Sweden during the pandemic. PCR/person in relation to age group, *Source*: Graph by the author. Data provided on request by Maria Thorlund from FHM. Children have had limited access to PCR testing, even when testing was recommended. Testing of children under the age of 6 was never recommended.

One man contacted me and told me about his family, where both his wife and his 92-year-old mum who lived with them were in a risk group. They kept their children home from school, to protect the family from falling ill in Covid-19, which they feared could kill one or both of them. Together, they home educated their children as well as they could, the mum being a teacher herself, but received no help from school. The principal of the school claimed that their environment is safe and reported them repeatedly to social services for the children not attending school. The school refused to grade the children, and with that, their future educational possibilities were destroyed. The family was also forced to pay fines. When they appealed against the fines, they were told that it is the job of the legal guardian of children to make sure they attend school and that duty weighs heavier than the rights of children to decide for themselves. With that, lawyer fees came on top of fines and the family has now paid over $10,000 for not sending their children to school. In a final exchange, he writes that his mum still got Covid-19 from a health care aid they had. She sadly passed away, but he is thankful because at least his children know that it was not they who infected their grandma and caused her death.

This is just the story of one family, but it is important to tell, as it demonstrates the societal stance in Sweden during the Covid-19 pandemic.

try to socially distance. For small children it was even asserted that socially distancing was impossible, establishing a low ambition level throughout the school system. Information about how schools would go about socially distancing in buildings often too small for their number of students already before the pandemic was not provided either. To this day the FHM denies asymptomatic and airborne spread as a major routes of Covid-19 disease transmission, which means that measures such as facemasks and regular airing out of rooms have not been recommended or used in general in *the whole Swedish society*.

To be physically present in school is compulsory from age 6. This law was fully enforced even during the pandemic, or maybe even especially so. Even children from families with confirmed Covid-19 at home were obliged to attend school in the beginning of the pandemic and until 1 December 2020,[2] which includes the entire first wave and the whole rise of the second wave. At the same time, children from families where someone was in a risk group were not exempted from the rule that all children should go to school.[3] Open schools became an issue of national pride – and parents who broke the law and kept their children at home were often reported to social services and some were even fined (see textbox).

In summary, children were legally bound to attend school during the entire pandemic. At the same time, no preventative measures were put in place such as recommending facemasks or increased ventilation. This led to a situation where parents were not free to protect their children, and in extension, their families, from being infected with SARS-CoV-2. One can wonder why parents and society would accept such a situation, and I will argue here that the reason they did so is because they were told from an early stage that this disease is not dangerous to children. A mantra was reiterated time and time again that "Children very rarely get seriously ill, and they do not spread the disease."[4] In fact, we were told this before anyone could possibly know the consequences of children having been infected with this new virus. In this chapter I will first analyze the origins of this statement and then try to spell out some of the consequences of establishing this myth in society early in the pandemic.

A scientific house of cards is built

The earliest articles in Swedish media about children's role in the pandemic focused on children not transmitting the disease to adults. On 1 March 2020, there was a story in several large Swedish newspapers where the FHM divulged information from a WHO delegation who had visited China to better understand the new coronavirus and gather information from the early stages of the community spread there. The newspapers presented interviews with the senior staff of the FHM. Karin Tegmark Wisell, who has since become the General Director of the FHM, was interviewed in an article titled "The Governmental Agency: Children Do Not Spread the Virus."[5] The article stated, "In the WHO study, it has not been possible to find any examples of cases where the infection has spread from child to child, nor from child to adult." However, what the WHO report stated was quite different:

> From available data, and in the absence of results from serologic studies, it is not possible to determine the extent of infection among children, what role children play in transmission, whether children are less susceptible or if they present differently clinically (i.e. generally milder presentations). The Joint Mission learned that infected children have largely been identified through contact tracing in households of adults. Of note, people interviewed by the Joint Mission Team could not recall episodes in which transmission occurred from a child to an adult.[6]

Tegmark Wisell was quoted to say "Do not let fear take over" and that it would be "completely disproportionate" to hold healthy children that had spent their sport vacation (late February) in areas with societal spread of the virus at home from school as a precaution in the light of this report.

The same day, another article with the title "The Public Health Agency: Children Do Not Transmit to the Same Extent as Adults" came out.[7] In there, the now famous State Epidemiologist Anders Tegnell said: "This [the WHO] report strongly supports our basic assessment: Closing schools and keeping children at home is not a reasonable measure." He continued, "The risk of transmission in school is extremely small, that is not where the virus is." Sweden had at that point a total of 14 identified cases.[8]

Tegnell continued repeating the mantra that children very rarely get seriously ill and they do not spread the disease. In an in-depth article in Sweden's largest broadsheet newspaper *Dagens Nyheter* Tegnell and a paediatrician, Jonas F. Ludvigsson, explain how children's immune systems protect them from getting severely ill in Covid-19.[9] This was echoed through society and for example, no facemasks were used in close care with premature babies during the entire spring 2020.

In the article Tegnell is cited as saying

> But the probability is high that children are not very infectious. There are extremely few examples where children have been infected by adults. There are Icelandic studies where very thorough reviews have been made where no cases of infection from children to adults have been found, says Anders Tegnell.

Despite searching, no such Icelandic studies have been found. In fact, even to the knowledge of Tegnell, there were no such studies in May 2020, which we know from his email exchanges.

In Sweden, emails of civil servants are public information and can be requested. On the 14th of May 2020 Tegnell sends an email to his Icelandic colleague Thorolfur Gudnason in preparation for this news article. Tegnell asks Gudnason if he has anything published on children and Covid-19. Gudnason replies the same day, "Nothing published. Only preliminary data from viral genetic analysis." Yet,

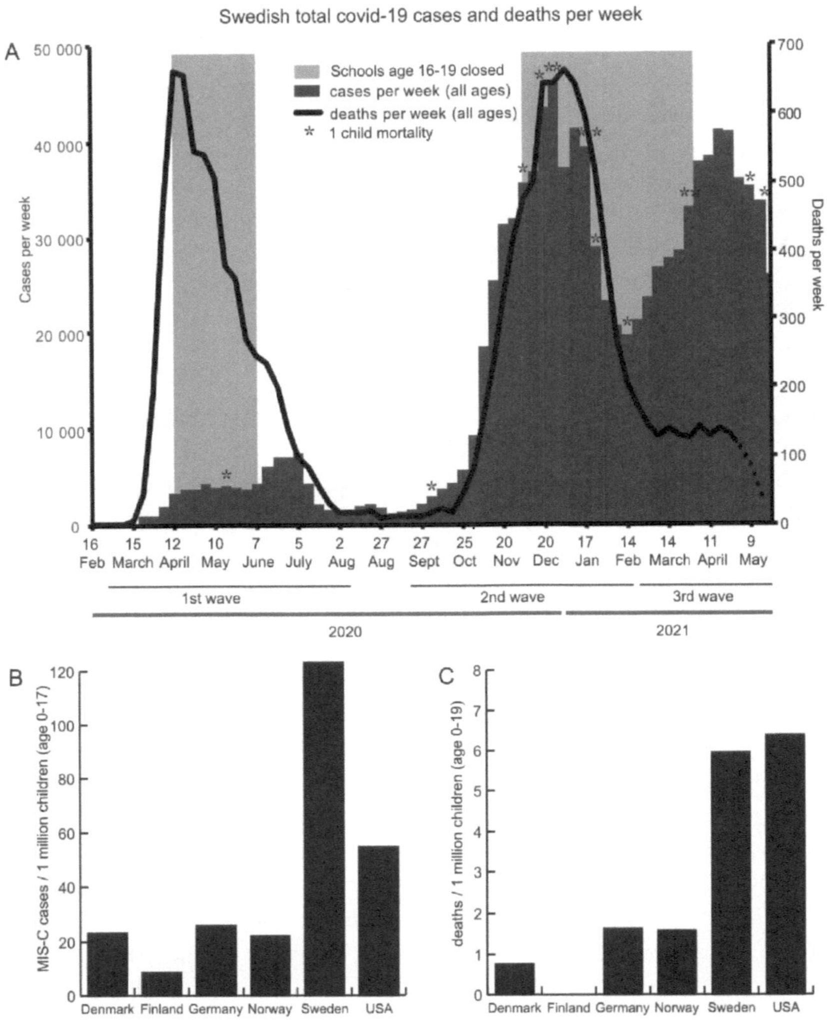

FIGURE 9.2 Health and mortality of Swedish children during the Covid-19 pandemic February 2020 to June 2021. *Source*: Three graphs by the author, based on public data from FHM (A), and on data from the sources in note 51 (B) and note 52 (C). A) This graph illustrates the first three waves of Covid-19 infections that Sweden has experienced. The black line illustrates the weekly total mortality and grey histograms show identified cases. Due to limited testing during the first wave of the pandemic, the mortality compared to number of cases is relatively high. Stars illustrate a registered child (age 0–19) death. The light grey squares show when schools (age 16–19) were closed proactively. This is the only age group for which schools were closed on a national level. B) Comparative number of MIS-C cases per million children in the Scandinavian countries, Germany and USA (ages 0–17). C) Comparative number of child mortalities per million in the same countries (age 0–19).

Tegnell still allows the quote about "Icelandic studies" (plural) to be published in our largest broadsheet newspaper five days later, on May the 19th. The editor in chief of the newspaper, Peter Wolodarski, has been shown these emails. However, the newspaper article remains unaltered online, still spreading scientific misinformation.

The other person cited in that article, the paediatrician Ludvigsson, came to play a large part of the information being spread on the topic of children and Covid-19 in Sweden. He is a paediatrician with a specialty in celiac disease and a former chair of the Swedish Society of Paediatrics. On his own YouTube channel he posted a video where he gives a presentation on the 16th of March 2020 for a layman audience in a church.[10] In this presentation he shows slides and tells the audience that "no children will get seriously ill," "Herd immunity – Good if all children get the disease? The virus dies out faster," "children do not die from coronavirus," "Pregnant? – No, not risk group". Ludvigsson also went on to become one of the 43 co-signers of the Great Barrington Declaration, where herd immunity via infection is the goal, and they suggest that schools should be left open to achieve it.[11] I will now analyze the scientific basis for each one of the statements Ludvigsson made in his presentation in mid-March.

"No children will get seriously ill."

Two days after his presentation in the church, Ludvigsson researched a review article "Systematic Review of COVID-19 in Children Shows Milder Cases and a Better Prognosis Than Adults" that was published in the middle of April.[12] There, Ludvigsson writes that over 90% of children had either asymptomatic, mild or moderate disease. The Chinese study Ludvigsson cited as the source for this information was the largest to that date and used data from the Chinese CDC, which at that point contained 2143 children with suspected Covid-19.[13] However, only 34.5% of children had confirmed Covid-19 with PCR. This is of course a caveat when using these numbers. From a more cautious perspective maybe attention should have been paid to the 5.9% of children who had severe or critical disease and the one child who had died, which was also presented in that same Chinese study.

"Herd immunity – good if all children get the disease? The virus dies out faster."

The herd immunity via infection approach was never official in Sweden, but often mentioned as a potential by-product of the strategy of keeping society open (see Emil J. Bergholtz's chapter). Yet from everything that was done, it is hard to not conclude that herd immunity via infection was their goal. Why else would they continuously update the percentage of people with antibodies in the population and repeatedly come up with new dates (usually another month or so away) when herd immunity would be reached?

On March the 14th, 2020, Tegnell wrote an email to his Finish colleague Mika Salminen where he suggests: "One point would be to keep the schools open to reach herd immunity faster."

Two years later, it is clear to see that this strategy didn't work as herd immunity has not been achieved here, or elsewhere, yet. However, to even suggest a strategy that involves the use of children to spread disease is immoral (not to mention that it goes totally against the idea that this disease does not spread among children and in schools). Since when do we expose our children to something we don't know is dangerous for them or not? Today we know of long-Covid, MIS-C (hyperinflammation), neurological effects and increased risks of developing diabetes after children have been infected with SARS-CoV-2, but even if these had never been discovered, it would have been wrong of us to expose children to an unknown virus. If the school cafeteria served a new wild mushroom that they think were very unlikely to harm your children, would you allow them to eat it? Just like with wild mushrooms, we know that some viruses can cause lasting damage to our bodies (e.g. herpes that stays in our bodies and later causes cold sores, human papilloma virus that can cause cancer and herpes zoster virus that first causes chickenpox but can come back later in life as shingles). These long-term effects of a SARS-CoV-2 infection couldn't be known in the spring of 2020. There were however warning signals from the previous SARS pandemic, where both psychiatric and physical morbidities such as PTSD, depression, reduced lung and exercise capacity were shown in survivors.[14] For that reason alone, the strategy of transmission of an unknown virus amongst children should never have been allowed. I leave it to the other authors of this book to discuss all the other scientific and ethical problems of the herd immunity via natural infection strategy, see for example the chapter by Lapo Lappin.

The 19th of May 2020, Ludvigsson repeats his message and publishes in the Swedish scientific journal *Acta Paediatrica*: "Children are unlikely the main drivers of the Covid-19 pandemic – a systematic review." In this review there is a quote from Tegnell: "So far, there have been no reports of major Covid-19 outbreaks in Swedish schools (personal communication, Anders Tegnell, State Epidemiologist, Sweden, 12 May 2020)."

In an email from Ludvigsson to Tegnell sent on the 12th of March 2020, we can see that in fact, this statement is written by Ludvigsson himself. Because of the limited testing of school children that I will discuss later, few school outbreaks were reported during the first wave, but a voluntary organization called "Covid-19 schools and children" registered 30 outbreaks (confirmed by either newspaper article, picture of positive PCR or principals' note to parents) during March and April 2020. Several of these outbreaks in the community spread had been reported in the national news.[15] *The burning question is if Tegnell and the FHM were not informed of any of these 30 school outbreaks and no one of them read about it in the news?* The emails studied for this publication do not show the reply from Tegnell, which leaves another possibility – that he never approved the quotation. However, the *Acta Paediatrica*'s editor-in-chief confirms that Tegnell had approved the personal communication in his name. The editor also wrote that Ludvigsson has already been investigated for research fraud and acquitted. Ludvigsson was investigated for research fraud due to this omission of the over-mortality of school children, but also because he had stated that there had been no major outbreak in schools and that he had failed to mention a conflict of interest as he was one of the 47 co-signers of the Great Barrington Declaration. Ludvigsson was acquitted on the grounds that "no data appears to have been omitted in a manner that is falsification according to the law."[16]

"Children do not die from coronavirus."

Even though children in general do not get as ill as elderly when infected with a coronavirus, there were reports of children dying of coronavirus before the Covid-19 pandemic started,[17] making this statement an uncareful generalization. It could have been possible that on the 16th of March Ludvigsson had not heard of the one child that had died in the previously discussed Chinese study. However, later that year, on August the 8th, 2020 Ludvigsson is on national TV saying: "Even if we have had so many dead and had two million children in school, it is exceedingly few children that have been severely ill in Covid-19 and no child has died." In the official Covid-19 statistics from the FHM there had been three child deaths registered in April and May 2020, one of which was also reported about in the news,[18] but two deaths were later removed. That means that there was child mortality in the Swedish death statistics when Ludvigsson made his claim of the opposite on Swedish TV. Internationally, there had certainly been reports of children dying[19] and a scientific briefing about the hyperinflammation (later called MIS-C) that may come after Covid-19 infection in children was published by the WHO in May 2020.[20] Reports about children dying from that hyperinflammation came as early as April 2020.[21]

There are also reasons to believe that more children died of Covid-19 in that first wave. Ludvigsson wrote an email to Tegnell as he prepared a new manuscript that was later published in *New England Journal of Medicine*: "unfortunately we see a clear indication of excess mortality among children ages 7–16 old, the ages where kids went to school." He goes on "For the years 2015 through 2019, an average of 30.4 children in that age group died in the four spring months; in 2020, 51 children in that age group died, = excess mortality +68%." He also noted that the younger age group, that didn't have to go to school, had a decreased mortality compared to the previous years. Ludvigsson with colleagues published their article "Open Schools, Covid-19, and Child and Teacher Morbidity in Sweden" in *NEJM* on January the 6th, 2021.[22] They state:

> The number of deaths from any cause among the 1,951,905 children in Sweden (as of December 31, 2019) who were 1 to 16 years of age was 65 during the pre-Covid-19 period of November 2019 through February 2020 and 69 during 4 months of exposure to Covid-19 (March through June 2020).

Thus, he did not split up the mortality rates of children between those who had mandatory school presence and those who did not. Further, they choose to compare child mortalities to the previous three months rather than the same months in previous years, like he did in the email. Thus, the over-mortality in school children that Ludvigsson had discovered and written to Tegnell about was no longer apparent.

The journal *Science* highlighted this issue in an article "Critics Slam Letter in Prestigious Journal That Downplayed COVID-19 Risks to Swedish Schoolchildren" and approached Ludvigsson for a comment before publication.[23] The day before the *Science* article was published, Ludvigsson answered two printed responses to his article published in *NEJM*.[24] In the response he added, without any of the written critiques asking him to: "I would also like to provide additional information on mortality . . . [the missing information]. . . . The Supplementary Appendix of our published letter (available at NEJM.org) has been updated with additional mortality data." However, in Swedish media coverage of the affair Ludvigsson stated "that his critics are wrong – the data about the over-mortality amongst school age children have not been hidden but are there in an online appendix to the text in that published in NEJM."[25] With that, he presumably refers to the data he added to the appendix three days prior after the interview with *Science*, both versions of the appendix are shown here.[26] The child mortality was also higher during subsequent Covid-19 infection waves of a similar size, strengthening the hypothesis that they were missed during the first wave.

"Pregnant? No, not risk group."

We now know that infection with SARS-CoV-2 when pregnant is a risk both for the mother and the child she carries.[27] So why did Ludvigsson claim it was not? Early in the pandemic, the sources of information were of course scarce and in his April review Ludvigsson also cites the previously mentioned WHO report about the risks during pregnancy. In the WHO report, it does say "women do not appear to be at higher risk of severe disease." The authors base this on 147 pregnant women, but again, this data included 56% suspected, not confirmed, Covid-19 cases. They note that 8% of cases were severe and 1% critical, which is lower than the average risk of severe disease reported in the whole population in that report (13.8%). However, the report mentions age as a risk factor for getting severe Covid-19. Therefore, a comparison of women in the same age group as the pregnant women could potentially have given an early warning to shield pregnant women rather than to inform them that they are not at risk. There were also reasons to be extra careful, as the previous SARS pandemic had caused high incidences of spontaneous miscarriage, preterm delivery and intrauterine growth restrictions.[28]

Taken together, a scientific house of cards had been built where weak and sometimes non-existent scientific evidence was used to deviate from the precautionary principle.

Swedish children have had limited access to testing

The Swedish Government convened a commission to investigate and analyze Sweden's response to the pandemic. In the commission's second report they concluded that it was a "wreckage" that testing and tracing did not start until after the first wave.[29] This is true, the testing was so low in Sweden during the first wave that it is barely detectable if one looks at a graph of the numbers of cases. If one instead looks at the number of dead, it is clear that the first wave in spring 2020 was almost as big as the second wave that autumn (Figure 9.2A). The termination of testing suspected cases was a formal decision announced on a press conference held by the FHM on March the 12th, when the societal transmission of the disease had been confirmed.[30] After this date, symptomatic persons were only tested if an intervention, such as hospitalization, was planned. The population was told to stay at home when ill, and maybe a couple of days extra to make sure one was no longer contagious when going back to work/school. Therefore, there was next to no testing, tracing and isolation during that first wave, a dereliction that was claimed to go against Swedish law.[31] In fact, isolation was not even imposed on family members of a confirmed Covid-19 case if they were not symptomatic themselves before October 2020,[32] and even then, children were exempted from that rule until December 1st, 2020.[33] This meant that children from families with confirmed Covid-19 were mixed freely with other children in school for the first and part of the second large wave of Covid-19 transmission in Sweden.

On top of the almost non-existent testing during the first wave, children in Sweden have received less access to testing than the rest of society (Figure 9.1). Long after the problems with starting up the testing, FHM decided to recommend testing of symptomatic schoolchildren from September 2020.[34] The reasons for the lower testing of children have been many. First, FHM has not recommended that children younger than 6 years should be tested during the entire pandemic, if not hospitalized. In fact, on occasion, the national health information and health care workers have presented it as abusive to test young children.[35]

Second, older children have also had difficulty getting tested, as they were completely exempted in some regions (e.g. in the region *Östergötland* where everyone below 13 was denied testing).[36] A third reason why testing for children was difficult to come by, was that teenage children without a digital ID could not book a test using that same health service line.[37] A digital bank ID can only be given by a physical visit at a bank, which you can't do if you have symptoms. Finally, when the testing capacity was reached, it was decided to deprioritize children. The situation was worsened by schools not informing parents when there were outbreaks, with staff saying that they have been told not to speak.[38] In parts of Sweden, it appears that not telling parents about Covid-19 community spread on schools was a pronounced rule from the municipality.[39] Thus, parents and children have not known when there was Covid-19 in their school and close environment, which made shielding of children impossible.

In this way, the children, their families and the teachers were excluded from partaking in the common struggle against the pandemic. This has led to increased anxiety, exclusion of the children from the society and a less effective protection against the contagion. As a 14-year-old child expressed it to the Children's Ombudsman: "They say children are not afflicted, but, like, I am a child and I have really been afflicted, hello? Why do they never say anything about that in their meetings? It feels so warped, really warped."[40]

Schools as a central for disease transmission

FHM claims in their text "Covid-19 in children and adolescents – a knowledge summary," (version 2) that Covid-19 transmission occurs mostly within families and not within schools. To support this they cite two studies,[41] both of which were conducted when schools were closed. The authors of *The Lancet Infectious Diseases* study writes:

> At the time of the COVID-19 outbreak, all schools were on the spring festival holiday, which might have prevented children from exposure to transmission sources. However, the school community is a place that can enhance rapid spread of the highly infectious SARS-CoV-2.

A similar concern is written in the second study. This poses the question if FHM read the articles at all or if they were deliberately being misleading. It is also interesting to note that both studies mention a high proportion of asymptomatic children testing positive in contact tracing situations, since asymptomatic spread is obviously not considered in the "stay at home when you are ill" directives from FHM to school children.

FHM's knowledge summary also has a paragraph that says "the contagion appears to spread more in the free time than in school." Here, they claim no studies have shown large spread of the disease in schools and "Rather, the infection seems to spread in leisure time, in sports contexts where you have close contact, and in other social contexts, for example at parties or camps." The whole paragraph does not contain any citations.

One way of being able to say that there have been no Covid-19 school outbreaks is not to ask to be informed. An official request to report school outbreaks to the FHM was first made in September 2020. School outbreaks were then included in the FHM weekly reports. In mid-December 2020, outbreaks in schools made out more than 75% of all public community spread (outside of health care).[42] Shortly thereafter, reporting of school outbreaks was discontinued.

In a large Indian study of Covid-19 transmission where over 50 000 index cases and their over half a million contacts were followed,[43] showed that school age children (5–17 years old) infected around 12% of their contacts. This translates to each positive child infecting three classmates in a class of 25 students. The FHM refers to this article in their text that was published just after the Indian study in

November 2020.[44] NPR made a clip about the article called "Kids and Superspreaders Are Driving COVID-19 Cases in India – Huge Study Finds."[45] *The Science Hour* at BBC also made a feature titled "Are Children the Biggest Covid-19 Spreaders?"[46] In FHM's knowledge summary (version 2), they say the Indian study "summarizes the dispersion dynamic in two Indian states" and imply that the study might not be relevant to high-income countries.

In February 2021 an elegant study was published where Vlachos et al. compared the disease transmission in Swedish parents and teachers to pupils ages 14–16 (open schools) with pupils ages 17–19 (distance education) during that first wave of the Covid-19 pandemic.[47] The study showed a small increased risk of being diagnosed with Covid-19 in parents to children in open schools. For teachers, the risk of getting infected doubled if working in an open school in comparison to a closed one. Moreover, being a partner of a teacher in an open school increased the risk of getting Covid-19.

In hindsight, it was an epidemiologically wise thing to close schools and other educational institutions, as several studies have shown that this was the second most effective non-pharmaceutical intervention that could be done to stop the spread of Covid-19.[48] In April 2020, the results from a massive American online survey were published in the esteemed journal *Science*.[49] The study showed that having children attending school in person increases the risk of contracting Covid-19, but if the school applied seven or more different mitigation measures (i.e. masking, social distancing and closed extracurricular activities), it could completely eliminate that risk.

In summary, the evidence that Covid-19 didn't spread in schools was always weak and by the winter of 2020 it was completely disproven. Despite this, and despite the fact that Swedish schools had not introduced any effective measures against disease transmission, Tegnell states on the national news 12 of January 2021: "There is no evidence that schools should be more dangerous than other work environments."[50]

Taken together, there is strong evidence that open schools have played a considerable part in disease transmission in Sweden and later, also outside of Sweden, when schools opened internationally.

Consequences of the strategy on paediatric physical health

As the Swedish strategy had failed on one level after another, and our death tolls rose well above our neighbouring countries, the fact that schools had stayed open remained something of a national pride. Yet, when the FHM has done antibody testing of small population samples, children have had as much, or more, antibody positivity as the adults, showing how we have completely failed to protect them from the disease. I gathered data in the end of June 2021, comparing the levels of MIS-C among children of the different Scandinavian countries, Germany and USA.[51] Sweden had then seen more than twice as high rates of hyperinflammation in children as the USA, who had the second highest rates (Figure 9.2B). In comparison to its closest neighbours, Sweden had MIS-C incidences of between four to 12 times as high. In this comparison of countries, Sweden and USA had the highest levels of child mortalities, which was over seven times as high as the average of the other Scandinavian countries (Figure 9.2C).[52]

As of this writing, the number of children who have passed away in Sweden has risen to 23, but a further six children have been removed from the FHM's statistics for unknown reasons.[53] In Finland, who has approximately half as many children as Sweden, but is otherwise very similar in terms of population density, there has still not been any child passing away from Covid-19. 2750 of our 2.13 million children and youth (age 0–18) have been hospitalized with Covid-19 and 166 have been in intensive care.[54] That is to be compared with Norway that has had 500 children in hospital and 39 in intensive care to date.[55] When compensated for the number of children of that age in each country, Sweden's numbers are more than double that of Norway's (2.6 times as many hospitalizations and 2 times as many children in intensive care), a country that is extremely comparable to our own.

Several studies have also shown that children also have might have long-term consequences, often called long-Covid or PASC, after having had Covid-19.[56] To this day, we have no insight into the numbers of children who suffer from this condition in Sweden, and the published international studies show a wide range of incidences. The need for more scientific studies centred on paediatric long-Covid is much requested[57] and on-going.[58]

Therefore, my conclusion must be that the strategy of keeping schools open, at the same time as propagating a myth that children are not affected by Covid-19, nor contribute to its transmission, and making it hard or impossible for them to test themselves, has yielded a result far worse for children's physical health than other countries achieved. How did this affect individuals, our country and the international community?

Consequences of the strategy on psychological health and education

One of the most presented arguments for children attending school in person has been mental health – going to school is good for children. As a scientist and educator, I do not disagree, but I also think children are adaptable, can learn well in many ways and that protecting their physical health is also important to psychological health. In FHM's knowledge summary they say that

> Studies show that children and adolescents have been adversely affected by school closures (3). There has been learning loss, and negative effect on mental and physical health. The negative consequences have also hit hardest the children who are most at risk, such as children with disabilities, children with underlying diseases, children in socio-economically disadvantaged groups and children living in social vulnerability and poverty.

Note that even if they speak about several studies, they only cite one. The cited study is a Norwegian publication where they introduce guidelines and considerations before reopening their schools.[59] Even by researching the sources inside of the article cited by FHM, I could not find evidence for the claims in their text.

Svaleryd and Vlachos investigated the psychological health of children for the Corona Commission.[60] Like in their PNAS article, discussed earlier, they used the fact that children aged 13–15 had to be physically in schools whilst older children were distance educated. In this comparison it was clear that the younger students being taught in school had more mental health problems than the distance educated children (that showed a decrease to an otherwise increasing trend of mental health problems).

In a report from the Swedish Children's Ombudsman (*Barnombudsmannen*), interviews with children of different ages stated many ways in which children have suffered psychologically by the Swedish strategy.[61] Some children live with someone belonging to a risk group and have been under constant fear of bringing the virus home from school. Other children have been long-term ill after Covid-19 infection or have parents or siblings that are. Long-term ill children shared an experience of not being listened to by health care professionals and that this was worsened by the fact that they were not tested for Covid-19 when they were ill, so it is harder for them to get a retrospective diagnosis. It has also been hard for them to get schools to understand the severity of their health issues and get help to adapt their schooling as to receive continued education. In fact, the report concludes that many aspects of The United Nations Convention on the Rights of the Child that became a Swedish law in January 2019 were breached during the pandemic, among those the right of survival and best achievable health. Many children had to experience their friends, family members and teachers getting sick, and many suffered when school classes in an acute chaotic process had to be shut down for a while. Did the state abandon the individual children and overburden them alone with the consequences of the on-going spread?

Of course, educating children is the main task of schools and a very important one indeed. However, teachers and principals witnessed a chaotic school situation during the pandemic, with both teachers and students being ill.[62] How much this has affected the teaching is hard to examine, but one study was performed by the company Lexplore that first investigated the knowledge gap that had occurred in UK schools during the pandemic. In the UK they have had distance education and indeed, the children's reading development had not developed normally.[63] However, when Lexplore did the same investigation on children's reading progression in Swedish schools, they had been held back twice as much as the British pupils, showing that in a situation where you got to choose between two evils, flexibility in school forms during a pandemic might lessen the detrimental effects on education.

Another reason often argued in defence of open schools is that not all children are well cared for in their homes or they are from poor backgrounds. School provides daily meals, and, hopefully, a safe environment where children have daily contact with adults that they can turn to for help should they need it. The

Children's Ombudsman report agrees that children in already troubled environments were disproportionately hit by the pandemic. This is of course an extremely serious matter, but the argument also opens the question what the official role of the school system should be. Other countries – such as Spain, Japan, South Africa (cf. the World Food Programme's "Special Report from the State of School Feeding Worldwide 2020") – kept school kitchens open so that children/families could come and pick up their lunches even when attending distance education. That leaves the emotional care for children as a major reason for keeping schools open. I would argue that a necessary precaution for similar crises in the future is that we strengthen other social services in our community so that children are well cared for in all situations.

Consequences of the strategy for society

Sweden is at the time of writing in the middle of the fourth, and so far, most widely spread wave of Covid-19. Even the staunchest supporter of the Swedish strategy is very likely to have seen occasions where a child has brought the disease into their families. The original message of children not contributing to the spread of the disease pretended a situation of a "house of cards," a message that should never have been allowed as much space as it was given. It appears, however, to be very hard to change this mind set now, and even if the evidence is in, Swedish schools continue to be open with little to no mitigating measures in place to halt the transmission of Covid-19. An official decision not to recommend vaccination of children aged 5–11 years old was taken in January 2022. This means that parents in Sweden have no access to vaccinating their children even if the vaccine is approved by the EMA. At the same time child hospitalizations have skyrocketed to a level over 16 times higher than the average since the pandemic started (Figure 9.3). On February the 15th, 2022, as many children had been in intensive care during this year as during the entire 2021.

It is my firm belief closing schools while investigating a new virus would have been a reasonable precaution and would have instilled a sense of seriousness of the situation in society. See Jens Stilhoff Sörensen's chapter on the other European countries' methods of including schools into the pandemic response. Instead, the situation became absurd when parents are told not to socialize with people outside of their household, but their children are spending full school days with their 25–30 classmates, to then be joined into larger groups for after school day-care and eat school lunch in a dining hall with hundreds of other students. School activities such as mother tongue language education, where the teacher often travels between schools continued. Children were also still allowed to participate in sports and other free-time activities where students from different schools mixed. In that situation, it can be hard to see the reasons not to meet with friends for dinner. I therefore consider the open/unmitigated schools a major reason why people might not have been so compliant with the restrictions that were eventually introduced.

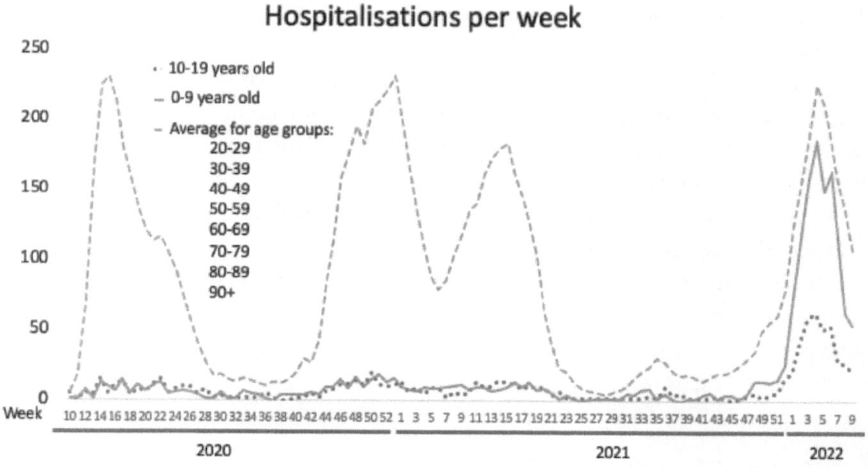

FIGURE 9.3 The number of hospitalizations in small children (age 0–9), children and adolescents (10–19) compared to the average of all other age categories. The same numbers of children were hospitalized in the two age groups of children up until the omicron wave in the beginning of 2022. At that time, approximately 60% of 12–17 year olds had been fully vaccinated. FHM have not advised vaccination of younger children, which means no Swedish parents can vaccinate their younger children even though a vaccine is approved by EMA for age 5–11.

Scurce: Data from Socialstyrelsen. *Vård och covid-19* (2022), www.socialstyrelsen.se/statistik-och-data/statistik/statistik-om-covid-19/statistik-om-slutenvard-av-patienter-med-covid-19/.

A very serious effect of a governmental institution spreading scientific misinformation and even contradicting themselves trying to cover that up is that the people sooner or later stop trusting the Government. One example is when the FHM published a report saying that teachers are not an above-average exposed occupation.[64] Later, when their own statistics indicated that over 75% of the community spread happened in schools, their weekly report claimed that it was mostly teachers infecting each other – not the children.[65] Thus, teachers managed to both not be more than averagely infected with the virus, but still stand for over 75% of the community spread. Later, both a scientific publication and the corona commission showed that Swedish teachers, especially pre-school teachers, were amongst the professional group most infected by SARS-CoV-2. Pre-school teachers were even comparable with medical doctors. A second example is during a press conference on the 13th of March when Johan Carlson first said children do not drive the pandemic and they are less contagious when infected.[66] Just seconds later, he said that one reason why schools cannot close is because grandparents would then be asked to provide day-care for their grandchildren. This would not be good as we need to protect the elderly. So, it appeared as if the Public Health Agency was saying that children do not transmit the disease in schools, but they do when they meet their grandparents.

There has also been disparity between what the Government says and what it does. For example, the Swedish Government has never recommended facemasks in society as a whole, and certainly not at all in schools. However, when the Government met again in person there was a demand on facemask usage and Minister of Education Anna Ekström used an FFP2 protection, which is a more advanced kind of facemask that also protects the user.[67]

Letting a disease spread over a population is of course also very expensive and the number of days taken off work to care for sick children have skyrocketed during the pandemic. In April 2020, there was an all-time monthly high of over 1 300 000 days registered.[68]

Future perspectives

The pandemic has revealed severe weaknesses in the Swedish society. One of them is that the FHM, called an "expert authority," was allowed to stipulate the Swedish pandemic strategy almost unchallenged by media or the Government, on pre-decided dogmas rather than international peer-reviewed science. FHM did not act according to the precautionary principle (cf. the introductory chapter and Jens Stilhoff Sörensen's chapter). This has now also been the one of the major conclusions by the Corona Commission.[69] In my opinion, they placed all Swedish children in harm's way by doing so. How this has changed our society is already apparent to some extent, but the consequences will unravel for years to come.[70]

In the future, I wish there would be more flexibility in the system, allowing parents to decide what is best for their children and family. For example, the law to physically attend school could be relaxed under such special circumstances. Instead, what happened was cruel, as many parents now were forced to choose between breaking the law and maybe risking a loved one's life. Around half of the world's countries, including all the other Scandinavian countries, allow home schooling as an alternative all the time.[71] Many of the countries that normally do require physical school presence relaxed this demand during the pandemic.[72] This forced some to keep their children at home illegally, under fear of being reported to social services and experiencing judgement from society. For these families, there was no support during an already trying time as being in a risk group during a pandemic is no laughing matter. On the biopolitical abandonment of this group, see also Lapo Lappin's chapter.

In many cases, parents had to act as teachers to their children while at the same time handling their normal jobs, as there were no distance education alternatives offered for children ages 6–15. Maybe at-risk teachers would have been happy to teach pupils online? New classes could have formed, with children and teachers that could connect over being in a similar situation. Instead, the isolation of these children became total. Other ways we could have been flexible would have been to push the semester schedules around a little, so that children and their teachers didn't have to be in school during the worst peaks of viral spread in society.

It is also worrisome that we have a society where the school is the one lifeline for many children from troubled families. Is this the role of schools? Where is the social welfare system? If this is a reason not to switch to distance education during a blazing pandemic, then why are these children left to fend for themselves for ten weeks every summer holiday?

Future research will show how detrimental distance education, and the pandemic, have been for the children's learning and life, but some of our children may prefer to be taught this way, pandemic or not.[73] The pandemic has caused a lot of added work for employees working within the educational system, but it has also caused a wealth of new pedagogical tools that need to be evaluated and maybe perfected in the years to come providing a whole new set of educational approaches to our arsenal.

This pandemic has revealed how children are still neglected citizens in the Swedish society. It is my sincere hope that during the next crisis, I can sit back and watch how society will first and foremost care for those who cannot care for themselves. This was not the case this time – again.

Notes

1 Svärdkrona, Z. "225.000 människor omkom i tsunamin", *Aftonbladet*, 22 August 2005.

2 FHM, *Symtomfria barn bör stanna hemma om någon i familjen har covid-19*, 1 December, 2020, www.krisinformation.se/nyheter/2020/december/symtomfria-barn-bor-stanna-hemma-om-nagon-i-familjen-har-covid-19 .

3 FHM. *Pressträff om covid-19 (coronavirus)*, 29 April 2020.

4 Harr, T. "Anders Tegnell: 'Liten risk att barn drabbas'", *Svenska Dagbladet*, 17 March 2021; Silverberg, J. "Tegnell: Barn smittar väldigt sällan vuxna", *Göteborgs-Posten*, 16 August, 2020; Regeringskansliet. *Digital pressträff med utbildningsministern, Folkhälsomyndigheten och Skolverket*, 2021; "Tegnell: inte mycket talar för att barn sprider smittan", *Sveriges Television*, 1 May 2020, www.svt.se/nyheter/inrikes/tegnell-om-skolstangingar-stangda-skolor-drabbar-barn; Canoilas, V. "Skolbarn driver inte epidemin – skolor fortsatt öppna", *Dagens Nyheter*, 13 March 2020; FHM. *Pressträff om covid-19 (coronavirus)*, 13 March 2020; Fernstedt, N. "Myndigheten: Barn sprider inte viruset", *Aftonbladet*, 1 March 2020; Tenitskaja, A.C. "Folkhälsomyndigheten: Barn smittar inte i samma utsträckning som vuxna", *Dagens Nyheter*, 1 March 2020; Peter Letmark, S.R. "Så kan barns immunsystem skydda dem från att bli allvarligt sjuka i covid-19", *Dagens Nyheter*, 19 May 2020.

5 Fernstedt. "Myndigheten: Barn sprider inte viruset".

6 WHO. *Report of the WHO-China Joint Mission on Coronavirus Disease 2019 (COVID-19)*. 2020.

7 Tenitskaja. "Folkhälsomyndigheten: Barn smittar inte i samma utsträckning som vuxna".

8 FHM. *Bekräftade fall av covid-19 i Sverige*. 2020 [cited 25 March 2022]; FHM's webpage containing statistics of confirmed Covid-19 cases, intensive care patients and deaths, www.folkhalsomyndigheten.se/smittskydd-beredskap/utbrott/aktuella-utbrott/Covid-19/statistik-och-analyser/bekraftade-fall-i-sverige/ .

9 Peter Letmark. "Så kan barns immunsystem skydda . . .".

10 Ludvigsson. *Information om Covid-19 med läkare Jonas Ludvigsson.*

11 Kulldorff, Martin, and Jay Bhattacharya. *Great Barrington Declaration*, 2020, https://gbdeclaration.org .

12 Ludvigsson, J.F. "Systematic Review of COVID-19 in Children Shows Milder Cases and a Better Prognosis Than Adults", *Acta Paediatrica* 109:6 (2020): 1088–1095.

13 Dong, Y., X. Mo, Y. Hu, X. Qi, F. Jiang, Z. Jiang, and S. Tong. "Epidemiology of COVID-19 Among Children in China", *Pediatrics* 145:6 (2020): e20200702.

14 Mak, I.W., C.M. Chu, P.C. Pan, M.G. Yiu, and V.L. Chan. "Long-Term Psychiatric Morbidities Among SARS Survivors", *General Hospital Psychiatry* 31:4 (2009): 318–326; Ngai, J.C., F.W. Ko, S.S. Ng, K.W. To, M. Tong, and D.S. Hui. "The Long-Term Impact of Severe Acute Respiratory Syndrome on Pulmonary Function, Exercise Capacity and Health Status", *Respirology* 15:3 (2010): 543–550.

15 Lindblom, F. "Vasaskolan i Göteborg stänger efter coronasmitta", *Göteborgs-Posten*, 13 March 2020; Sjögren, A. "Coronasmitta på skola – föräldrar informerades inte", *Aftonbladet*, 4 April 2020; Trus, H. "Lärare dog i covid-19 – var fjärde i personalen smittad", *Aftonbladet*, 2 May 2020; Olsson, E. "Anställd på Danderydsskola död i corona", *Läraren*, 27 April 2020; "Förskolan Sörgård i Brunflo öppnar igen på torsdag", *Sveriges Television*, 26 May 2020, www.svt.se/nyheter/lokalt/jamtland/forskolan-sorgard-i-brunflo-oppnar-igen-pa-torsdag; Hagström, J. "Kålltorpsskolan trotsar förvaltningen – bekräftar coronasmitta", *Göteborgs-Posten*, 17 April 2020; "Elev coronasmittad – Kunskapsskolan i Nacka stänger", *Sveriges Television*, 6 March 2020, www.svt.se/nyheter/lokalt/stockholm/elev-smittad-skola-stanger; "Prinsessan Estelles skola stängs efter coronasmitta", *Sveriges Television*, 5 March 2020, www.svt.se/nyheter/lokalt/stockholm/estelles-skola-stangs-efter-coronasmitta; "Alléskolan i Hallsberg hålls stängd – personer smittade av coronavirus", *Sveriges Television*, 8 March 2020, www.svt.se/nyheter/lokalt/orebro/alleskolan-i-hallsberg-halls-stangd-personer-smittade-av-coronavirus; Svensson, Olof, and H.Trus. "Prinsen besökte skola som nu är stängd efter coronasmitta", *Aftonbladet*, 12 March 2020.

16 Ström, M. "Oredlighetsnämnden friar Jonas F Ludvigsson", *Läkartidningen*, 29 June 2021.

17 Al Hajjar, S., S. Al Thawadi, A. Al Seraihi, S. Al Muhsen, and H. Imambaccus. "Human Metapneumovirus and Human Coronavirus Infection and Pathogenicity in Saudi Children Hospitalized with Acute Respiratory Illness", *Annals of Saudi medicine* 31:5 (2011): 523–527; Konca, C., G. Korukluoglu, M. Tekin, Mehmet, H. Almis, I.H. Bucak, İbrahim, H. Uygun, A.B. Altas, and F. Bayrakdar. "The First Infant Death Associated with Human Coronavirus NL63 Infection", *Pediatric Infectious Disease Journal* 36:2 (2017): 231–233; Thabet, F., M. Chehab, H. Bafaqih, and S. Al Mohaimeed. "Middle East Respiratory Syndrome Coronavirus in Children", *Saudi Medical Journal* 36:4 (2015): 484–486.

18 "Swedish Doctors Investigate Whether Young Child Died from Coronavirus", *The Local*, 6 May 2020; Malmqvist, Matilda Aprea, and John Granlund. "Ett barn kan ha dött i Sverige av covid-19", *Aftonbladet*, 6 May 2020.

19 Ries, Brian, and Elizabeth Joseph. "Cuomo Warns of 'Entirely Different Chapter' as 5-Year-Old NYC Boy Dies from COVID-Related Complications", *CNN*, 8 May 2020; Barmore, J. "5-Year-Old with Rare Complication Becomes First Michigan Child to Die of COVID-19", *The Detroit News*, 19 April 2020; Canty, J., R. Pires, and J. Lennox. "11-Year-Old Miami-Dade Boy Dies from COVID-19 Amid Rise in New Cases", *7 News Miami*, 2 July 2020; Campbell, D. "Five Children Have Died of Coronavirus in UK, Study Reveals", *The Guardian*, 23 June 2020; Staff, W. "ADPH: Second Child Under Age 5 Has Died from COVID-19", *WSFA12 News*, 24 June 2020; Ombour, R. "Kenya Confirms First Death of Minor from COVID-19", *VOA News*, 6 April 2020; Gripenberg, P., and M. Holmgren. "12-årig flicka från Belgien är Europas yngsta dödsoffer i covid-19", *Dagens Nyheter*, 1 April 2020.

20 WHO. *Multisystem Inflammatory Syndrome in Children and Adolescents Temporally Related to COVID-19*, 2020, www.who.int/news-room/commentaries/detail/multisystem-inflammatory-syndrome-in-children-and-adolescents-with-covid-19 .

21 Faulconbridge, G., and K. Holton. "UK Says Some Children Have Died from Syndrome Linked to COVID-19", *Reuters*, 28 April 2020.
22 Ludvigsson, J.F., L. Engerström, C. Nordenhäll, and E. Larsson. "Open Schools, Covid-19, and Child and Teacher Morbidity in Sweden", *New England Journal of Medicine* 384:7 (2021): 669–671.
23 Vogel, G. "Critics Slam Letter in Prestigious Journal That Downplayed COVID-19 Risks to Swedish Schoolchildren", *Science*, 2 March 2021.
24 Takefuji, Yoshiyasu, Lonni Besançon, David Steadson, and Antoine Flahault. "Replies to the Correspondence 'Open Schools, Covid-19, and Child and Teacher Morbidity in Sweden'", *New England Journal of Medicine* 384 (29 April 2021): e66.
25 Delin, M. "Forskare anklagas ha dolt överdödlighet bland barn under pandemin", *Dagens Nyheter*, 4 March 2021.
26 MarieF_GG writes: "On Ludvigsson paper. Here are 2 appendices. The original (left) and the one published March 1st after critics on the paper and request for clarification from *Science Magazine* GretchenVogel. The added data from March 1 show 68% increased mortality for the same period. 2021 March 5th", https://twitter.com/MarieF_GG/status/1367818969919455233?s=20&fbclid=IwAR3miRNEb6VlS6wI9cn1ZtMPsScckLFbUTlLdUH9Nl85BA2U92ZpKKPo0SY .
27 CDC. *Covid Data Tracker – Pregnancy Data*, 2022, https://Covid.cdc.gov/Covid-data-tracker/#pregnancy-data; Stock, S.J., D. McAllister, E. Vasileiou, C.R. Simpson, H.R. Stagg, U. Agrawal, C. McCowan, L. Hopkins, J. Donaghy, L. Ritchie, C. Robertson, A. Sheikh, and R. Wood. "COVID-19 in Pregnancy in Scotland (COPS): Protocol for an Observational Study Using Linked Scottish National Data", *BMJ Open* 10:11 (2020): e042813; Howard-Jones, A.R., D.P. Burgner, N.W. Crawford, E. Goeman, P.E. Gray, P. Hsu, S. Kuek, B.J. McMullan, S. Tosif, D. Wurzel, A.C. Bowen, M. Danchin, A. Koirala, K. Sharma, D.K. Yeoh, and P.N. Britton. "COVID-19 in Children. II: Pathogenesis, Disease Spectrum and Management", *Journal of Pediatrics and Child Health* 58:1 (2022): 46–53.
28 Wong, S.F., K.M. Chow, T.N. Leung, W.F. Ng, T.K. Ng, C.C. Shek, P.C. Ng, P.W. Lam, L.C. Ho, W.W. To, S.T. Lai, W.W. Yan, and P.Y. Tan. "Pregnancy and Perinatal Outcomes of Women with Severe Acute Respiratory Syndrome", *American Journal of Obstetrics and Gynecology* 191:1 (2004): 292–297.
29 Corona Commission. *Delbetänkande 2 – Sverige Under Pandemin SOU 2021:89*, 2021.
30 FHM. *Pressträff om covid-19 (coronavirus)*, 12 March 2020.
31 Alvner, Johan, Lars Eriksson, Peter Galatius, Peet Tüll, and Petra Östergren. "Experter: Sveriges smittskyddslag har inte efterföljts", *Altinget*, 30 September 2021.
32 Westling, E. "Nu införs familjekarantän i Västra Götaland: 'Viktig åtgärd'", *Sveriges Television*, 28 October 2020.
33 FHM. "Symtomfria barn bör stanna hemma . . .".
34 FHM. "Barn och unga med symtom på covid-19 rekommenderas PCR-testning för snabbare återgång till skolan", 31 August 2020.
35 Larsson, E. "Avråddes att testa sin 6-åring: '1177 sa att det vore ett övergrepp'", *Sveriges Television*, 2 December 2020; "Läkare: Barn kan uppleva coronatestet som ett övergrepp", *Upsala Nya Tidning*, 13 May 2021.
36 Sousa Mestre, Lillemor, and Johan de Sousa Mestre. "Varför covidtestar man inte barn i Region Östergötland?" *Corren*, 10 September 2021.
37 Haglund, M. "1177 låter inte vårdnadshavare boka covidtest för unga", *Sveriges Television*, 11 December 2020.
38 Sjögren, A. "Coronasmitta på skola – föräldrar informerades inte", *Aftonbladet*, 4 April 2020.
39 Hagström. "Kålltorpsskolan trotsar förvaltningen – bekräftar coronasmitta".
40 Barnombudsmannen. *Covid-19 pandemins konsekvenser för barn*, 2021, www.barnombudsmannen.se/aktuellt/covid-19-pandemins-konsekvenser-for-barn/ .

41 Su, L., X. Ma, H. Yu, Z. Zhang, P. Bian, Y. Han, J. Sun, Y. Liu, C. Yang, J. Geng, Z. Zhang, and Z. Gai. "The Different Clinical Characteristics of Corona Virus Disease Cases Between Children and Their Families in China – the Character of Children with COVID-19", *Emerging Microbes & Infections* 9:1 (2020): 707–713; Qiu, H., Junhua Wu, Liang Hong, Yunling Luo, Qifa Song, and Dong Chen. "Clinical and Epidemiological Features of 36 Children with Coronavirus Disease 2019 (COVID-19) in Zhejiang, China: An Observational Cohort Study", *The Lancet Infectious Diseases* 20:6 (2020): 689–696.

42 FHM. *Veckorapport om covid-19, vecka 50*, 2020.

43 Laxminarayan, R., B. Wahl, S.R. Dudala, K. Gopal, B.C. Mohan, S. Neelima, K.S. Jawahar Reddy, J. Radhakrishnan, and J.A. Lewnard. "Epidemiology and Transmission Dynamics of COVID-19 in Two Indian States", *Science* 370:6517 (2020): 691–697.

44 FHM. *COVID-19 in Children and Adolescents*, 2020.

45 Baubien, J. "Kids And Superspreaders Are Driving COVID-19 Cases in India, Huge Study Finds", *NPR*, 1 October 2020.

46 Peace, R. "Are Children the Biggest Covid-19 Spreaders?" *BBC, Science in Action*, 2 October 2020.

47 Vlachos, J., E. Hertegard, and H.B. Svaleryd. "The Effects of School Closures on SARS-CoV-2 Among Parents and Teachers", *PNAS* 118:9 (2021): e2020834118.

48 Haug, N., L. Geyrhofer, A. Londei, et al. "Ranking the Effectiveness of Worldwide COVID-19 Government Interventions", *Nature Human Behaviour* 4:12 (2020): 1303–1312; Brauner, J.M., S. Mindermann, M. Sharma, D. Johnston, J. Salvatier, T. Gavenčiak, A.B. Stephenson, G. Leech, G. Altman, V. Mikulik, A.J. Norman, J.T. Monrad, T. Besiroglu, H. Ge, M.A. Hartwick, Y.W. Teh, L. Chindelevitch, Y. Gal, and J. Kulveit. "Inferring the Effectiveness of Government Interventions Against COVID-19", *Science* 371:6531 (2021): eabd9338; Li, Y., H. Campbell, D. Kulkarni, A. Harpur, M. Nundy, X. Wang, and H. Nair. "The Temporal Association of Introducing and Lifting Non-Pharmaceutical Interventions with the Time-Varying Reproduction Number (R) of SARS-CoV-2: A Modelling Study Across 131 Countries", *The Lancet Infectious Diseases* 21:2 (2021): 193–202.

49 Lessler, J., M.K. Grabowski, K.H. Grantz, E. Badillo-Goicoechea, C. Metcalf, C. Lupton-Smith, A.S. Azman, and E.A. Stuart. "Household COVID-19 Risk and In-Person Schooling", *Science* 372:6546 (2021): 1092–1097.

50 "Statsepidemiolog Tegnell om smittan bland elever: Barnens bästa väger tyngre", *Sveriges Television*, 12 January 2021.

51 *Sveriges Barnreumatologiregister, Årsrapport 2020*, K. Palmblad, Editor (2021), https://barnreumaregistret.se/media/v4hbz0t0/korr3_barnreumarapport_2020_211021.pdf .

Personal communication: Greve-Isdahl, M., Amount of MIS-C cases in Norwegian children up to 5th July 2021, J. Höög, Editor. 2021: email.

"Amount of MIS-C cases in Norwegian children up to 5th July 2021", author's mail correspondence with MD Margrethe Greve-Isdahl, Norwegian Institute for Public Health (FHI), 2021.

Holm, M., U.B. Hartling, L.S. Schmidt, J.P. Glenthøj, A. Kruse, M.H. Rytter, M.S. Lindhard, M.C. Lawaetz, T. Zaharov, J.J. Petersen, R.M. Andersen, G. Lemvik, P. Marcinski, J. Thaarup, L.H. Jensen, L. Borch, A.B. Nielsen, N.H. Vissing, K. Schmiegelow, and U. Nygaard. "Multisystem Inflammatory Syndrome in Children Occurred in One of Four Thousand Children with Severe Acute Respiratory Syndrome Coronavirus 2", *Acta Paediatrica* 110:9 (2021): 2581–2583. "Number of Danish children with MIS-C until 30th of June 2021", author's mail correspondence with U. Nygaard, 2021.

"Number of Finish children with MIS-C", 2021. Author's email correspondence with E. Sarvikivi, 2021.

CDC. *Health Department-Reported Cases of Multisystem Inflammatory Syndrome in Children (MIS-C) in the United States*, https://covid.cdc.gov/covid-data-tracker/#mis-national-surveillance .

Deutsche Gesellschaft für Pädiatrische Infektiologie, PIMS-Survey-Update, 2021, https://dgpi.de/pims-survey-update/ .

52 FHM. *Bekräftade fall av covid-19 i Sverige*, 2020, FHM's webpage containing statistics of confirmed Covid-19 cases, intensive care patients and deaths, www.folkhalsomyndigheten.se/smittskydd-beredskap/utbrott/aktuella-utbrott/Covid-19/statistik-och-analyser/bekraftade-fall-i-sverige/ .

Norwegian Institute of Public Health and The Norwegian Surveillance System for Communicable Diseases, Number of children who have died with Covid-19 in Norway. 2021. Author's email conversation with Eirik Olsen.

Statens Serum Institut (SSI). *Ugentlige opgørelser med overvågningsdata*, 2021, https://covid19.ssi.dk/overvagningsdata/ugentlige-opgorelser-med-overvaagningsdata?fbclid=IwAR1yUYugxWLA9yhDTl2NPRhw_6D3AjJnqbQe1FTA2RaMQpRiLJA9PioMxkc .

Finish Institute for Health and Welfare, *Konstaterade coronavirusfall (COVID-19) i Finland*. 2021, https://experience.arcgis.com/experience/2b4648368532409788966d21e9c1e840 .

CDC. *Demographic Trends of COVID-19 cases and deaths in the US reported to CDC*, 2021, https://covid.cdc.gov/covid-data-tracker/#demographics .

Robert Koch Institut (RKI), *Täglicher Lagebericht des RKI zur Coronavirus-Krankheit-2019 (COVID-19)*, 2021, www.rki.de/DE/Content/InfAZ/N/Neuartiges_Coronavirus/Situationsberichte/Gesamt.html .

53 FHM. *Bekräftade fall av covid-19 i Sverige*, 2020, FHM's webpage containing statistics of confirmed Covid-19 cases, intensive care patients and deaths, www.folkhalsomyndigheten.se/smittskydd-beredskap/utbrott/aktuella-utbrott/Covid-19/statistik-och-analyser/bekraftade-fall-i-sverige/ .

54 Socialstyrelsen. *Vård och covid-19*, 2022, www.socialstyrelsen.se/statistik-och-data/statistik/statistik-om-covid-19/statistik-om-slutenvard-av-patienter-med-covid-19/; FHM. *Bekräftade fall av covid-19 i Sverige*, 2020.

55 Folkhelseinstittutet. *Ukerapport* – uke 11, 2022, www.fhi.no/contentassets/8a971e7b0a3c4a06bdbf381ab52e6157/vedlegg/2022/ukerapport-uke-11-14.03–20.03.22.pdf .

56 Thallapureddy, K., E. Zerda, et al. "Long-Term Complications of COVID-19 Infection in Adolescents and Children", *Current Pediatrics Reports* (2022): 1–7.

57 Munblit, Daniel, Frances Simpson, Jeremy Mabbitt, Audrey Dunn-Galvin, Calum Semple, and John O. Warner. "Legacy of COVID-19 Infection in Children: Long-COVID Will Have a Lifelong Health/Economic Impact", *Archives of Disease in Childhood* 107:3 (2022): e2.

58 Stephenson, T., R. Shafran, B. De Stavola, N. Rojas, F. Aiano, Z. Amin-Chowdhury, K. McOwat, R. Simmons, M. Zavala, C. Consortium, S.N. Ladhani, and CLoCk Consortium Members. "Long COVID and the Mental and Physical Health of Children and Young People: National Matched Cohort Study Protocol (the CLoCk Study)", *BMJ Open*, 11:8 (2021): e052838.

59 Johansen, Tone Bjordal, Elisabeth Astrup, Solveig Jore, Hege Nilssen, Bente Barton Dahlberg, Claus Klingenberg, Are Stuwitz Berg, and Margrethe Greve-Isdahl. "Infection Prevention Guidelines and Considerations for Paediatric Risk Groups When Reopening Primary Schools During COVID-19 Pandemic, Norway, April 2020", *Eurosurveillance* 25:22 (2020): pii=2000921.

60 Corona Commission. *Delbetänkande 2 – Sverige under pandemin SOU 2021:89*, 2021.

61 Barnombudsmannen. *Covid-19 pandemins konsekvenser för barn*, 2021.

62 Olsson, E. "Så säger lärarna själva om covid-läget", *Läraren*, 15 February 2022.

63 Seimyr, G.Ö. "Learning Loss From Sweden to England to the U.S.", 2021, www.lexplore.com/en/learning-loss-from-sweden-england-us/ .

64 FHM. *Förekomst av covid-19 i olika yrkeskategorier – delrapport 2*, 2021.

65 FHM. *Veckorapport om covid-19, vecka 50,* 2020.

66 FHM. *Pressträff om covid-19 (coronavirus)*, 13 mars 2020.

67 Medborgare, O. "Hej @Anna_Ekstrom! Vad bra att se att du har på dig ett FFP2 andningsskydd, som skyddar både din omgivning och dig själv. Varför fick inte varenda #lärare i #Sverige också ha det i 1,5 år av pandemi?" 2021, https://twitter.com/okuvad/status/1406919425396183051 .

68 Nilsson, M.M. "Försäkringskassan efter rekord-vab: En dag extra kostar en miljard per år", *Arbetet*, 4 February 2022.

69 Corona Commission. *Summary in English*, 2022, https://coronakommissionen.com/wp-content/uploads/2022/02/summary_20220225.pdf .

70 Munblit et al. "Legacy of COVID-19 Infection in Children".

71 *Homeschooling International Status and Statistics*, https://en.wikipedia.org/wiki/Homeschooling_international_status_and_statistics .

72 Höög, J. "How Have Children Been Protected in Other Countries", 2021, www.youtube.com/watch?v=sx3nUkb3sWg .

73 Singer, N. "Online Schools Are Here to Stay, Even After the Pandemic", *New York Times*, 11 April 2021; Lockee, B.B. "Online Education in the Post-COVID Era", *Nature Electronics* 4:5–6 (2021).

10

THE BIOPOLITICS OF HERD IMMUNITY

Lapo Lappin

In the first spring of the new decade – when the pandemic spread of SARS-CoV-2 kicked off the "boring twenties" – Sweden became almost synonymous with herd immunity. To the great dismay of the Swedish public, of course, at least so long as herd immunity was thought of as something negative.[1] Yet within the borders of the northern kingdom, the Swedish strategy was received with a mixture of obviousness and inevitability; there was a refusal to understand that there could be any other way to deal with health and politics.

Back in the seventies, the French philosopher Michel Foucault opened a field of reflection on precisely the intersection between politics and health: "biopolitics". Foucault's analyses and predictions, it has lately been argued, have aged badly. Much has since changed in both ambits, and his all-too sketchy reflections about biological power are no longer applicable to the complex nexus of contemporary health policies that the pandemic has laid bare. Recent events have shown that there is some truth to this evaluation. Where biopolitical thought has been deployed in Europe during the pandemic, the analysis resulted in simplistic and quasi-conspiratorial platitudes.[2] But while a critical biopolitical analysis rings shallow when targeting the lockdowns or vaccination programmes that have punctuated the pandemic, Foucault's grim predictions prove prescient in the case of Sweden. In particular, Foucault's reading can help us to understand how modern biopolitics allows the exclusion of certain people (or certain kinds of people) whose lives are considered not worth protecting.

The first section of this essay is therefore a plea for a renewed biopolitical reflection on the pandemic, underpinned by an explanation of the core concepts laid out by Foucault. After that, in the second section, the role of herd immunity in the Swedish strategy will be outlined. As a result of a deliberately ambiguous communication strategy on the part of FHM, the precise bearing of herd immunity on their overall policy remained opaque. I here attempt to clarify the role of

DOI: 10.4324/9781003289364-11

herd immunity, and identify two aspects of FHM's communicative strategy: first, an unclear distinction between the "goals" of a strategy and the outcomes of a strategy, second, taking objection to the very term "herd immunity" rather than herd immunity as such. Particular attention will be given to the discourse around the pandemic, especially concerning institutional communication. As I will argue, the abandonment of certain people is preceded by an abandonment at the level of language.

In the third section, I examine the justification for Sweden's *Sonderweg*. It has been claimed that the strategy builds upon a utilitarian calculus. Drawing upon Foucault's reflections on biopolitics, I show how the idea of maximising utility at the population level is linked with the conceptual apparatus that views the population as a statistical unit. In the fourth section, I investigate how this conceptualisation justifies thinking of losing lives for the greater good. In doing so, I borrow the biopolitical concept of the "including exclusion" (as theorised by Roberto Esposito and Giorgio Agamben), by which the State abandons the biological life it normally tends to protect. I see this mechanism at work among two demographics in the Swedish pandemic: the elderly and risk-group parents of school-children.

Death to biopolitics?

In a 1976 lecture at the Collège de France, Michel Foucault introduced the concept of "biopolitics" as a way to conceptualise the ways in which the modern State exercises power over biological life. "Biopolitics deals with the population", Foucault writes, "a problem that is at once scientific and political".[3] In his *History of Sexuality* (1976) Foucault provides a further piece of the puzzle. At the dawn of the modern era a transformation of sovereign power took place. In the pre-modern paradigm, the figure of the sovereign concentrated power over life and death, like the sword-wielding figure on the cover of Hobbes's *Leviathan*. It was the "ancient right to *take* life or *let live*", to execute or spare life. The biological stratum of life thus surfaced only in rare but fateful moments, when life itself was negotiated *vis-à-vis* the monarch.[4]

In the modern paradigm, by contrast, the biological aspect of life becomes the very object of sovereignty. Biological life is something to be constantly monitored and policed. A new kind of power emerges: the technological power to administer and uphold biological life, on the one hand, and to withhold such administration, on the other. As Foucault writes, it is no longer the power to take life, but rather "to *foster* life or *disallow* it".[5] As an example of fostering biopolitics, one can pick freely from the myriad screenings, check-ups and vaccinations that make up modern public health policy.[6] As an example of lives that can be disallowed – and the construction of the category of "lives that do not deserve to be lived"[7] – one could pick the dental health experiments with disabled patients, sponsored by the sugar industry, at the psychiatric hospital of Vipeholm in Lund.[8] In the early 1940s, for instance, the mortality rate suddenly tripled under mysterious circumstances. The institution had decided not to treat its patients, cutting down on their food intake and allowing nature to take its course.[9] The lives of the patients were thus abandoned, not in the manner of a pre-modern execution, but as a withdrawal of the care the State would otherwise have administered.[10]

Incidentally, the roots of the term biopolitics stretch further back than Foucault's lectures. Originally, the concept was coined by the Swedish conservative philosopher Rudolf Kjellén, with whom Foucault came into contact during his infelicitous spell at Uppsala University. In Kjellén's biopolitics (*biopolitik*), individuals are sucked up into an organicist collective, like cells in a living, breathing organism: the State, which flails around in search of sustenance and *Lebensraum* (another of Kjellén's fateful neologisms).[11]

Notwithstanding its early success, the Covid-19 pandemic seemingly put an end to the pertinence of biopolitical reflection.[12] According to Slavoj Žižek, biopolitical critique has outlived its usefulness,[13] a feeling echoed by the Swiss historian Philipp Sarasin,[14] as well as by the French philosopher Jean-Luc Nancy.[15] The American theorist Benjamin Bratton goes as far as to argue that the entire tradition "needs to be shelved".[16] These reactions are not entirely unprovoked. As soon as the pandemic broke out, the chief theorists were absorbed by what – when stripped of their glossy jargon – one would be inclined to regard as conspiracy theories.

In Germany, for instance, philosopher Peter Sloterdijk prophesied a "medical-collectivistic dictatorship",[17] while Byung-Chul Han described the West's reaction as a "biopolitical quarantine society that permanently restricts our freedom".[18] But the cautionary tale remained that by Italian philosopher Giorgio Agamben, in what Bratton described as "the most cataclysmic and grotesque self-owns in the history of philosophy".[19] In columns and interviews, subsequently collected in the florilegium *A che punto siamo?* (2021), Agamben railed against the "invention of a pandemic",[20] dredging up colourful parallels to the 1930s.[21] "When a biopolitical philosophy was most needed", Bratton comments, "the author went mad".[22]

Whether or not Agamben actually strayed too close to the edge, there is reason to challenge Bratton's bleak diagnosis of biopolitics. If there is anything striking in Agamben's interventions, it is rather the *lack* of biopolitical reflection. Interviewers – including on Swedish State Radio[23] – managed to tease out some gnomic pronouncements on "bare life" (the mere biological existence down to which we have been stripped, according to Agamben, when divested of all social or psychological dimensions by lockdown).[24] For the most part, however, the reflections deal with the illegitimacy of the state of exception,[25] infringements of civil rights and the alleged advent of a novel, fear-fuelled totalitarianism. On the West's collective thanatophobia, Agamben writes, "one can only erect a dictatorship, a monstrous Leviathan with an unsheathed sword".[26]

Agamben's critique thus attacks a sovereignty grounded in violence, leading us back into the jaws of Leviathan; on the Foucauldian dyad sketched earlier, a resolutely "old" form of sovereign power, legitimised by exhibitions of brute force.[27] For Foucault, however, biopolitics arises precisely when the violent interpositions of the sovereign's repressive and juridical power are transcended, when the State's power over biological life melts into the ever present yet invisible background.[28]

What Foucault described as biopolitics is not the Hobbesian totalitarianism feared by Agamben, but a particularly *liberal* (or even neo-liberal) form of governmentality.[29]

It would therefore be wrong to conclude, with Bratton, that Agamben's fall from grace is an unavoidable culmination of the biopolitical tradition. It is rather a subversion – and betrayal – of the foundational insight of biopolitics. If Foucault is right that the shape of modern biopolitics is found in the *continuous* support and withdrawal of life-support, rather than any earth-shattering state of exception, we should expect to find these mechanisms at work in those pandemic strategies that style themselves as explicitly liberal, that claim to be simply an extension of business as usual. One such strategy stands out: that of Sweden.

Talk of the troll: herd immunity and the Swedish strategy

At the centre of Sweden's strategy was the hope of achieving herd immunity.[30] The virus was allowed to spread through the population, curbed just enough to keep the health-care system afloat. In the early months of the pandemic, mentions of herd immunity cropped up everywhere, like a *lupus in fabula*, a chimaera always only a month away.[31] As a consequence of considerable institutional trolling, however, the exact role of herd immunity in the strategy became increasingly unclear (on the failures of institutional communication see Bergholtz's and Edvinsson's chapters in this volume). Gradually, it was relegated to a mere "rumour".[32] This obnubilation, I argue, was predicated on two aspects. First, a distinction between "goals" of a strategy, on the one hand, and mere desirable effects, on the other. Second, that these "effects" were to be passed over in silence, and were best left undiscussed.

In the early days of March 2020, the Swedish State Epidemiologist Anders Tegnell claimed that the Swedish strategy was the same as the British one. The latter, he declared in the same comment, was to achieve herd immunity.[33] When pressed by journalists, Tegnell recoiled: herd immunity was not a *part* of the strategy. The strategy was simply to allow the virus to spread at a speed the health services could keep pace with. While herd immunity is well and good, it was not the explicit *goal* of the Swedish strategy (although Tegnell also stressed that it was "not in conflict with" the strategy).[34]

In April 2020, Johan Giesecke, previously State Epidemiologist and subsequently advisor to FHM, was featured on the British news site *UnHerd*, an outlet aiming to "push back against the herd mentality".[35] The interview garnered over a million views, making Giesecke into an internationally acclaimed spokesman for the herd immunity line. Giesecke at first attempts to draw the same distinction as Tegnell: herd immunity is a *consequence*, not a strategy in and of itself. Yet as the interview unravels it becomes progressively obvious that this distinction was never especially clear-cut. In the end, Giesecke says that the strategy "essentially" is to allow the virus to pass through the population. He summarises it in two words: "herd immunity".[36]

The first sophism was thus a putative distinction between goals and effects. Herd immunity was a desired yet inexorable outcome of the strategy[37] – indeed, the only way to get rid of the virus at all. But it is not an official "part" of the strategy, nor was it an explicit "goal". Only a "consequence" or an "effect".[38] While no one provided a definition of these terms, they were treated as a panacea. Tegnell foists this distinction *ex post facto* onto a laconic email to the Finnish professor of Health Security, Mika Salminen: "An argument would be to keep schools open in order to [*för att*] more quickly achieve herd immunity". Tegnell glossed it in hindsight as suggesting "a possible effect" of keeping schools open, not the reason for doing so.[39] This interpretation pushes not only the limits of credibility but the limits of language itself – "in order to" simply does not indicate a side-effect or vague possibility.

An offshoot of the definition of herd immunity as a possible (yet at the same time inevitable) consequence was that it should no longer be talked about. Tegnell took objection to the very term "herd immunity" rather than with a *strategy* of herd immunity. Tegnell confessed he was "wary of using the word because it evokes the idea of surrender".[40] Or as Johan Carlson expressed it in an untranslatable turn of phrase: "*Det där med flockimmunitet har det gått lite troll i*."[41] The discussion thus shifted from herd immunity to the shibboleth "herd immunity", which Carlson explicitly forbade his employees from using in public.[42]

Among those who got the memo was the Left Party leader Jonas Sjöstedt, who also bought into the distinction between ends and consequences of a strategy. On Twitter, he recounts that although "many [in Parliament] realised" that the virus would rip through the population as "an effect" of the Swedish strategy, the "Government did not *say* that a greater spread was an end in itself".[43] Sjöstedt's concession captures the apophatic, unspeakable nature of the Swedish strategy. It can be gleaned between the lines yet should never be asserted. The linguistic exclusion, as will become clear later on, mirrors a deeper exclusion.

The same exclusion can be seen in the ruling Social Democratic Party's revision of the document outlining the Swedish strategy of controlled spread several months after publication. The original version contained the admission that they did not want "too many people to be infected at the same time". Later on this purple passage was conveniently elided from the document. The edit was later attributed to "a mistake".[44] In any case, the Minister for Social Affairs Lena Hallengren denied that herd immunity was the strategy. According to Hallengren, there was never a strategy at all.[45] A similar vacuum was almost palpable when Hallengren declared that there were no extant minutes for the 149 meetings between FHM and the Government.[46] In hindsight, one can see how the strategy was pocked with absences, with *in*actions, exclusions and omissions: by cordoning off areas of language one cordons off areas of reality (see the fourth section).

Nevertheless, the denial that herd immunity was a core component in the Swedish strategy became impossible after the surfacing of a batch of emails between Tegnell and infection doctor Peet Tüll, who presented three alternatives: lockdown, track-and-trace or herd immunity. The last one would lead to deaths in the thousands, which Tüll considered "unacceptable" (and "headless" and "defeatist"). Tegnell answered that he had already sifted through the options and had opted firmly for herd immunity.[47]

A last stand is attempted in journalist Amina Manzoor's *Pandemier!* (2021), which makes the case that "herd immunity" was never a part of the Swedish strategy. The evidence she adduces for this is Tegnell's occasional denials. Confronted with Tegnell's emails to Peet Tüll, Manzoor claims that this too is a misconception: FHM allegedly provided the correct context, that Tegnell viewed both lockdown and track-and-trace as unviable alternatives. Exactly how this means that Tegnell did not actually endorse the herd immunity alternative is something Manzoor fails to explain.[48] In any case, the reader is left with the unmistakable impression that the whole "herd immunity" allegation was a conspiracy spearheaded by none other than Donald Trump. Thanks to a rhetorical *legerdemain*, the whole issue is dispelled.

It cannot be said that Manzoor's *book* withstood the test of time particularly well. Only two weeks after its publication, it was eclipsed by another overview of the Swedish pandemic, *Flocken* ("The Herd"), authored by Swedish journalist Johan Anderberg. Building on over 100 interviews with the main actors of the Swedish pandemic, Anderberg builds an incontrovertible case that herd immunity was on the cards from the very outset.[49]

On herds and morality

Given that the Swedish strategy was to allow the virus to spread in the hope of reaching herd immunity, one should pose the further question of how this strategy was justified, especially when the entire project was considered highly controversial from an international perspective. The WHO declared that seeking herd immunity "is simply unethical", due to the unnecessary loss of lives and the long-term effects of Covid illness.[50] Ireland's Chief Clinical Officer lashed out at Giesecke's suggestion that herd immunity should also be pursued in Ireland, claiming such a course of action is not "acceptable in a civilised society".[51] All of which begs the question: how could an entire country flock to a strategy that others found instinctively repulsive?[52]

It has been suggested that utilitarianism provides the ethical underpinning for the Swedish strategy.[53] In line with utilitarian reasoning, the Swedish strategy seemed to pick the greatest good for the greatest number, the good of the herd even at the cost of individual lives. Also in line with utilitarian reasoning, the values embodied by the Swedish strategy come close to the utilitarian idea of goodness as utility (that is to say, pleasure or well-being).[54] The Swedish strategy gave precedence to the economy and the general well-being of the population (affirming the right to go to the pub so as to keep morale high). The godfather of Swedish utilitarianism, Torbjörn Tännsjö, praised the Swedish strategy for its implicit utilitarian character;[55] the only possible alternative to Sweden's approach to the pandemic was, according to him, "magical thinking".[56] In contrast to other ethical approaches, such as Kantian ethics or virtue ethics, utilitarianism sees no special value in human life: life is one among many competing aspects that generate utility.[57] If the scales are balanced right, it may even become just to take life: as utilitarian philosopher Peter Singer argues, some lives are worth so little that it is morally imperative to take them.[58]

Unsurprisingly, Singer was the guest of honour at a seminar hosted by the Swedish National Council on Medical Ethics (SMER) about health-care in the pandemic.[59] In the Swedish strategy, even though some lives are lost, the sum of well-being generated by keeping society rolling outweighs this human cost.

But the question remains of why the utilitarian approach – the herd immunity strategy – seemed to be the obvious choice for policy-makers. The proof, as they say, is in the pudding: to be precise, in the word *herd*. While it is hardly a term of art in modern statecraft, it has a venerable history. From the first glimmerings in antiquity through the use of pastoral imagery in Jewish poetry and Christianity, the metaphor of the shepherd and the sheep-herd has dominated Western political thought. At least, that is the essence of Foucault's ruminations on the subject. This "pastoral power", according to Foucault, builds on the image of the shepherd and his flock. The pastoral imagery allows the conceptualising of the collective as a flock, considered a homogenous whole that can be herded in different directions by its leaders.[60] In time, the herd evolved into the "population"[61] – an innovative modern concept that opened up an entirely new level of abstraction. The concept of "population" presents the sum of bodies as a unified mass, capable of being controlled and manipulated through "forecasts, statistical estimates, and overall measures".[62] The conceptual apparatus of the "population" brings with it an interest in the "health" of the population, which is achieved by collecting information about bodies in a territory and subsequently compounding it into a quantifiable mass of utility.

Already in its embryonic form, the issue of conceptualising persons was at the base of epidemiology – epidemic derives, after all, from the Greek *epi* ("on") and *demos* ("people", "crowd", "rabble").[63] It is this biopolitical conceptual apparatus that constitutes the ground for the utilitarian reasoning of the Swedish strategy. The pastoral image of the herd evolved into the concept of the population *as one thing*, as a "global mass",[64] a totality that subsumes and compounds all biological data into a homogenised *quantum*. One need only turn to *Folkhälsomyndigheten* – literally the Authority of *population health*[65] – to see how this conceptual mechanism is cashed out. In the pandemic plan from 2015, for instance, three guiding principles are proposed: "the negative effects on society should be as small as possible", "population health should be impacted as little as possible" and "trust in the State ministries and healthcare system should be upheld".[66] The first point in FHM's plan constitutes the kind of biopolitical totality we are treating: the goal is to minimise the negative effects on "society", a vacuous totality, left nebulous and indeterminate (and therefore all-encompassing). The second principle dovetails onto the first: "population health" (*folkhälsa*), a second biopolitical totality, is another example of a sum abstracted from its parts, composed of abstract variables that are bundled into a whole.

As the Swedish historian of ideas Karin Johannisson has argued, the project of *folkhälsa* ("population health") was not only a medical but an overwhelmingly social and political project, an offshoot of the organicist discourse of society as a living body over and above its members.[67] *Folkhälsa*, Johannisson writes, "became a metaphor for an entire political project":[68] the conceptualisation of population as a *unit*, seen from above.[69] This image of the population, as "Folk", was a requirement for the Social Democrat project of social engineering. *Folkhälsa* is intimately related to the concept of *folkmaterialet* or *befolkningsmaterialet*, the conceptualisation of the population as a lump of raw material, malleable and kneadable in the hands of social engineers.[70]

While the 2015 framework is no longer officially in place, it continues to exert an influence.[71] The principle of population health was dropped in the new pandemic strategy (2019). Nonetheless, the term "population-health perspective" (*folkhälsoperspektivet*) came into broad currency as a description of the Swedish strategy. FHM General Director Johan Carlson explains it strikingly: the pandemic strategy assumes its particular shape because it is seen in "broader population health perspective".[72] This perspective was allegedly more holistic, more attuned to the needs of the entire population than a myopic fixation with "lives" to be saved. Carlson further identifies the public health perspective as a weighing of different values against each other (and in line with consequentialist ethics these options are only evaluated in terms of their "effects").[73] After Carlson's exquisitely timed retirement, his successor Karin Tegmark Wisell echoed the same sentiments.[74] Yet the details of how such a calculation was tallied, what parameters were weighed, how "effects" were calculated, if ethical dimensions were considered – we will probably never know. What is important for our purposes here, however, is the rhetorical strategy of "putting into perspective" within a larger panorama of "public health" (whether veridical or fictitious). It is the paroxysm that gripped apologists of the official line, that the Swedish strategy had wider lenses, which maximised well-being at the level of the population.[75]

Luckily enough, others stepped in to fill the absence of ethical justification in FHM's strategy. Part of the task of providing this window-dressing fell to the Swedish National Council on Medical Ethics (SMER), in the report *Etiska vägval i pandemin* (Ethical Choices in a Pandemic). Here too, we find the same biopolitical conceptual apparatus at work. In an international seminar in summer of 2020, a representative of SMER connected the Swedish strategy to the Social Democrat notion of *folkhemmet*, the home of the "Folk", the People.[76] (Incidentally, *folkhemmet* also just happens to be a term of Kjelléan provenance.) *Folkhemmet*, in the Social Democratic mythopoeia, represents the State, painted as a homely abode for a homogenous population – a big happy family.

In the document, SMER plots a conflict of values between two perspectives: on the one hand, individual rights and freedoms (freedom of movement and association, privacy, etc.); on the other hand, what is shiftingly termed "population health",[77] "the collective"[78] and "society as a whole".[79] The individual marks a limit that cannot be trespassed, but only approached asymptotically. The whole is the domain of population health, where the name of the game is to "maximise the good" (something which is obtained by optimising different statistical variables).

The value of human life is not included in SMER's first category, that of inalienable rights. Instead, it is placed in the second category, the maximisation of the good on the level of population health. Human lives are just one of the many values that make up the *totum* that is population health (alongside physical and psychological well-being, feelings of alienation, economic factors,[80] and – SMER underscores the importance of this aspect – trust in the State).[81] This positioning entails several consequences. First, an individual human life is no longer a human life *as such*, but becomes conglomerated with a number of other lives. SMER only mentions *lives* (in the plural) as bundles of numbers: 720 against 350, 500 against 500, etc. These quantities are then tempered against other quantities. Thus, human lives are placed in the "population-health perspective" and become dominated by what SMER calls (in utilitarian-tinged language) the principle of "maximising the good". The problem is this: from the perspective of maximising population health (and its concomitant economic dimension) some lives are well lost; they are too expensive, too brittle or simply not conducive to greater well-being for the whole. In some cases, it could even be good to thin out the ranks (for example, of the elderly who overwhelmed Swedish population statistics). This observation is not to claim that this reasoning was in place (or endorsed by SMER); it is rather to draw out the logical conclusions of this line of argument. The protection of life is not a question of rights (unlike going to the pub), but only one among many biological facets of population health.

A more interesting and blatantly apologetical contribution was authored by four researchers affiliated with the Institute for Future Studies. At the beginning of the pandemic, they published a debate article pleading for the institution of an "ethical council" at FHM. The authors' mission to create an ethical council culminated in a chapter on the ethics of pandemics in a Government investigation and a convivial seminar with Anders Tegnell.[82] Reassuringly, the authors explain how the institution of their council would be a way to counter corruption.[83]

The authors' chapter, "Etiska avvägningar i pandemitider" (Ethical choices in times of pandemic), expands on the same themes broached by SMER. Two of the authors, Gustaf Arrhenius and Krister Bykvist, happen to be experts in utilitarian "population ethics".[84] Here, too, freedom is placed within the sphere of rights,[85] while life is but one value among many others – a calculus in which some lives are simply worth more than others.[86] In an important passage, the authors weigh the lives saved by imposing restrictions against the lives lost as a consequence of not shopping at the mall.[87] This conflict of value, however, should not be framed as a choice between lives and the economy, the report declares. "The economy" is also a discourse about life. The same point was made by Kerstin Hessius (who was crowned with the epithet "our hero" by a Social Democrat minister),[88] director of the Third Swedish National Pension Fund: the economy is, at the end of the day, "about lives", "about people".[89] The authors of the report likewise hypostatise the economy into a biopolitical abstraction. The economy, they claim, should not be viewed as mere faceless fluctuations of capital. It is about *life*. But life cannot be made into the subject matter of the economy (as with population health) without, at the same time, being reduced to a vague shadow of what actual life is. Entirely sublated into a totalising economic/utilitarian calculation, it can only itself become an economic abstraction.[90]

To conclude this section, the utilitarian approach of the Swedish strategy builds on the biopolitical conceptual apparatus of "population", in all its permutations. We saw an unexpected renaissance of the term *herd*, awoken from its cryogenic sleep, alongside all its historical descendants: the *population*, "the collective", "*folkhemmet*", "population health", "society as a whole", "the economy".[91] The totalising view of the population and its "health" cannot but place human lives within a morass of biological variables. A telling offshoot of this discussion is the unexpected return of the old biopolitical *motif* of the "body politic" (*samhällskroppen*).[92] References to the *samhällskropp* – to depict the overarching concern with broad biopolitical systems, instead of the reductive focus on individual bodies – sprouted up like mushrooms in the Swedish discourse.[93] A few scalpel-knocks underneath, for the archaeologically inclined, lie the relics of Kjellén's organicism.

Immunity: the biopolitics of abandonment

We turn now to the second pole of the Swedish strategy: that of *immunity*. As the Italian philosopher Roberto Esposito has pointed out, immunity is the key-term of biopolitics. Immunity is from its inception a double concept, denoting at once biological immunity as well as legal or political immunity. In this coincidence of the biological and political, Esposito sees an entire "immunitarian paradigm". Politics, Esposito argues, has often been imagined on the model of biological immunity: external threats are conceptualised as poisons or maladies that can be combated by a sort of immunisation. By assimilating a portion of the threat one can better defend against it. Just as a small dose of poison can immunise the body from an otherwise lethal dose further down the line, politics also works according to the logic of this "including exclusion". By including part of a threat, the threat can be repelled.[94]

The Swedish strategy follows this immunitarian logic closely. Instead of shutting the virus out, the virus is allowed to spread *in order to fight the virus*.[95] Covid-19 is included precisely in order to exclude it. The aim is to immunise the societal body. But Esposito's insight is that this including exclusion is at work on all levels of biopolitics, not only at the level of society but also that of individuals. Recall Foucault's two faces of biopolitics: the upholding of the biological functions of the population (which was explored in the previous section) and the abandonment of the life of certain individuals. In this section I will show how the second aspect is at work in the Swedish strategy. The maximising of utility for "society" entailed the abandonment of certain kinds of people.

This abandonment took the shape of an including exclusion. For this purpose, it is worth turning to the early biopolitical work of Giorgio Agamben. Agamben tracks the biopolitical mechanism of the including exclusion back to its very beginnings. He identifies this beginning with the figure of the *homo sacer* (literally: the sacred human), an obscure figure in ancient Roman law. The *homo sacer* was someone who had been banished from the political community. As a consequence of this expulsion, the *homo sacer* could be killed without any legal repercussions. He/she no longer enjoyed any legal protection and was thus reduced to mere natural life, stripped of any political rights or duties. The *homo sacer* is thereby placed outside the realm of the law. At the same time, however, it is *the law itself* that places him/her outside the law. Agamben points out this double movement: on the one hand, the *homo sacer* is excluded from the political community; on the other hand, political power must first include the person to be able to exclude him. The original structure of biopolitics, according to Agamben, consists in an *abandonment*. Agamben couples this phenomenon etymologically to the further figure of the *bandit*, who is banned from the polity and outlawed by the law. Nevertheless, it is the law itself that, prior to this exclusion, includes the bandit into the realm of the law.[96]

This motif of the including exclusion remains a constant in the history of politics. It culminates in the abandonment of biological life of modern biopolitics. The abandonment of certain people which was carried out in the Swedish management of the pandemic is precisely the same kind of abandonment. As Foucault describes it, there are cases in which the State's usual activity of upholding biological life is arbitrarily rescinded, in which biological life is abandoned. This exclusion, however, is made possible by a prior inclusion. Although it is not, as Agamben describes in the case of the *homo sacer*, at the juridical level, by being stripped of legal rights. It happens instead at a societal level: such people are forcibly included in the workings of society (in the vaporous and general biopolitical sense of the word), and thus abandoned at the level of biological life, since their life is no longer protected.

The first, and obvious, demographic that was the target of this abandonment were the elderly. As soon as the pandemic broke out, Stockholm Region issued (utilitarian)[97] guidelines for prioritisation between patients. Among those who were to be denied treatment were patients with COPD, a BMI over 40, pacemakers, as well as alcoholics, drug addicts,[98] those with dementia[99] and elderly people more generally. Even though maximum capacity was never reached in ICU, the hospitals still made severe priorities.[100] According to the Health and Social Care Inspectorate (IVO), 20% of the patients in a care home with suspected or confirmed cases of Covid-19 were administered palliative care without an individual check-up by a doctor, some not even by a nurse.[101] Rather than oxygen, they were dosed with morphine.[102]

There was certainly an *exclusion*: the biological life of the elderly is deemed as not worth saving. These lives, from a population health perspective, were of little value. But there was also an *inclusion*: the lives were included into a strategy that allowed the virus to pass through the population. The deaths among the elderly were proportionate to the spread of the virus in society.[103] The inclusion in this grand plan presupposed their exclusion from the State's protection of biological life: once they had been included in the spread, they were abandoned by the health-care system, filled up with morphine, and sent on their way.

But the *including exclusion* is also at work in the biopolitical abandonment of another (less discussed) group: the parents of school-age children. This group received considerably less attention than the elderly.[104] This "forgetting" is highly relevant: as was sketched before in the case of Jonas Sjöstedt and Lena Hallengren's sins of omission, an abandonment at the level of discourse mirrors and permits an abandonment in society.

Let us wind back to the first days of the pandemic: Emma Frans, one of the main commentators of the pandemic in the media, was interviewed by CNN in late March 2020.[105] The interviewer wondered why Sweden had decided to keep its schools open. In particular, the interviewer highlighted the mismatch between keeping schools open, on the one hand, and the explicit goal of "protecting risk-groups", on the other. Children are after all bound to get infected at school and thereafter pass the infection on to their parents. Many of these belong to those risk-groups Sweden is allegedly invested in protecting. "The strategy in Sweden is not to stop the virus from spreading", Frans explains, "but instead to slow down the process". She also assures that it is easier to isolate the elderly since "*it is not as common* to live in large families" in Sweden. This statement in itself is already an admission of abandonment. Those (predominantly foreign) households that span generational gaps are written off as a statistical aberration. Their marginalisation resulted in high levels of deaths in immigrant communities where living together in intergenerational households was still the norm. But more importantly, Frans refuses to answer the question. Her answer about controlled spread fails to answer the question of what will happen to vulnerable risk-group parents. The point is precisely that this question is *omitted*, that it is not even granted existence as a concrete issue. When Frans uploaded the CNN clip on Twitter, the part dealing with the issue of parents was edited out completely.[106] Nowhere in Frans's other writings is this question acknowledged.[107]

In her podcast *Hjärta och Hjärna* (Heart and Brain), aired on Swedish Radio, Frans answered a similar question from a teacher worried about getting infected in school. What is important to understand, says Frans, is that we must "weigh different values against one another", in accordance with the population health perspective. She assures that "most people under seventy will do very well". What about those teachers who have died, and the many more who have fallen gravely ill? These cases are also left unmentioned, not even worthy of an acknowledgement. What is important, Frans stresses, is rather that the biopolitical totality of "society continues to carry on [*samhället fortsätter att pågå*]" – whatever that means, whatever the price.[108]

Frans is not alone. The Minister of education, Anna Ekström, also embodies the same kind of abandonment. Nowhere, to my knowledge, was this question brought up at any of the many press-conferences that punctuated the pandemic. In an interview in the Swedish newspaper *Dagens Nyheter*, Ekström was pressed on this matter. The Minister gave a laconic answer: "It was never an option to take away compulsory school attendance [*skolplikt*]. This obligation is uncompromisable."[109] Ekström follows the pattern in refusing to answer the query; she also lays bare the philosophical bedrock: the legal principle of *skolplikt*, which states clearly that all healthy children must be physically present in school (thus excluding as illegal any kind of alternative education from the State-provided one),[110] is an imprescriptible principle that cannot budge.[111] The same argument was made by Peter Fredriksson, General Director of the Swedish National Agency for Education (*Skolverket*), on the subject of parents keeping their children home to avoid infection: "It may sound harsh, but in school there is *skolplikt*. That's all one can say to them."[112] Nothing more.

The linguistic abandonment at the level of language culminates in an abandonment at the level of reality. And parents were abandoned: 800 children lost a parent as a consequence of the pandemic.[113] Yet as a biopolitical abandonment, it is important to realise that this exclusion has an including aspect. The legal precept of *skolplikt* provided the mechanism for the forced inclusion of these groups into society. Those parents who broke *skolplikt* faced astronomical fines. In a report from the Ministry of Education, school principals describe how they contacted parents daily to explain the importance of being physically present in school, even going to their homes in person.[114] The infringement of *skolplikt*, apart from fines, could also mean that Social Services could take over custody of the child(ren) in question.[115]

The including exclusion of parents was achieved through the forced inclusion of their children into the "continuation of society" – in this case, the obligation that all children be physically present within certain walls. The workings of the society these individuals were coerced into participating in also presupposed the spread of a dangerous disease, which they would in all likelihood be unable to avoid.

Or rather, perhaps better, a disease they *should* be infected with. It was arguably a part of the strategy that quick contagion in schools would speed up the advent of the promised herd immunity. The previous FHM State Epidemiologist, Annika Linde, described FHM's strategy as permitting the "slow spread of the disease among school-children *and their parents* so as to build up herd immunity".[116] The same argument was made by the influential paediatrician Jonas Ludvigsson,[117] endorsed by FHM's "patriarch" Johan Giesecke,[118] as well as by Tegnell himself, in the email to Mika Salminen quoted earlier. Parents were thereby abandoned – they were excluded from the normal protection of life offered by the State, and they were left at the mercy of unfettered spread. At the same time, this exclusion is worked by means of an inclusion: they are sucked into the strategy, as pawns to reach herd immunity.

The biopolitical abandonment, by which the protection of life is rescinded and persons are left bare in front of potentially lethal threats, takes the form of an including exclusion. It is not just an abandonment, by which the State leaves some citizens behind. Prior to this abandonment, the State coerces them into participation, including them in the vaporous "continuation of society" for its own sake, as well as dragged into a strategy that presupposes that a vast majority will be infected. I have pointed out how this biopolitical mechanism is deployed in the cases of two demographics: the elderly and parents of school-children. This is by no means supposed to be understood as an exclusive classification: other groups fall into similar patterns, for example, teachers and essential workers whose protection of life is rescinded for societal gain,[119] the disabled,[120] already marginalised immigrant groups[121] and those otherwise healthy, both children and adults, who were hit by long-Covid (and subsequently abandoned, pathologised and denied proper diagnoses or sick-leave).[122]

Conclusion: the invisible pandemic

In lieu of a conclusion, allow me to summarise the main trajectories of the argument, and gesture to some possible further directions. The concept of herd immunity – however blurred in the rhetoric – was at the core of the Swedish strategy to manage the Covid-19 pandemic. Its ethical justification is found in a utilitarian calculus. This kind of utilitarianism is, in turn, strongly implied in the conceptual apparatus that views the "population" as a thing, a bundle of biological statistics that should constantly be maximised. The focus on the support of the biological functions and health of this "whole" (the herd) is closely linked (as Foucault describes it) to the possibility of taking away the biological protection for certain individuals. I investigated two cases where this abandonment takes place: the lives of the elderly and parents of school-age children. The form of this abandonment is that of an "including exclusion", of the kind Roberto Esposito links with an immunitarian biopolitical paradigm.

One of the chief advantages of a biopolitical reflection is that it allows us to deal with passivities: it enables the conceptualisation of when the State abandons the biological life of its citizens. A difficulty in dealing with this issue has been characteristic of the discussion of the Swedish pandemic. This can be gleaned in Peter Baldwin's foreword to this volume, which falls back on the image of the "sacrifice" of the elderly.

The fundamental insight, I think, is correct, although it leaves itself open to contradiction. Sacrifice requires someone to draw the knife, to which the critic can answer: there is no evidence that there was a nefarious plan to weed out the weak. It was all a matter of unfortunate side-effects we can put behind us.

Biopolitical analysis allows us to side-step this impasse. The question is not so much on the level of how the State acted but the State's *in*action, how it refused to act. Of who was excluded, eliminated or abandoned. We are dealing with passivities, inactivities, omissions, which by their very nature tend to easily become invisible. One can hardly think of a better description of the Swedish predicament than the title of Johan Giesecke's article in *The Lancet*: "The Invisible Pandemic".[123] Much of the Swedish line was invested precisely in rendering this pandemic invisible, remaining passive in the face of suffering, denying all evidence in favour of a convenient myth.

But even passivities, though translucent, can nonetheless be intentional. They have desired goals (or "effects"). This is precisely what biopolitical reflection tries to pinpoint: we are dealing with a case where the upholding of biological life is rescinded, and the citizen is abandoned.

A further aspect that surfaced in our biopolitical investigation is a crisis within the discourse of human rights, arguably the dominant ethical idiom of our time. As we saw in the (official) ethical reflection on the Swedish pandemic, the language of rights was the only bulwark against an all-encompassing utilitarianism of "populations".[124] Yet at the same time this discourse was deployed in very particular (and highly selective) ways.[125] Rights were synonymous with freedoms for the individual: the right to association, right to movement and so on.[126] The "right to education" was the reason why schools could not move online,[127] while "rights to privacy" provided the excuse for not pursuing proper tracking.[128]

But there are, one could argue, also other rights, which were not mentioned at all: rights to know whether one is carrying a potentially lethal disease, the arguably fundamental "right to life", right to the *protection* of life (which is the function of modern biopolitics).[129] Instead, these values were encysted by the broader utilitarian calculation of population health. The discourse of rights has turned against itself: in the name of rights, the liberal tradition attacks other, more foundational rights (such as the State's duty to protect life). Something like an autoimmune condition is afflicting the liberal tradition.

Finally, one could ask what alternatives present themselves to the Swedish style of biopolitics. The conceptual apparatus of "populations", with the statistical mechanisms of monitoring and policing health, is hardly going away soon. A modern State requires this kind of control to protect the life of its citizens. This formula is in any case what proponents of a "positive biopolitics" (such as Esposito or Bratton) have argued against the negative biopolitics championed by Agamben. Perhaps they are right: biopolitics is here to stay, and the challenge is to formulate a more life-affirming and just biopolitics.

Yet while biopolitics is arguably inescapable in our current predicament, the utilitarian population-perspective that characterises Swedish biopolitics is not. Other principles than the blind maximisation of utility can undergird the State's duties and interests *vis-à-vis* biological life. In Germany, Spain and Italy, for instance, the bioethical discourse repudiated the utilitarian point of view due to its incompatibility with the inalienable dignity of every human being.[130] The "worth" of a person cannot be calculated on the basis of their societal contribution or their standard of life. *The principle of human dignity* precludes the option of abandoning people as was done in Sweden, in the hope of cutting one's losses.[131]

Moreover, the appeal of utilitarianism, that it offers a global approach, that deals with entire communities rather than isolated individuals, is chimerical. The biopolitical unit of the population is a fundamentally misguided way of viewing the political community. The common good is something more than GDP growth and healthy average BMI. Communities are more than herds. Instead of utilitarianism, a guiding principle should be solidarity and the human dignity of every single person independent of age, race, gender, education, etc.: the realisation of our particular responsibility in relation to each other and the most vulnerable among us.

Notes

1 On the other hand, science journalist Emma Frans tweeted: "Isn't flockimmunitet [*herd immunity*] the most beautiful word in the Swedish language?" https://twitter.com/DrEmmaFrans/status/1493989947686141961 .

2 See the following discussion, as well as: Scaldaferro, Maikon. "A biopolítica da pandemia: Agamben e Bolsonaro entram em um bar (The Biopolitics of the Pandemic: Agamben and Bolsonaro Walk into a Bar)", *Griot-Revista De Filosofia* 21:3 (2021): 319–335.

3 Foucault, Michel. *Society Must Be Defended: Lectures at the collège de France, 1975–1976*, London: Picador, 2003: 245.

4 Foucault, Michel. *The History of Sexuality, Vol. 1: The Will to Knowledge*, London: Penguin, 1979: 136.

5 *Ibid*., 138–139. Cf. Foucault. *Society Must Be Defended*, 247.

6 Cf. Foucault, Michel. "The Birth of Social Medicine", in Foucault, Michel et al. (eds.). *The Essential Foucault*, New York: The New Press, 2003: 319–337; see especially 319–321.

7 See Pereira, Gomes, and Pedro Paulo. "In and Around Life: Biopolitics in the Tropics", *Vibrant: Virtual Brazilian Anthropology* 10:2 (2013): 13–37, 16.

8 Gustafsson, Bengt E., Carl-Erik Quensel, Lisa Swenander Lanke, Claes Lundqvist, Hans Grahnén, Bo Erik Bonow, and Bo Krasse. "The Effect of Different Levels of Carbohydrate Intake on Caries Activity in 436 Individuals Observed for Five Years", *Acta Odontologica Scandinavica* 11:3–4 (1953): 232–364.

9 https://sverigesradio.se/avsnitt/65245 .

10 Vipeholm has incidentally also become a *topos* in the Swedish pandemic debate: see Gustavsson, Gina. *Du stolta, du fria: Om svenskarna, Sverigebilden och folkhälsopatriotismen*, Stockholm: Kaunitz-Olsson, 2021: 175, 180, 336–337. Sweden's history of social-Darwinist biopolitics has also been mentioned as a background for the herd immunity strategy by Roberto Esposito, in an interview in *Svenska Dagbladet*, 22 April 2020, www.svd.se/installning-i-sverige-de-bast-anpassade-overlever .

11 Gunneflo, Markus. "Rudolf Kjellén: Nordic Biopolitics Before the Welfare State", *Retfærd: Nordisk juridisk tidsskrift* 35:3 (2015).

12 See a discussion in Esposito, Roberto. *Immunità comune*, Turin: Einaudi, 2022: 188.

13 Caffo, Leonardo, and Slavoj Žižek. "A Conversation with Slavoj Žižek: Why Only a Super-Anthropocentrism and the Reading of Hegel Can Save Us", *Public Conversation*, 20 October 2021. Cf. Žižek. *Pandemic!* OR Books, 2021: 73–76.

14 Sarasin, Philipp. "Mit Foucault die Pandemie verstehen?" *Geschichte der Gegenwart*, 5 March 2020, https://geschichtedergegenwart.ch/mit-foucault-die-pandemie-verstehen/ .

15 Nancy, Jean-Luc. "La sindrome biopolitica", *Micromega* 8 (2020): 57. See also the critical editorial in the same issue: Flores D'Arcais, Paolo. "Gli inganni di Foucault", *Micromega* 8 (2020): 7.

16 Bratton, Benjamin. *The Revenge of the Real*, New York: Verso Books, 2021: 100. Cf. *ibid*., 18, 39, 93, 97–98, 101–103.

17 www.lepoint.fr/politique/sloterdijk-le-systeme-occidental-va-se-reveler-aussi-autoritaire-que-celui-de-la-chine-18-03-2020-2367624_20.php .

18 Han, Byung-Chul. "Viviremos como en un estado de guerra permanente", *EFE*, 12 May 2021, www.efe.com/efe/espana/destacada/byung-chul-han-viviremos-como-en-un-estado-de-guerra-permanente/10011-4244280 .

19 Bratton. *The Revenge of the Real*, 92.

20 Agamben, Giorgio. *A che punto siamo? L'epidemia come politica*, Macerata: Quodlibet, 2021: 11.

21 Agamben. *A che punto siamo?* 37–38: the control exerted by tracking mobile phones, Agamben avers, "greatly exceeds any form of control exerted by totalitarian regimes, like fascism or nazism", my translation. Cf., *ibid*., 64–65, 75–76, 103.

22 Bratton. *The Revenge of the Real*, 93–94.
23 https://sverigesradio.se/avsnitt/1479820 .
24 Agamben's distinction between "bare life" (Latin: *nuda vita*) and biological life (Greek: *zoe*) is not always clear-cut: see Mills, Catherine. "Biopolitics and the Concept of Life", in *Biopower*, 87–88; Agamben, Giorgio. *Homo Sacer: Sovereign Power and Bare Life*, Stanford: Stanford University Press, 1998: 3.
25 Granted, Agamben holds that every state of exception is necessarily biopolitical (*Homo sacer*, 6) – indeed that politics *simpliciter* has been biopolitics "from the very beginning". (*Homo sacer*, 181) (cf. *A che punto siamo?* 26–27). However, one could subscribe to all Agamben's points on the pandemic while rejecting the entire biopolitical project – Agamben himself hardly connects the two.
26 Agamben. *A che punto siamo?* 23.
27 The critique of Agamben's choice of totalitarianism as the paradigm of modern biopolitics is also found in Rabinow, Paul, and Nicholas Rose. "Biopower Today", *BioSocieties* 1 (2006): 195–217.
28 On the difference between Foucault and Agamben's conceptions of biopolitics: Patton, Paul. "Agamben and Foucault on Biopower and Biopolitics", in Calarco, Matthew, and Steven DeCaroli (eds.). *Giorgio Agamben: Sovereignty and Life*, Stanford: Stanford University Press, 2007: 203–218.
29 Foucault, Michel. *The Birth of Biopolitics*, New York: Macmillan, 2008: 19–20. See also Stilhoff Sörensen, Jens. "Utilitarian Life: Shifting Biopolitics and the Life – Economy Nexus", *Arena* 51–52 (2018).
30 Cf. the introductory chapter and Emil J. Bergholtz's chapter.
31 Lindström, Martin. "The New Totalitarians: The Swedish COVID-19 Strategy and the Implications of Consensus Culture and Media Policy for Public Health", *SSM – Population Health* (14 June 2021): 100788, www.sciencedirect.com/science/article/pii/S235282732100063X .
32 Irwin, Rachel Elisabeth. "Misinformation and De-Contextualization: International Media Reporting on Sweden and COVID-19", *Globalization and Health* 16:62 (2020): 4–5. See also Lindström. "The New Totalitarians", 3.
33 www.aftonbladet.se/nyheter/a/6j7vaO/anders-tegnell-hyllar-brittisk-tanke-kring-flockimmunitet-dit-vi-behover-komma .
34 www.svd.se/tegnell-flockimmunitet-inte-huvudtaktiken , https://svenska.yle.fi/artikel/2020/04/04/nej-sveriges-strategi-ar-inte-flockimmunitet-men-flockimmunitet-ar-enda-sattet .
35 https://unherd.com/about-unherd/ .
36 Cf. Anderberg, Johan. *Flocken*, Stockholm: Bonnier, 2021: 189.
37 https://svenska.yle.fi/artikel/2020/04/04/nej-sveriges-strategi-ar-inte-flockimmunitet-men-flockimmunitet-ar-enda-sattet, www.svt.se/nyheter/inrikes/kontroversiell-strategi-kan-minska-spridningen .
38 Similar oracular pronouncements were made by the Swedish ambassador to the United States, Karin Olofsdotter, in a panegyric for the Swedish strategy on Fox News: "It's not a strategy to get herd immunity, but it's something we want to get", https://video.foxnews.com/v/6154832181001#sp=show-clips .
39 www.expressen.se/nyheter/qs/interna-radslaget-om-flockimmunitet/ .
40 Although Tegnell also said in the same breath that herd immunity "is where we need to get to. There is no other way to control this." www.aftonbladet.se/nyheter/a/6j7vaO/anders-tegnell-hyllar-brittisk-tanke-kring-flockimmunitet-dit-vi-behover-komma .
41 For the literally inclined: Trolls have walked in herd immunity. (The "trolls" in question are those of Scandinavian folklore; the idiom expresses that a certain subject has become infected and problematic, presumably due to the nefarious influence of these supernatural critters). Anderberg. *Flocken*, 196.
42 *Ibid.*
43 https://twitter.com/jsjostedt/status/1349503516352548868 . Emphasis mine.

44 https://emanuelkarlsten.se/regeringen-andrar-i-dokument-om-coronastrategi-raderar-mening-om-kontrollerad-spridning/ .

45 www.gp.se/nyheter/sverige/regeringen-saknade-formell-coronastrategi-1.44377808 , cf. Jens Stilhoff Sörensen's chapter.

46 www.dagensmedicin.se/vardens-styrning/politik/coronakommissionen-nekas-ta-del-av-regeringens-underlag/; the pattern repeated itself with other documents that were withheld from public scrutiny, www.svd.se/hemliga-dokument-avslojar-strategin .

47 www.svd.se/fhms-tidiga-strategi-var-flockimmunitet .

48 Manzoor, Amina. *Pandemier! Från spanska sjukan till covid-19*, Stockholm: Fri tanke, 2021: 160.

49 See especially: Anderberg. *Flocken*, 108–111, 113–114, 141, 144, 155. For a more extensive description and discussion of Anderberg's book see the introductory chapter.

50 www.who.int/director-general/speeches/detail/who-director-general-s-opening-remarks-at-the-media-briefing-on-covid-19–12-october-2020 .

51 www.irishexaminer.com/news/arid-40053920.html . A similar reaction took place in Germany, www.faz.net/aktuell/gesellschaft/gesundheit/coronavirus/corona-pandemie-drosten-und-kollegen-warnen-vor-konzept-der-herdenimmunitaet-17010496.html .

52 Cf. Bergmann, Sigurd. "Sweden's Experiment with Herd Immunity Is Unethical and Undemocratic – and Reveals an Underlying Political Pathology", *ABC*, 14 October 2020, www.abc.net.au/religion/the-ethics-of-swedens-herd-immunity-strategy/12764868 .

53 See Bergmann, Sigurd. "Navigating Ethics in a Pandemic – Contempt for the Weak Versus Love of Neighbor in a Swedish Lens", *Dialog*, 7 November 2021, https://doi.org/10.1111/dial.12697; Lappin, Lapo. "The Justice of Gold: The Philosophical Roots of Sweden's Pandemic Strategy", *Macrina* 6 (20 February 2021), https://macrinamagazine.com/issue-6-general/guest/2021/02/20/the-justice-of-gold-the-philosophical-roots-of-swedens-pandemic-strategy/ .

54 The question of what specific *kind* of utilitarianism we are dealing with is left open: let it just be noted that, in the philosophical discussion, there seems to be a convergence between both preference utilitarians (like Peter Singer) and hedonistic utilitarians (like Torbjörn Tännsjö). To closer determine what kind of utilitarianism FHM can be associated with one would need to know the specifics of how they "calculated" the stakes in question, something we do not know (*vide infra*).

55 Lappin, Lapo, and Åke Gafvelin, *Filosofi och pandemi*, Skellefteå: Norma, 2021: 32–34.

56 www.dn.se/ledare/replik-fran-torbjorn-tannsjo-magiskt-tankande-och-faktaresistens-ar-inget-alternativ/ .

57 On the use of utility maximising reasoning within health-care prioritisation see Fagerström, Erica. *Svensk pandemisk beredskap i organisationsetisk belysning*, Stockholm: Institute for Future Studies, 2021: 67–68, 71, 81–82, 89.

58 Singer, Peter. *Practical Ethics*, 2nd ed., Cambridge: Cambridge University Press, 1999: 185–186.

59 https://smer.se/calendar/award-winner-seminar-2021-priority-settings-in-healthcare-in-pandemics-and-other-situations-of-mass-casualties/ . For a critical discussion see, https://kvartal.se/artiklar/foresprakare-av-spadbarnsmord-pa-etikseminarium/ , and the rejoinders.

60 Foucault, M. "Omnes et singulatim: Towards a Criticism of Political Reason", in Foucault, Michel et al. (eds.). *The Essential Foucault*, New York: The New Press, 2003.

61 Foucault. *The History of Sexuality*, 139. See also Dean, Mitchell. *Governmentality: Power and Rule in Modern Society*, London: Sage, 1999.

62 Foucault. *Society Must Be Defended*, 246. On statistical power, see Hacking, Ian. "Biopower and the Avalanche of Printed Number", in Cirsney, Vernon, and Nicolae Morar (eds.). *Biopower: Foucault and Beyond*, 65–81; for Sweden in particular, see *ibid*., 72, 74.

63 Martin, Paul M.V., and Estelle Martin-Granel. "2,500-Year Evolution of the Term Epidemic", *Emerging Infectious Diseases* 12:6 (2006): 976–980. doi:10.3201/eid1206.051263.

64 Foucault. *Society Must Be Defended*, 242–243.

65 Although more usually translated as Public Health Agency. On the difference between the concept of public health and "population health"/*folkhälsa* see Stenius, Kerstin. "Public Health Is Not an Innocent Concept", *Nordic Studies on Alcohol and Drugs* 35:2 (72018): 100–103. For further discussion of the difference between the concepts see: Berg, Annika. *Den gränslösa hälsan: Signe och Axel Höjer, folkhälsan och expertisen*, Västerås: Edita Västra Aros, 2009: 24.

66 Folkhälsomyndigheten. *Planering för beredskap mot pandemisk influensa*, 13.

67 Johannisson, Karin. "Folkhälsa: Det svenska projektet från 1900 till 2:a världskriget", *Lychnos* (1991): 139–195, 172, 155, 145.

68 *Ibid.*, 145.

69 "The concept of *folkhälsa* is formulated (as with other terms comprising the suffix "*folk-*") *from above*." Johannisson. "Folkhälsa", 154.

70 *Ibid.*

71 So much so that the Ethical Board of State (SMER) mistakes it for FHM's *current* strategy. *Etiska vägval*, 25. As do others, for example Arrhenius et al. "Etiska avvägningar i pandemitider", *I en tid av pandemi – en ESO-antologi med samhällsvetenskapliga reflektioner*, *ESO* (2021): 1.

72 Folkhälsomyndigheten. *Folkhälsans utveckling – årsrapport 2021*, 3; cf. *ibid.*, 10, www.folkhalsomyndigheten.se/contentassets/39ef6af33177445bb6d2ad88829cc5ce/folkhalsans-utveckling-arsrapport-2021.pdf .

73 Folkhälsomyndigheten. *Folkhälsans utveckling*, 10.

74 https://lakartidningen.se/aktuellt/nyheter/2021/03/karin-tegmark-wisell-vissa-utgar-fran-att-vi-har-en-dold-agenda/ , https://tt.omni.se/smittspridningen-okar-i-sverige-allvarligt/a/wePdbn, https://sverigesradio.se/artikel/tegmark-wisell-forsvarar-coronastra tegin-avgorande-att-vi-tittat-pa-helheten .

75 See for instance: Manzoor, *Pandemier!* 166; Frans, Emma. *Alla tvättar händerna*, Stockholm: Volante, 2020: 48.

76 www.youtube.com/watch?v=QTnTlxBSovw .

77 SMER. *Etiska vägval i pandemin*, 39–40, https://smer.se/wp-content/uploads/2020/06/smer-2020_3-rapport_webb.pdf .

78 *Ibid.*, 40.

79 *Ibid.*, 41.

80 *Ibid.*, 44. Cf. Hultkrantz, Lars. "Värdet av ett statistiskt liv och covid-19", *Ekonomisk Debatt* 48:8 (2020): 46–54.

81 *Ibid.*, 43, 48.

82 www.youtube.com/watch?v=4TcAP8ELqjY .

83 Arrhenius et al. "Etiska avvägningar i pandemitider", 71. Cf. *ibid.*, 62, which includes a bizarre commendation of Tegnell's vaccination fiasco during the swine-flu epidemic.

84 See for instance Arrhenius, Gustaf. *Population Ethics: A Challenge for Moral Theory*, Uppsala: Reprocentralen Ekonomikum, 2000.

85 Arrhenius et al. "Etiska avvägningar i pandemitider", 65–66.

86 "Etiska avvägningar i pandemitider", 60–61.

87 *Ibid.*, 61.

88 Anderberg. *Flocken*, 160.

89 www.expressen.se/nyheter/kerstin-hessius-vi-ar-pa-vag-in-i-en-katastrof/ . Cf. Anderberg. *Flocken*, 157.

90 The predominantly economic nature of this utilitarian approach surfaces in other places in an exchange with Tegnell in Viktor Nordenskiöld's documentary *Bakom den svenska modellen*: "A disease that impedes many people from working for several months, is potentially much worse for society [*samhället*] than a lethal disease", www.svtplay.se/video/34250462/bakom-den-svenska-modellen .

91 This totalising discourse of the "population" is necessarily linked to nationalism; on the awakening of nationalist sentiment in the Swedish pandemic, see Lindberg, Helen. "Inflexion Points", *ArkDes*, 2022.

92 For the relevance of the image of "the body politic" in biopolitics see Esposito, Roberto. *Immunitas: The Protection and Negation of Life*, Cambridge: Polity Press, 2017: 126–136, 143–152. For the history of the body politic in Sweden cf. Berg. *Den gränslösa hälsan*, 25, especially note 32.

93 A handful of examples among many: Karlsten, Emanuel. "Pandemin hotar hela samhällskroppen", *Sändaren*, www.sandaren.se/nyhet/pandemin-hotar-hela-samhallskroppen; Nerbrand, Sofia. "Pandemin skadar även samhällskroppen", *Opulens*, 5 May 2020; Stakston, Elisabeth. "Farlig virusinfo infekterar samhällskroppen", *Blankspot*, 2 April 2020; Åkesson, Nils. "Risk att vi aldrig kommer tillbaka till "det normala"", *Dagens Industri*, 14 December 2021; Åhlund, Arvid. "Varning för corona-infodemin", *Kristianstadsbladet*, 25 March 2020.

94 Esposito, Roberto. *Immunitas: The Protection and Negation of Life*, Cambridge: Polity Press, 2017: 23–26, 136–143.

95 *Ibid.*, 84–86.

96 Agamben. *Homo sacer*, 34.

97 Fagerström. *Svensk pandemisk beredskap i organisationsetisk belysning*, 67–68, 71, 81–82, 89.

98 https://kvartal.se/artiklar/hardare-prioriteringar-gors-redan-trots-att-iva-platser-startomma/; see also www.dn.se/kultur/varfor-fick-de-aldre-do-utan-lakarvard/ , www.sydsvenskan.se/2021-06-08/vardskandalen-vaxer-aldre-i-hela-skane-portades-fran-sjukhusvard-under-pandemin , www.sydsvenskan.se/2021-06-09/erik-dog-efter-hemligt-coronabeslut .

99 https://kvartal.se/artiklar/hardare-prioriteringar-gors-redan-trots-att-iva-platser-startomma/ , www.dn.se/sthlm/karolinska-kritiseras-for-brister-vid-prioritering-inom-covid-iva/ .

100 www.dn.se/kultur/varfor-fick-de-aldre-do-utan-lakarvard/ .

101 Manzoor. *Pandemier!* 155.

102 https://yle.fi/uutiset/3-11433976; www.cbsnews.com/video/sweden-sees-high-virus-mortality-rate-after-resisting-lockdown/ .

103 As was determined beyond reasonable doubt by the Corona commission: "We find it most likely that the single most important factor behind the major outbreaks and the high number of deaths in residential care is the overall spread of the virus in the society", https://coronakommissionen.com/wp-content/uploads/2020/12/summary.pdf .

104 Cf. Johanna Höög's chapter, which highlights the invisibility of children and their families in the pandemic.

105 www.youtube.com/watch?v=7_aJfas51BY .

106 https://twitter.com/dremmafrans/status/1244575569318154240 .

107 See Frans. *Alla tvättar händerna*, 118.

108 https://urplay.se/program/216911-skola-hemma-experterna-27-mars-emma-frans-om-barn-och-smittspridning . Frans. *Alla tvättar händerna*, 61.

109 "Utbildningsminister Anna Ekström: Skolplikten rör vi inte", *Dagens Nyheter*, 4 June 2020, www.dn.se/nyheter/utbildningsminister-anna-ekstrom-skolplikten-ror-vi-inte/ .

110 In contrast to neighbouring Finland, which has instead opted for "compulsory learning" (*läroplikt*), rather than compulsory physical attendance: children have the duty to gain knowledge, and can also be taught according to the national syllabus from home if necessary.

111 Another staunch defender of *skolplikt* was Johan Giesecke, whose reason for doing so – according to journalist Johan Anderberg – is in line with the biopolitical discourse outlined in the previous section. See *Flocken*, 79: "Schools were a part of Society, of that system that nations of the world had built centuries ago to uphold [*upprätthålla*] population health".

112 https://skolvarlden.se/artiklar/foraldrar-som-corona-trotsar-skolplikten-riskerar-boter .

113 Cf. Jens Stilhoff Sörensen's chapter in this volume.

114 Skolinspektionen. *Utbildning under påverkan av pandemin,* www.skolinspektionen.se/aktuellt/nyheter/ny-rapport-utbildning-under-paverkan-av-coronapandemin-i-gymnasieskolan/ .

115 www.socialstyrelsen.se/globalassets/sharepoint-dokument/artikelkatalog/ovrigt/2021-1-7155.pdf, 5.

116 www.facebook.com/monica.renstig/posts/10156765899140178 .

117 www.youtube.com/watch?v=NXCcSF1IYQk&t=2254s .

118 Anderberg. *Flocken*, 104.

119 www.science.org/content/article/keeping-schools-open-without-masks-or-quarantines-doubled-swedish-teachers-covid-19?

120 Cf. Chapter 2 (Timeline), note 106.

121 Gustavsson. *Du stolta, du fria*, 11. Immigrants, as well as being the demographic hit the hardest, were also scapegoated and blamed for the spread of the virus, see *ibid.*, 52–53, 146–159.

122 Another aspect of the abandonment of the victims of the virus is of course the abandonment on the level of memory: see Bergmann, Sigurd. "*Memoria Passionis Subversiva*: The Moral Power of Remembrance in the Pandemic – in a Swedish Lens", in Erbele-Küster, Dorothea, and Volker Küster (eds.). *Between Pandemonium and Pandemethics: Responses to Covid-19 in Theology and Religions*, Leipzig: EVA, 2022: 101–121.

123 Giesecke, Johan. "The Invisible Pandemic", *The Lancet* 395:10238 (30 May 2020), www.thelancet.com/journals/lancet/article/PIIS0140-67362031035-7/fulltext .

124 Giritli Nygren, Katarina, and Anna Olofsson. "Swedish Exceptionalism, Herd Immunity and the Welfare State: A Media Analysis of Struggles Over the Nature and Legitimacy of the COVID-19 Pandemic Strategy in Sweden", *Current Sociology Monograph* 69:4 (2021): 529–546; see especially 539–540.

125 In addition to the rights mentioned here, there has been a further discussion about the right to religious freedom, which critics have claimed was infringed upon by the Swedish pandemic restrictions: see Rudenstrand, Jacob. *Den första rättigheten: Frihet till religion, frihet från religion*, Stockholm: Timbro, 2022: 10–13, 221–223.

126 The sudden preoccupation with rights is, from the point of view of the history of ideas, a peculiar one. Swedish Social Democrat ideology has traditionally been suspicious of any discourse involving human rights: Schultz, Mårten. "På rättsstatens grund", *Axess* 5 (2020), www.axess.se/artiklar/pa-rattsstatens-grund/ . Cf. Grill, Kalle. "Frihet under pandemin: Två liberala perspektiv på generella frihetsbegränsningar", *Tidskrift för politisk filosofi* 25:1 (2021): 30–47.

127 Gustavsson. *Du stolta, du fria*, 73.

128 For the outlines of the ethical discussion see: SMER. *Etiska vägval*, 49–51.

129 As well as in accordance with the second article of the European declaration of human rights, www.echr.coe.int/documents/convention_eng.pdf . Cf. note 57 in the introductory chapter .

130 Palazzani, Laura. "The Pandemic and the Ethical Dilemma of Limited Resources: Who to Treat?" *Bioethics Update* 6:2 (2020): 67–79.

131 Cf. Fagerström. *Svensk pandemisk beredskap i organisationsetisk belysning*, 89, who concludes that the principle of human dignity, equal worth, security (*trygghet*), equality and solidarity were almost absent from the policy documents in action during the pandemic.

11

COLLABORATORS, SUPPORTERS, AND SCIENCE JUDGES

How trust in the Public Health Agency's messaging was achieved

Kajsa Klein

Access to health information is widely seen as a human right.[1] To communicate the true mode of transmission of the virus (SARS-CoV-2) correctly, to those living in Sweden, is unquestionably the duty of the Swedish Public Health Agency (FHM). Yet, two years into the pandemic, the agency has failed still to do so. If one were to visit the Covid-19 recommendations section of their website, one would be offered a poster with handwashing instructions.[2] Facemasks are not mentioned, and not a single word is said about making indoor environments safer by filtering or cleaning the air. What about the section on recommended measures in health and social care settings? The same: *zilch*, not a single word to indicate that the virus is airborne.[3]

The FHM continues to stress the importance of "basic hygiene routines" to prevent the spread of infection but says nothing about the importance of clean air. It is as if they, in 2022, are still in denial about some of the fundamental facts of SARS-CoV-2. While it is true that Sweden is not alone in understating the importance of airborne transmission, it has been more extreme in its science denialism than many other comparable countries.[4] Research by Bengt Johansson et al. suggests a strong link between blind trust in the Swedish Government and frequent hand washing. Another conclusion is that those who trusted the message of the FHM were also *less* likely to wear facemasks.[5]

As the UN points out, trust in public institutions is essential for the functioning of society.[6] During the pandemic, the FHM has been proven wrong many times, but is still largely seen as legitimate among the general public and Government institutions. How has this situation, with a powerful Government Agency repeatedly misinforming the public, and denying them important health information, been allowed to take place? Why is it still happening, even now, after criticism from the Royal Swedish Academy of Sciences[7] and after the Corona Commission presented its findings?[8] This chapter discusses some of the key actors who throughout the pandemic have upheld the legitimacy of the FHM; they have also

DOI: 10.4324/9781003289364-12

significantly contributed to spreading the Agency's message in Sweden and beyond. It is an eclectic mix of people (and institutions), ranging from members of Facebook groups dedicated to combatting online hate and fake news, to university professors and Government representatives. Drawing on literature about promotional culture[9] and research on trust and critical information assessment three categories are identified (that should not be understood as clear-cut): the *collaborators* transmitting and promoting the FHM message, the *supporters* expressing public health patriotism, and, finally, the *science judges* who punish the critics and award decision makers and loyal public health patriots.[10]

Pandemic narratives travel across the public sphere through different genres and contexts. The media landscape has developed considerably in recent years which has enabled new forms of communication. The Government now has its own channels (including on social media) in which to put out crisis information. Still, the news media remain important. Lisa Bjurwald, who analyzed Swedish media coverage during the first pandemic year, concluded that, with a few notable exceptions, journalists acted as Government megaphones.[11] Of special interest is a particular kind of journalist, the influential science journalists who choose what actors to frame as trustworthy and who to brand as less knowledgeable. They are examples of what in this chapter is referred to as "science judges". Here, inspiration is taken from media theorist Daniel Dayan and his sociology of collective attention.[12] Another recurring theme is the relationship between Sweden and the wider world. Sweden was not and is not as isolated as one is led to believe, if one consumes the many reports containing streaks of Swedish exceptionalism. Attempts were for example made by different Swedish actors to influence pandemic management in other countries.

Sweden and the WHO

"The cure should not be worse than the disease", the WHO Strategic and Technical Advisory Group for Infectious Hazards (STAG-IH) wrote in a letter to the WHO Director-General on 12 May 2020.[13]

The starting point for the FHM back in early 2020 was the Influenza pandemic preparedness plan. This plan assumed that a virus would be spread primarily by contact and droplet transmission. Consequently, the FHM chose to communicate that the virus was transmitted after the first symptoms came; "stay home if you are ill and have symptoms" is a mantra that has been repeated ever since. The public was also urged to wash their hands and to keep their distance from each other. This approach was, however, hardly cautious enough. It was a new virus, and aerosol transmission could not be ruled out. According to the Corona Commission, the FHM should have instead followed the precautionary principle.[14] It would have been wise to listen to and be inspired by East Asian countries such as Japan or Taiwan with a different level of knowledge and tradition of infection control against airborne respiratory viruses such as SARS-CoV-1. The information from China could also have been more carefully interpreted.[15]

One possible explanation for the FHM's reliance on the old plan and the stubborn denial of airborne infection, is the strong position of hygiene specialists and surgeons in Sweden and elsewhere. Trisha Greenhalgh et al. have shed light on the struggle between different disciplines and actors involved in the airborne versus droplet debate within the WHO and in Canada, Japan and the UK.[16] One example they relate is when, at the beginning of the pandemic, the WHO made the mistake of appointing an infection control expert group consisting of several handwashing specialists but zero experts on airborne infection. With such a composition of experts, it is not surprising that the hegemonic grip of the droplet orthodoxy was maintained, for quite some time.[17] Gradually, however, the WHO changed its messaging on transmission modes, and, in comparison to Sweden they have been quick to emphasize the importance of masking and ventilation, precisely because airborne transmission could not be ruled out.[18] For people in Sweden who followed international news, this difference was perplexing. Why did Sweden, a WHO member, not follow WHO's advice?[19]

When discussing Sweden versus WHO, it is worth pointing out that not only is Sweden a member, it is among the organization's top donors. The current Swedish WHO strategy emphasizes the importance of "continuous and consistent bilateral dialogue with WHO at both the policy and officer level", and further, that Sweden should make use of opportunities to influence the WHO, "for example by proposing candidates for strategic posts".[20] Indeed, Sweden has had some success in placing its people on committees. Johan Giesecke (a former State Epidemiologist and Karolinska Institute professor) was appointed to STAG-IH (WHO's advisory group for infectious hazards) and State Epidemiologist Anders Tegnell is included as advisor in the WHO Covid-19 IHR emergency committee.[21]

Sweden's pandemic messaging was never confined to the national context. Representatives of Swedish authorities actively tried to influence other countries' pandemic management. One documented example was when Anders Tegnell in March 2020 called on the ECDC to remove their facemask recommendation, since it would imply that the virus was airborne, which would harm communication efforts.[22]

The collaborators

"The importance of establishing trust in Sweden and Swedish competencies goes as a guiding principle through all SI's activities", the Swedish Institute/SI (a Public Agency under the auspices of the Ministry for Foreign Affairs) writes in its Mission statement.[23]

The Ministry for Foreign Affairs has coordinated its Covid-19 communications with the FHM, but how, and to what degree, needs to be further investigated. Diplomacy involves image management.[24] Was the Swedish strategy a burden or an asset in promoting the image of Sweden?[25] How should it be presented internationally? One rhetorical choice the Ministry made was to describe the Swedish

Covid-19 strategy as *more scientific*,[26] thus praising themselves, rather than engaging others.[27]

In spring 2020, the Ministry for Foreign Affairs produced a number of film clips for its website and social media, featuring amongst others the Ambassador for Global Health, Anders Nordström. Asked about the global impact of the Covid-19 outbreak at the end of April 2020, the Ambassador noted that it had caused a lot of concern but that it, from a health perspective, was actually not so significant (in relation to what normally affects people).[28] Anders Nordström is a man with a lot of international connections. He is also a former WHO executive who, a few months into the pandemic, was appointed to head The Secretariat of the Independent Panel for Pandemic Preparedness and Response (IPPPR) tasked by the WHO to evaluate the world's response to the Covid-19 pandemic.[29] Like Tegnell, Nordström has publicly criticized other countries' infection control work and argued that restrictions can be more harmful than the disease itself. He is not, judging from his public statements, a fan of facemasks:

> I usually jokingly say that the best thing about facemasks is perhaps that people do not smoke and eat so much.
>
> *(Anders Nordström, interviewed in Omvärlden, 31 August 2020)*[30]

What did the Karolinska Institute (KI) have to say on matters such as mode of transmission and masking? Here, it is important to recall that the KI consists of a large and diverse group of scholars with different competencies (including contributors to this book). There is a plurality of views. Still, some KI professors are more influential and well connected than others. When The National Board of Health and Welfare saw the need to educate Swedish healthcare professionals about the new virus, the task went to the professor in disaster medicine and surgeon Johan von Schreeb. His team worked fast, according to information on KI's website; two online training courses were launched as early as March 2020. The course material was based on recommendations from the FHM and the local hygiene specialists of *Health Hygiene Stockholm*,[31] which helps explain the emphasis that the courses placed on hand-washing. This is also how KI in 2020 ended up teaching that the SARS-CoV-2's mode of transmission was primarily fomite and droplet. And they still do; no major update of the course materials has been made since that time. The courses are still open and recommended by the KI. Many Swedes with care professions have been asked by their employers to participate. So far, more than 160,000 people have taken the courses.[32]

Another collaborator who helped transmit and promote the FHM's misleading messages was The Swedish Civil Contingencies Agency (MSB). They were directed by the Government to carry out a Covid-19 information campaign targeted at the public. Several goals were set, one effect goal (to reduce the spread of infection) and then subordinate communication goals (e.g. to motivate individuals to follow current advice).[33] Central to the strategy was to build confidence in the FHM recommendations. People were told that "source trust" was important and that "confirmed" Government information was what they should look out for (and by that they meant *Swedish* Government information). Unfortunately, there were significant goal conflicts, the goal of reducing the spread of infection was too often lost at the expense of the communication goals. For communicators at the MSB, this resulted in difficult trade-offs. Sometimes the FHM advice went against international expertise and risked being classified as misinformation by social media companies. Here is an example taken from the MSB account *Krisinformation's* Twitter feed (11 August 2020):

> The Swedish Public Health Agency refrains from recommending masks to the public as a mask that itches and slides below the nose contributes to the hands often touching the mouth, eyes and nose, which can increase the risk of transmission.

No, the use of facemasks will not increase the risk of spreading the airborne virus; that statement is false. It is certainly not what the WHO, the ECDC, or other national public health authorities say about facemasks. Could the Swedish expert authority be wrong? Were they not trustworthy? And if they were, then what about the WHO and the others? At the same time as MSB was working to strengthen the confidence in the FHM, they were damaging people's trust in other authorities, including the WHO, the most important actor fighting the *infodemic.*[34]

These were just a few examples of the FHM's collaborators, but in reality the list is much longer.[35] The details of the collaborations and how the misleading messages were shaped remain to be studied. The assumption here is that they include the aforementioned Giesecke, Nordström, Tegnell, and von Schreeb. Karolinska Institute has several important ties to the FHM and contributed greatly to the legitimacy of the agency's messaging regarding issues such as mode of transmission and relevant protections, not least through its courses.

The supporters

There are many different examples of supporters of the FHM during the pandemic. The focus here is on how support was expressed in text on social media, mainly on Facebook. Unfortunately, there is no room to get into the rich visual culture of "Tegnell idolatry" off- and online; let's just say that it was significant, particularly during 2020. First, however, a look at Twitter. Occasionally, that platform has, just like Facebook, been marked by heated debates about Sweden's strategy and the FHM. The tone has sometimes been vicious, but there have also been elements of fact-checking and dissemination of high-quality information. Researchers have generously shared their insights, but it has not always been easy to distinguish between the relevant, the less relevant, and the harmful. As Jevin D. West and Carl T Bergstrom point out, scientists are not immune to echo chambers and filter bubbles and they too depend to a certain extent on social media for information.[36]

An interesting phenomenon that appeared during the pandemic was the truth-seeking communities emerging around issues such as "Covid is airborne". This is how Eliot Higgins, the citizen journalist and founder of *Bellingcat*, describes the truth-seekers:

> These are the internet users who want to inform themselves while guarding against manipulation by others. . . . What's important about these communities is that they react quickly to information being put out by various actors, including states.[37]

In Higgins' view, they are an example of the power of the crowd and a strong defense against disinformation. When Government deception and hypocrisy cause a moral injury, truth-seekers step in. To do so is, however, not without its risks. In Sweden, the Government had strong support, and the critics, whether truth-seekers or disinformation agents, met a lot of resistance, sometimes in the form of hate speech and bullying. Deeply problematic were also personal attacks on Twitter targeting Government representatives. Whereas a certain amount of parody and the Bakhtinian *carnivalesque*[38] is healthy and maybe even necessary in open democracies, things can easily spin out of control online.[39] To call for a Government representative to step down is one thing; to harass and incite violence is quite another. Even though toxic discourse and violent memes were in the minority, Government authorities felt that the situation was serious enough for them to heighten security around certain individuals. The critics, some of whom were also threatened, received no such protections.

What has received less attention than the debate climate on Twitter, is what happened early during the pandemic on Facebook. When the authorities failed to explain the strategy in an exhaustive way (with factual basis), individual users took on the role of interpreter. Pseudo-experts with influencer status supporting the Swedish strategy went on to explain concepts such as "natural immunity" and "herd immunity" to a growing number of followers. Whether what was said was based on correct facts or not was difficult for many users to determine. The virus was new and there was a considerable information void, especially due to the lack of transparency on the part of the FHM. Even more significant than the individual pseudo-experts were the Facebook groups.[40] The already existing ones like *#jagärhär* (I'm here) with about 70,000 members, and *Källkritik, fake news och faktagranskning* (source criticism, fake news and fact-checking) with about 20,000 members, to name two particularly influential groups.

The former group was founded in 2016 to combat online hate, misinformation, and harassment.[41] They claim to support the "targeted and victimized" in the comment sections in social media and say that they sustain each other by "sticking together". Among those who have previously benefited from love-bombing is Greta Thunberg and LGBT+ activists.[42] During the pandemic, the group came to influence Swedish public opinion by repeatedly backing the FHM's representatives. When a news article featuring Anders Tegnell drew critical (sometimes hateful) comments, the group intervened to love-bomb Tegnell.[43] This happened several times in the spring of 2020 and there were enough *#jagärhär*-counter-speak comments to push down the critical voices. This was hardly planned. It was what the members chose to focus on that spring, especially after FHM Director-General Johan Carlson told the press about a supposed hate storm against FHM representatives.[44] More surprising was how one-sided the love-bombing was; not once did a FHM critic (also under attack) receive a similar treatment. The *#jagärhär* membership is pre-dominantly female and consists of a great number of human rights activists, journalists, politicians (mainly center-left), and teachers. Suddenly, they found themselves positioned against the international scientific consensus, against the WHO's recommendations, and for the male clique spreading its peculiar machismo attitude toward public health interventions.[45]

The second Facebook group, dedicated to source criticism and fact-checking, had developed into an important resource for Swedes interested in various aspects of critical information assessment. It covers recent research and assembles several of the country's top experts in the field. The group was, however, rather strictly moderated throughout the pandemic, in fact, increasingly so. Comments that touched on controversial aspects of the Swedish authorities' strategies and messaging quickly disappeared – only a certain kind of fact-check was in practice allowed. A turning point was when in fall 2020 a debate on facemasks nearly broke the group apart. From then on, pro-mask truth-seekers critical of the FHM saw their efforts at fact-checking vanish in cyberspace. Another challenge was antivaxxers who tried to get their message out through the Facebook group, and they too saw their comments being deleted. Sometimes the moderators did their own research which they posted in the group. When the hash tag *#Sparka Tegnell* (fire Tegnell) appeared on Twitter, the moderators tried to trace its spread and draw conclusions on who was behind it. Notably lacking, were, however, efforts to scrutinize the FHM-supporters' smearing of the critics. The truth-seekers on Twitter mentioned earlier never gained the group's attention. Instead, the moderators acknowledged and even praised Amina Manzoor, an award-winning but not uncontroversial science journalist known for her FHM-friendly editorial choices, including denial of the benefits of masking.[46]

The groups were characterized in different ways and to varying degrees by Government loyalty and source trust, with the FHM as the trusted source. For the third group, We Support Anders Tegnell & Co (FHM), it can be argued that that was the whole point, the *raison d'être*. The group were among the new groups that popped up during the pandemic, it quickly gained 90,000 members (roughly 1% of the population, some of whom were also active in the two groups previously discussed). This is how the group was presented on Facebook:

> We, who are the members of this group, support the Public Health Agency and their front people, who meet the international press and the Swedish people every day with relevant facts and wise recommendations about Corona and Covid-19.

In an opinion piece published in *Dagens Nyheter*, 25 February 2021, the moderators clarified:

> We believe that in this situation we need to stick together. That is why we support the Swedish Public Health Agency. We support them when they are right, we also support them when they were wrong. Signed by the moderators of *We Support Anders Tegnell & Co (FoHM)*.[47]

Members of the group were invited to assume the role of supporter, or to use terminology taken from Gina Gustavsson's book *Du stolta, du fria*, to act as *public health patriots*.[48] Government officials were love-bombed and praised by members of the group, and critics were heckled. The initiator and public face of the group was a local Social Democratic politician; other members included politicians, Government representatives (e.g. ambassador Anders Nordström), and journalists, which further contributed to its impact. For many, group membership likely became a way to show commitment during the early phase of the pandemic. In a difficult situation, people wanted to show that they were prepared to follow good advice and do their part to help stop the spread of the virus. In the early days, the untrustworthiness of the FHM was likely not a factor. However, in time this became a dilemma for at least some of the members. Because the FHM's communication contained errors and unsubstantiated claims, it so happened that the group contributed to the spread of misinformation, including such misinformation that was reminiscent of, but not identical to, Government communication. The FHM was against masking, toned down the risks to children and young people, and opposed lockdowns. Several messages were eerily similar to what was said by the signatories of the Great Barrington Declaration (GBD)[49] and its Swedish counterpart, *Läkarupppropet*.[50] Therefore, it was hardly a coincidence that some Swedish signatories of the GBD and *Läkarupppropet* also came to participate in the support group on Facebook, often with hundreds, sometimes thousands of likes as a reward. This also meant that the "facts" that are associated with the GDB and *Läkarupppropet*, but which are regarded by the wider scientific community as problematic, came to be normalized. The moderators of the support group, who did not necessarily want to be associated with antivaxx themselves, were given an even more difficult challenge when the vaccines arrived, as GBD and *Läkarupppropet* increasingly merged with the international antivaxx movement. What to do when someone like the Swedish GBD co-author Martin Kulldorff spread the Great Resist conspiracy or when *Läkarupppropet*-Sven Román called on people to break restrictions? The result was a kind of compromise, where there was greater tolerance in the Facebook group for arguments against vaccine certificates and child vaccinations (not unlike the FHM's argumentation at certain times). The leaders of *Läkarupppropet* posted Sweden-praising posts but were not given space to invite members to the antivaxx demonstrations.

The science judges

To be the judge of science, of who is trustworthy and who is not, and of what the shared facts are, is to exert power. Money and careers are also at stake. During the pandemic, there are examples of how judges punished the critics and awarded the decision makers and the loyalists; the most obvious category arguably being those judges who sat on prize committees and research councils with medals and research grants to distribute. Then there were those who were active on social media assessing scientists involved in the debates; a few were even employed by the Government as experts to analyze suspicious behavior and possible foreign interference. Last, but not least, the prominent science journalists, who distinguished between the trustworthy and those who were mere *hobby epidemiologists*, were influential partly because other journalists relied on their judgments.

But first, the awards. From 2020 and onwards, Swedish institutions gave various kinds of awards to Government representatives and debaters who spoke positively about the Swedish strategy and the FHM. Distinctions, medals, and prizes as proofs of excellence, that should mean that those recognized acted wisely and that their reasoning was based on good science, right? First out was Umeå University, which awarded Martin Kulldorff, known for the GBD and for his praise of the Swedish strategy, an honorary doctorate. Other recognitions: State Epidemiologist Anders Tegnell (Linköping University's alumni of the year), the FHM Director-General Johan Carlson (Uppsala's gold medal), science communicator Agnes Wold ("Göteborgare" of the year), science communicator Emma Frans (a royal medal by HM the King). Prominent science journalist Maria Gunther of *Dagens Nyheter* received a prize from the Swedish Academy, and Amina Manzoor (*Dagens Nyheter/Expressen*) got the Royal Swedish Academy of Engineering Sciences award for science journalism. In fact, even the source criticism Facebook group received an award. The list goes on, and the one-sidedness is clear, not a single Swedish critic was among those awarded.[51] This judgment on the part of the establishment made it even more difficult for people to resist public health patriotism.

> Being source critical means evaluating the information you find. Firstly, this means understanding that some sources have greater credibility than others, and secondly, being aware that the originator of the information has an objective.
>
> *(From the Krisinformation section of the MSB website)*[52]

The MSB has tried to impress the public that *källtillit* (source trust) is important, in particular trust in "confirmed" information from Swedish authorities. The concept was launched by information studies professor Olof Sundin in the years before the pandemic, but is now widely used by authorities and even schools in Sweden.[53] What the MSB also did, was warn against influence campaigns threatening Swedish democracy.[54] The fact that the pandemic happened in a climate of rising rightwing populism as well as Russian hybrid warfare was an unlucky coincidence. Yet, it unquestionably had an impact on the public debate. What if there were state actors who saw a window of opportunity? What if all that criticism of the Swedish Government and its authorities was orchestrated?

On social media, there was talk about how the critics who dared to question the FHM in a time of crisis were traitors. The associate professor in linguistics and GBD supporter Anna-Lena Wiklund, Lund University, tweeted that the security services better get involved. Lund University associate professor in strategic communication, James Pamment, had an article published in which he portrayed the critics' communications as bordering on the illegal and illegitimate. Russian propaganda was mentioned, and there was undoubtedly a portion of guilt-by-association.[55] Another variant that was fairly common on social media, was to cast those who wanted to have more protections as adherents of totalitarian ideology, under the influence of China. The scientists who argued for a temporary lockdown were contrasted with the macho epidemiologist Tegnell. One professor in intellectual history, Andreas Önnerfors, suggested that the critics were perhaps "claustrophiles" with a morbid desire to be shut in. This was a form of bullying; rarely were the critics met with factual arguments. The discourse was black and white, even calls for airborne protections such as masking and safe indoor air were sometimes equated with totalitarian restrictions.[56]

Evidently, there were times when the critics exaggerated, and some used language associated with the far right, which didn't help things in the eyes of the influence operation experts. "State media" was used instead of public service media, for example. Some speculated carelessly in social media posts about evil intentions on the part of the Government and the authorities, and there was some talk of "genocide" and "crimes against humanity" that caught the MSB's attention and led to accusations of radicalization. What the information specialists looking for patterns and coordination perhaps failed to understand was that there was a lot of genuine anger and despair, especially from those who had lost loved ones, and from the vulnerable most at risk, but also from the scientists who like Cassandra tried to get their message through and call out Government misinformation. Passionate feelings are often interpreted as unbalanced, and nuances tend to get lost when people are upset.[57] Were there extremists amongst the critics? Yes, a few, but they were a minority. And unlike the authorities, the critics didn't have access to professional communicators – they had nothing like the resources of the FHM and its collaborators, so they were essentially dissidents.[58]

In 2021, MSB published and promoted a mostly well-written, but not entirely unproblematic report on Covid-19 and conspiracy theories by Andreas Önnerfors. It is insightful when it comes to general characterization of conspiracy theories. Throughout history, various actors have used conspiracy theories to influence opinion and to tarnish the reputation of opponents. There is in the report a focus on antivaxx conspiracy thinking but also a section on conspiracy theories from the top down, exemplified with Trump's big lie on the "stolen" election. However, and far more controversially, the report describes conspiratorial pandemic narratives as "a horseshoe with two extremes that meet in the criticism directed at political measures based on public health science".[59] While Önnerfors has a point, if you read his text carefully, that horseshoe characteristic can nonetheless be misunderstood to include every critic, pro- as well as antivaxxers. Combined with MSB's other efforts to avert influence campaigns, the report became a tool in the hands of those who guarded the image of the Government and its authorities. The MSB again encouraged people to be suspicious. While it makes sense to call out antivaxxers for their harmful misinformation and their well-researched links to various interests (including state actors), it's a stupid idea to demonize scientists and concerned citizens advocating for conventional public health measures (e.g. to follow WHO recommendations) for their international connections.[60]

Remember how the official image of the Swedish pandemic response was "more scientific" than that of other countries? Now the Swedish critics were put against "public health science" (as if protections were somehow unscientific?), they were conspirators with an evil plan, to sow distrust and damage the image of Sweden, possibly with hidden links to Russia.[61] The accusations in social media posts of Government crimes against humanity were taken as proofs, and seen as particularly toxic and threatening, possibly leading to violent extremism.[62] It's arguably one thing to fail miserably at pandemic preparedness and response, and quite another to execute premeditated genocide (as some supercritical debaters have hinted at). Analysts who were experts in rightwing extremism and state propaganda were quick to draw conclusions once they noticed what they interpreted as patterns of illegitimate discourse. The reputation of the critics was effectively damaged. At least some of them were branded as radicalized members of a potentially violent sect. This is not to say that no conspiracy theory elements have ever existed in the discourse of the critics. But every value statement is not problematic, and not every call to bring those responsible of misconduct to justice is a threat to democracy, quite the opposite. Just because people are extremely upset does not mean that they are on the track of committing illegal acts. It moreover appears that the science judges in the form of influence campaign specialists (such as James Pamment) misread the truth-seeking communities on social media. They saw "coordination" to an extent that was frankly bordering on the conspiratorial. It was as if they themselves fell into the very trap they warned against.[63]

A final example of a category of science judges with significant impact on the perception of the FHM as trustworthy and the critics as less so, is the prestigious science journalists (some of whom were themselves awarded by other science judges for their efforts). Here, it is worth recalling Daniel Dayan and his view of the media as *reality pronouncing institutions* managing collective attention.[64] Dayan argues that professionalism can be used as a shield against discussion. Certain actors, such as prominent journalists, are to be trusted. The media validates statements and for a victim to challenge its media image is according to Dayan nearly impossible:[65]

> When non-journalists enter into debates with journalists concerning the establishment of current political-historical realities, journalists become both litigators and judges.[66]

It is common, but not always the case, that the science judges themselves have a background in science. In the case of the Swedish public radio, it is notable that the head of the science newsroom 2011–2021, Ulrika Björkstén, holds a PhD in physical chemistry. She is typical of influential Swedish science journalists in that she has expressed a rather narrow view of what is an acceptable research method. High standards are of course important, and it is good to be skeptical of pre-prints and the like, but during the pandemic a lot of relevant research, entire disciplines, were deemed as irrelevant. Sometimes, the science journalists would smear the publication forum of research they didn't feel matched the Swedish mainstream view, confirmed by the authorities. Like when in fall 2020 *Nature* published a news feature about the value of facemasks.[67] Suddenly, word spread that *Nature* wasn't such a reliable source, it wasn't as good as it used to be. Swedish radio was not alone in this. For award-winning Amina Manzoor, no amount of evidence for the benefits of masking seemed to be enough. There was also talk on how publications such as *Der Spiegel*, *Washington Post*, and *Le Monde* had it wrong in their news features about Sweden. To find research that supported the Swedish mainstream, science reporters sometimes looked in news outlets such as the *Washington Times* (where a *Dagens Nyheter* science journalist found a reference to one now infamous paper on lockdowns written by economists linked to libertarian think tanks).[68] Suddenly, the ribbon was not as high any longer.

To judge the quality of science demands a solid knowledge base as well as an openness to the world. When it is done in a parochial way it risks getting silly. Trustworthy, in Sweden? Swedish facts? A striking feature of the media coverage in general and science journalism in particular, has been an overreliance on Swedish expertise. Unless research on a certain aspect (e.g. whether the virus is airborne) has been conducted in Sweden, by Swedish scientists, preferably associated with the FHM, it is unlikely that the results will gain much attention. Moreover, some Swedish scientists were treated with respect, others were challenged or even met with contempt.[69] Critics of the FHM were too often either dismissed as unknowledgeable "hobby epidemiologists" or as representatives of partisan interests, "lobby groups".[70] Professors affiliated with, or sometimes even employed by the FHM were on the other hand portrayed as independent experts. Notable is how Swedish public radio chose to give a lot of space to Agnes Wold, a professor of clinical bacteriology and a popular media personality in Sweden. Wold even got her own podcast, *Ask Agnes Wold*, which was later named "breakthrough of the year 2021" by the Radio academy (*Radioakademin*). Wold has denied that the virus is airborne and blamed what she in a tweet dismissed as "the ventilation mafia" for trying to profit from the protections. She has repeatedly claimed that face visors are better than masks and has tweeted that young people do not need vaccines. Like the Swedish GBD profiles she interacts with on Twitter, she has criticized vaccine certificates for being totalitarian. Despite her record of spreading what is obviously misinformation, she was invited to be on a panel at the annual Gothenburg Book Fair in 2021 to assess the state of science journalism during the pandemic. The media, particularly television, has long had control over the possibility of appearing in public; they focus attention on certain facts and individuals and ignore others. Dayan sees this as an ethical issue. Attention can be diverted, subverted, or even perverted.[71] On social media, there is more of a freedom to control one's image, the message given off. In your own media, it is possible to appear in public (á la Hannah Arendt) as opposed to being shown, outed, and defamed.[72] It was not by coincidence that some of the critics (in the Science Forum Covid-19) decided to create their own channels. Yet, they still depended on the judgment of the science journalists.[73] Not only did the judges mentioned earlier contribute significantly to the demonization of the critics, the critics were also left without public acknowledgment of their science communication[74] and their efforts to battle Government misinformation in the spirit of WHO's infodemic work. It became mainstream to view the critics as out of touch, unknowledgeable, and generally suspicious.

The myth of the impartial mainstream

This chapter has outlined how powerful actors misinformed the public, and sometimes more specific target groups, such as health professionals. The responsibility for this is distributed; there were many collaborators and supporters amplifying the message, thus undercutting the global battle against the virus. It was a mainstreaming of misinformation on crucial issues such as mode of transmission. The fact that this was hardly planned communication, originating in some evil conspiracy, does not take away from the fact that the Swedish people were misled and that they have therefore not known how to protect themselves. As has been pointed out by aerosol expert Jose-Luis Jimenez: if the virus is airborne then it is not enough to place the responsibility for infection control on the individuals.[75] Unlike in some other countries, no major investments have been made in Sweden in things that could actually reduce virus levels in the air. Nor was it easy for individual actors in the public sector to disregard the FHM and choose to instead follow the recommendations of the WHO, the ECDC, or other national public health agencies. One reason was social pressure; confidence in the FHM was high in Sweden, and Government information was spread throughout the country – millions had been invested in spreading the message. The care workers had completed KI's training. If the healthcare professionals had been given correct information on the mode of transmission, it might have been more difficult to motivate them to work in environments without adequate infection control. Now, there was no reason for concern, or was there? Admittedly, many people did get sick at work and some died, but there was never public rebellion. Most stayed silent.

Lying in science is in some ways different from lying in politics, as Martin Jay has suggested.[76] Whereas truth and politics rarely stand on a common ground,[77] Government health information is in a country like Sweden expected to be accurate. To quote what the Corona Commission says in its conclusions: it [communication] "has to be honest, factually correct, as complete as possible, and at the same time easy to understand".[78] Public administration is, unlike political campaigning, supposed to be factual and impartial. Sadly, that was not always the case during the pandemic in Sweden. It is striking how the Covid-minimizing discourse of people like Giesecke, Nordström, and Tegnell was in some ways similar to that of right-wing populists such as Bolsonaro and Trump.[79] Gustavsson has pointed to the machismo involved, a treat that is otherwise not commonly associated with Swedish men.[80]

Globally, it has been fantastic to follow the rapid development of knowledge during the pandemic. But the progress has not come without conflicts, both within and between disciplines. Old rulers tend to want to keep the grip, which is understandable from a psychological perspective. But that does not make it reasonable to request other actors to disseminate information that is knowingly incorrect and out of date. Why have they persisted? Why has the FHM been so reluctant to tell people that they got it wrong? Were they afraid of losing credibility?[81] What is publicly circulated as the *truth* has long been problematized in media research. John Corner sees promotional activity as a defining characteristic of public life.[82] In recent years, however, there has been instances of what Corner views as a new *casualness* in the use of blatant falsehood (e.g. Trump).[83] This is worrying. That the FHM and its supporters sometimes ridiculed the Swedish proponents of public health measures in line with the WHO's recommendations was perilous and short-sighted since it also risked undermining the credibility of science.[84]

In an interview 17th April 2022, the director of the Swedish public radio, Cilla Benkö, talks about the "impartial mainstream".[85] Exactly what she means by this is unclear, but it speaks of a perspective that has become disturbingly common. If the mainstream is impartial, then the opposite must be true for that which goes against the stream which is how dissidents become suspicious in the view of journalists. What the critics said clearly deviated from the Swedish mainstream during the pandemic. In a climate of disinformation campaigns, a growing Public Relations industry, and new investments in psychological defense, it is more important than in a long time to maintain focus on facts and to critically assess information. Public health patriotism and other forms of blind source trust risks impeding the development of knowledge. The public sphere must be wide enough to accommodate speech that is uncomfortable for Government authorities.[86]

Notes

1 See for example this statement by the Pope, www.washingtonpost.com/world/2022/01/29/pope-coronavirus-vaccine-misinformation/ .

2 www.folkhalsomyndigheten.se/the-public-health-agency-of-sweden/communicable-disease-control/covid-19/how-to-protect-yourself-and-others-covid-19-recommendations/ .

3 www.folkhalsomyndigheten.se/the-public-health-agency-of-sweden/communicable-disease-control/covid-19/how-to-protect-yourself-and-others-covid-19-recommendations/control-measures/ . N.B. There are differences between the Swedish and English language versions; the Swedish is more extensive and if you dig deep enough you will find some material on facemasks under a "source control" header. Here, I have chosen to link to the English version.

4 Brusselaers, Nele, David Steadson, Kelly Bjorklund, Sofia Breland, Jens Stilhoff Sörensen, Andrew Ewing, Sigurd Bergmann, and Gunnar Steineck. "Evaluation of Science Advice During the COVID-19 Pandemic in Sweden", *Humanities and Social Sciences Communications* 9, Article number: 91 (2022), www.nature.com/articles/s41599-022-01097-5; Greenhalgh, Trisha, Mustafa Ozbilgin, and Damien Contandriopoulos. "Orthodoxy, Illusio, and Playing the Scientific Game: A Bourdieusian Analysis of Infection Control Science in the COVID-19 Pandemic", *Wellcome Open Research* 6 (2021): 126–126.

5 Brusselaers, Nele et al. "Evaluation of Science Advice During the COVID-19 Pandemic in Sweden", Johansson, Bengt, Jacob Sohlberg, Peter Esaiasson, and Marina Ghersetti. "Why Swedes Don't Wear Face Masks During the Pandemic – a Consequence of Blindly Trusting the Government", *Journal of International Crisis and Risk Communication Research* 4:2 (2021): 335–358, https://stars.library.ucf.edu/jicrcr/vol4/iss2/7/ .

6 www.un.org/development/desa/dspd/2021/07/trust-public-institutions/ .

7 www.kva.se/sv/publicerat/slutrapport-vad-kan-vi-lara-av-pandemin (2021).

8 https://coronakommissionen.com/wp-content/uploads/2022/02/summary_20220225.pdf (2022) .

9 Wernick's promotional culture concept captures how advertising, marketing, and branding now saturate the world. Bakir et al. argue that while useful, the approach underplays the importance of the state in what they call *minimization*, the opposite of promotion. Secrecy, misdirection, and strategic silence are also part of the picture and can be as detrimental and deceptive as lying. They view propagandistic organized persuasive communication within liberal democracies as a blind spot in research. Bakir, V., E. Herring, D. Miller, and P. Robinson. "Organized Persuasive Communication: A New Conceptual Framework for Research on Public Relations, Propaganda and Promotional Culture", *Critical Sociology* 45:3 (2019): 311–328.

10 On public health patriotism see Gustavsson, Gina. *Du stolta, du fria: Om Svenskarna, Sverigebilden och Folkhälsopatriotismen*, Stockholm: Kaunitz-Olsson, 2021.

11 Bjurwald, Lisa (ed.). *Maktens granskare eller maktens megafoner? Svensk journalistik under coronapandemin*, https://naringslivets-medieinstitut.se/wp-content/uploads/2021/05/Coronarapporten_2.pdf .

12 Dayan, Daniel. "On Whose Terms Are You Shown?" in Couldry, N., M. Madianou, and A. Pinchevski (eds.). *Ethics of Media*, London: Palgrave Macmillan, 2013: 161–177.

13 The advisory group (which includes Johan Giesecke) states that there is a risk that the WHO is perceived as accountable for the negative impact of lockdowns. STAG-IH, Letter to WHO director-general, 12 May 2020, https://cdn.who.int/media/docs/default-source/stag-ih/letter_to_dg_lockdown_11_may_rev9e5179ec-ae50-452e-ae34-ea42b4490544.pdf?sfvrsn=1a0094ae_1&download=true .

The STAG-IH's *Views of mask use in the general public* (published 25 May 2020) insisted that decision makers should explain that masking was a mere additional measure and that people should be trained in how to best remove, clean, and dispose of them. The starting point for STAG-IH was most likely contact and droplet transmission. The committee was in May 2020 still reluctant to full out recommend masks. In fact, the discourse was similar to how the authorities later would talk about masks in Sweden, www.who.int/publications/m/item/update-stag-ih-views-on-mask-use-by-the-general-public .

14 Corona Commission, *English Summary*, 2022, https://coronakommissionen.com/wp-content/uploads/2022/02/summary_20220225.pdf .

15 Tufekci, Zeynep. "How Millions of Lives Might Have Been Saved from Covid-19", *The New York Times*, 3 November 2022.

16 Greenhalgh et al. "Orthodoxy, Illusio, and Playing the Scientific Game", 126.

17 *Ibid.*

18 Cf. Lewis on why it took the WHO so long to acknowledge that the virus is airborne and how this affected national and local health agencies around the world. WHO's role is to be a cautious certifier of expert consensus; Lewis, Dyani. "Why the WHO Took Two Years to Say COVID Is Airborne", *News Feature, Nature* 604 (2022): 26–31. One

example of an influential WHO airborne denier is John Conly, who is also known for saying that masks cause harm, for example, acne, www.cbc.ca/news/health/canada-doctor-world-health-organization-airborne-1.5994889 .

19 Cf. also Martin Lindström's chapter.

20 Ministry of Health and Social Affairs. *Strategy for Sweden's Cooperation with the World Health Organisation (WHO) 2021–2025*, 17, www.government.se/articles/2021/05/strategy-for-swedens-cooperation-with-the-world-health-organization-who-20212025/ .

21 www.who.int/groups/covid-19-ihr-emergency-committee . Less successful were the efforts to secure a job for Tegnell at the WHO in March 2022, www.reuters.com/world/anders-who-who-has-no-job-swedish-health-agency-chief-2022–04–20/ .

22 Bjorklund, Kelly, and Andrew Ewing. "The Swedish COVID-19 Response Is a Disaster. It Shouldn't Be a Model for the Rest of the World", *Time*, 4 October 2020, https://time.com/5899432/sweden-coronovirus-disaster/ .

23 Swedish Institute mission statement, https://si.se/en/about-si/our-mission/ .

24 Cf. the Swedish Ministry for Foreign Affairs declaring 2017 in its *Strategy for the promotion of Sweden abroad 2.0*: "If we want the image of Sweden to continue to develop in a positive direction, all of us who represent the country must continue to do good things". https://sharingsweden.se/app/uploads/2017/09/strategy-for-the-promotion-of-sweden-abroad-2.0.pdf .

25 Falkheimer and Raknes have concluded that Sweden's international reputation has indeed taken a blow from its handling of the pandemic, but that it is still too early to say anything about its long-term effects. Sweden, they argue, framed itself as rational, the sole nation immune from global hysteria. This proved to be a risky choice. Falkheimer, J., and K. Raknes. "Nordic Neighbors in Pandemic Crisis: The Communication Battle Between Sweden and Norway", *Place Branding and Public Diplomacy* 18 (2022): 26–29, https://doi.org/10.1057/s41254-021-00234-2 .

26 Andrae, Cecilia, and Christina Nyström. "Svenskt samhällsstyre i fokus under coronapandemin", *Svenska Institutet* (2020), https://si.se/app/uploads/2020/06/pm-samhallsstyre-2020.pdf .

27 See Cull on how during pandemics, international relations, health, and reputation become intertwined. He has identified four different rhetorical strategies used by communicators associated with nation states. Cull, Nicholas J. "From Soft Power to Reputational Security: Rethinking Public Diplomacy and Cultural Diplomacy for a Dangerous Age", *Place Branding and Public Diplomacy* 18 (2022): 18–21. Cf. Simons, G. "Swedish Government and Country Image During the International Media Coverage of the Coronavirus Pandemic Strategy: From Bold to Pariah", *Journalism and Media* 1:1 (2020): 41–58.

28 Anders Nordström, Interview video, www.facebook.com/SwedenforGlobalHealth/videos/704671650343946/ .

29 https://theindependentpanel.org/about-the-independent-panel/#the-secretariat . It is notable that the whole debate around mode of transmission is lacking in the panel's report. Nothing is said about the importance of clean air in its 86 pages and the word "airborne" is absent.

30 www.omvarlden.se/nyheter/det-ar-inte-konstigt-att-who-omvarderat-sina-rad .

31 https://news.ki.se/karolinska-institutet-launches-covid-19-training-for-care-providers-and-medical-staff .

32 https://medarbetare.ki.se/people/johan-von-schreeb .

33 The Swedish Civil Contingencies Agency (MSB). *Delredovisning av regeringsuppdrag att "Samordna, stärka och utveckla kommunikationsinsatserna riktade till allmänheten med anledning av coronapandemin"*, MSB, 2021, www.msb.se/sv/aktuellt/pagaende-handelser-och-insatser/msbs-arbete-med-anledning-av-coronaviruset/vad-gor-msb/uppdrag-och-projekt-med-anledning-av-coronapandemin/ .

34 See Mosleh and Rand on elite misinformation on social media, including messages from public figures such as politicians and bureaucrats. Mosleh, Mohsen, and David G. Rand.

"Falsehood in, Falsehood Out: Measuring Exposure to Elite Misinformation on Twitter", *PsyArXiv*, 11 September 2021, https://psyarxiv.com/ye3pf/ .

35 One such actor worth mentioning is the PR agencies the authorities use for help with strategy work and crisis communication. The FHM has *Gullers group*, known for marketing the concept "strategic improvisation". This is also the theme for a book that Katarina Gentzel Sandberg, the person who signed the agreement with the FHM on behalf of Gullers, is a co-author of (with Falkheimer, J. *Nu: strategisk improvisation för effektiv kommunikation*, Malmö: Roos & Tegnér, 2017). In 2020, she participated in the breakfast seminar *Strategic Communication in the Corona Crisis* with the message that those who want to succeed should "nurture a culture where it is not so dangerous to make mistakes". Unfortunately, PR agencies tend to prefer to act in a shroud of secrecy, so exactly what they did to transmit and promote the messaging (including the misleading parts) is not known.

36 West, Jevin D., and Carl T. Bergstrom. "Misinformation in and About Science", *PNAS* 118:15 (2021): e1912444117.

37 Higgins, Eliot. "The Big Idea: How to Win the Fight Against Disinformation", www.theguardian.com/books/2022/apr/04/the-big-idea-how-to-win-the-fight-against-disinformation .

38 Bakhtin, Mikhail. *Rabelais and His World*, Cambridge, MA: MIT Press, 1968.

39 On different types of hate speech and on how YouTube users in the case of Covid comments in Italian skewed towards reliable content used a more toxic language than their counterpart see: Cinelli, Matteo, Andraž Pelicon, Igor Mozetič, Walter Quattrociocchi, Petra Kralj Novak, and Fabiana Zollo. "Dynamics of Online Hate and Misinformation", *Scientific Reports* 11: 22083 (2021).

40 The assessment on what took place in the Facebook groups is based primarily on observation (the author is a member).

41 For more on *#jagärhär*, including the International group, see, https://iamhereinternational.com .

42 www.theguardian.com/world/2019/jan/15/the-swedish-online-love-army-who-battle-below-the-line-comments .

43 *Love-bombing* circumscribes the disarming of someone with friendliness, and the term is used in the sociology and psychology of cult-like groups to describe expressions of apparent love targeted at someone who is being recruited by a cult. Here the term plainly aims at the practice of flooding an admired person with expressions of esteem and unlimited appreciation. Cf. Buerger, Catherine. "#iamhere: Collective Counterspeech and the Quest to Improve Online Discourse", *Social Media + Society* 7:4 (2021), https://doi.org/10.1177/20563051211063843 .

44 The FHM Director-General's press conference in March 2020, https://lakartidningen.se/aktuellt/nyheter/2020/03/johan-carlson-kritiken-mot-tegnell-ar-narmast-ovardig/ . On the difference between criticism and hate, see Ola Wong. "FHM drar hatkortet", *Kvartal*, 14 March 2021, [The FHM leads the hate card], https://kvartal.se/artiklar/fhm-drar-hatkortet/ .

45 On the machismo of Tegnell et al., see Gustavsson, Gina. *Du stolta, du fria*. Ironically, the *#Jagärhär* founder collaborated with the WHO in combatting the infodemic.

46 One of the group's moderators is the producer of *Digiteket's* online course about the Corona Infodemic, which promotes Government-loyal *source trust*. There is, moreover, talk about *information hygiene*, participants are encouraged to choose one or two news sources. Involuntarily comic is the final lesson (no. 19), where the content is summarized in a tweet from 2020 with a call for hand washing, hand disinfection, and advice that you should sit on your hands to avoid spreading misinformation. The course was updated in February 2022, but the mantra of hand washing as infection control against the airborne virus remains intact.

47 www.dn.se/insandare/svar-under-pandemin-maste-vi-svenskar-halla-ihop/ .

48 Gustavsson. *Du stolta, du fria*.

49 Cf. Emil J. Bergholtz's chapter.
50 https://lakaruppropet.se/ .
51 One notable exception to the rule: Trisha Greenhalgh's honorary doctorate at Jönköping University, 2021.
52 www.krisinformation.se/en .
53 Sundin, Olof. "Den pedagogiska bibliotekarien: Från källkritik till källtillit", in Hansson, J., and P. Wisselgren (eds.). *Bibliotekarier i teori och praktik: Utbildningsperspektiv på en unik profession*, Lund: BTJ Förlag, 2018: 103–123.
54 Manheim, who wrote a book about influence campaigns published in 2011, saw them as examples of manipulative strategic political communication. He suggests how best to form a strategic defense (a mix of deterrence, deflection, and minimizing of the campaigns). Manheim, Jarol B. *Strategy in Information and Influence Campaigns: How Policy Advocates, Social Movements, Insurgent Groups, Corporations, Governments and Others Get What They Want*, New York: Routledge, 2011.
55 Pamment, James. "Does Public Diplomacy Need a Theory of Disruption? The Role of Nonstate Actors in Counter-Branding the Swedish COVID-19 Response", *Journal of Public Diplomacy* 1:1 (2021): 80–110.
56 Another influential group of academics who contributed to this assessment were a group of utilitarian philosophers with good Government connections, in institutions such as The Swedish National Council of Medical Ethics (SMER) and the Institute for Futures Studies. They were against strict lockdowns but also skeptical to other forms of mandatory restrictions and precautions which they saw as illiberal and undemocratic. Cf. also Lapo Lappin's chapter.
57 Corner, John. "Passion and Reason: Notes on a Contested Relationship", *European Journal of Cultural Studies* 19:3 (2016): 209–217.
58 Håkan Lindgren discusses in *Svenska Dagbladet* in his review of Lena Einhorn's book (cf. the first chapter) why the critics of Sweden's way were perceived and treated as "dissidents", www.svd.se/a/G38Rj9/lena-einhorn-synar-pandemins-sverige-i-ny-bok .
59 Önnerfors, Andreas. "Conspiracy Theories and COVID-19: The Mechanisms Behind a Rapidly Growing Societal Challenge", *The Swedish Civil Contingencies Agency (MSB)* (2021): 13, www.msb.se/siteassets/dokument/publikationer/english-publications/conspiracy-theories-and-covid-19.pdf .
60 See for example Swedish Radio on *Mediawatchdogs Sweden (Mewas)*: "Private Facebook group attempts to influence Swedish interests abroad", https://sverigesradio.se/artikel/private-facebook-group-attempts-to-influence-swedish-interests-abroad .
61 Önnerfors. "Conspiracy Theories and COVID-19", 28.
62 *Ibid.*, 17.
63 *Ibid.*
64 Dayan. "On Whose Terms Are You Shown?" 161.
65 *Ibid.*
66 *Ibid.*, 162.
67 News Feature. "Face Masks: What the Data Says", *Nature*, 6 October 2020, www.nature.com/articles/d41586-020-02801-8 .
68 www.washingtontimes.com/news/2022/jan/31/lockdowns-had-little-or-no-impact-covid-19-deaths-/ , www.dn.se/vetenskap/forskare-nedstangningarna-raddade-nastan-inga-liv-alls/ .
69 In 2021 Swedish Radio published a story on the Swedish critics that many people felt amounted to smearing. Influence experts, including James Pamment participated. Ulrika Björkstén defended the publication and claimed to be neutral, www.dagensmedia.se/medier/radio-podd/sr-om-harda-kritiken-vi-ar-helt-neutrala/ . Cf. the second chapter's timeline, 9 February 2021 .
70 Virologist and writer Lena Einhorn analyzes in detail how Tegnell's rhetoric impacted on the journalists at the regular press conferences, by improvisation and dubious handling of facts, especially when "their" FHM facts were questioned, and "scientific smokescreens"

are put up. Einhorn, Lena. "Vetenskapliga dimridåer och en myndighet som drar en vals", [Scientific smokescreens and an Agency that fabulizes], *Kvartal*, 17 June 2021, https://kvartal.se/artiklar/vetenskapligadimridaer/ .

71 Dayan. "On Whose Terms Are You Shown?" 172.

72 Dayan, Daniel. "Sharing and Showing: Television as Monstration", *Annals of the American Academy of Political and Social Science* 625 (2009): 19–31; Dayan, Daniel. "Mothers, Midwives and Abortionists: Genealogy and Obstetrics of Audiences and Publics", in Livingstone, Sonia (ed.). *Audiences and Public: When Cultural Engagement Matters for the Public Sphere, Volume 2*, Bristol: Intellect Press, 2005: 43–76; Dayan. "On Whose Terms Are You Shown?"

73 Dayan writes about how what he refers to as publics (associated with certain opinions) have careers, and go through different stages including birth, growth, fatigue, aging, death (and sometimes resuscitation and hiding). They are both social realities and intellectual constructions. The media are screening agencies as well as abortionists, which is not least evident in the case of the treatment of op-eds where people who are too famous to be ignored are often prioritized over lesser known writers:

> But the media can also function as a screening agency, becoming no longer midwives, but "bouncers" of publics, or worse, abortionists. They can easily do so by rejecting op eds, by returning letters to the editor, by closing the gates of talk shows, by selecting for publication poorly-written letters with unconvincing claims, by conceding access to figures that are too famous to be silenced and then neutralising that access through character assassination. (Dayan. "Mothers, Midwives and Abortionists", 65.)

74 Among few exceptions is Karin Sörbring's article where a specialist in research ranking compares in a detailed list the poor merits of the FHM leaders and officers with 45 prominent critical scholars in the debates, many in the Science Forum Covid-19, ranked as leading international science experts, belonging to "the country's absolute research elite", www.expressen.se/nyheter/unika-listan-sa-rankas-svenska-coronaexperter/ .

75 Cf., www.thelancet.com/article/S0140-6736(21)00869-2/fulltext .

76 Jay emphasizes the dangers of the ideal of "the big truth" as mirror image to "the big lie". Some fictions are necessary (particularly in politics) and there is a constant need for ongoing debate and pluralism. Jay, Martin. *The Virtues of Mendacity: On Lying in Politics*, Charlottesville: University of Virginia Press, 2010: 179. See also Arendt, Hannah. "Lying in Politics", in Arendt, H. (ed.). *Crises of the Republic*, London: Penguin, 1973: 9–42; Wernick, Andrew. *Promotional Culture: Advertising, Ideology and Symbolic Expression*, London: Sage, 1991; Jay. *The Virtues of Mendacity*.

77 Hill, Samantha Rose. "Hannah Arendt and the Politics of Truth", *openDemocracy*, 25 October 2020, www.opendemocracy.net/en/transformation/hannah-arendt-and-politics-truth/ .

78 Corona Commission. *English Summary*, 22.

79 Cf. Lincoln, Martha. "Necrosecurity, Immunosupremacy, and Survivorship in the Political Imagination of COVID-19", *Open Anthropological Research* 1:1 (2021): 46–59, 54.

80 Gustavsson. *Du stolta du fria*.

81 News Feature. "Why the WHO Took Two Years to Say COVID Is Airborne", *Nature* 604 (2022): 26–31, www.nature.com/articles/d41586-022-00925-7 .

82 Corner, John. "Mediated Politics, Promotional Culture and the Idea of 'Propaganda'", *Media, Culture & Society* 29:4 (2007): 669–677.

83 Corner, John. "Fake News, Post-Truth and Media – Political Change", *Media, Culture & Society* 39:7 (2017): 1100–1107.

84 Antivaxxers and provaxxers arguing for more protections were by some seen as equal offenders and just as problematic. It got a bit absurd. It is unfortunate that the Corona Commission never investigated the Swedish vaccine campaign and FHM's communication regarding for example child vaccinations. Another theme that deserves more

attention is the nature of Swedish influence over the WHO's communications and strategic choices. Clearly, the relationship between Sweden and WHO is more complicated than is sometimes suggested.

85 *Söndagsintervjun*, https://sverigesradio.se/avsnitt/cilla-benko-om-temperamentet-vagvalen-och-stormarna .

86 This chapter offers a further developed reflection of my earlier text in Swedish: "Vådan av blind källtillit", *Biblioteksbladet*, 24 February 2022, [The trouble of blind source trust], www.biblioteksbladet.se/ideer/essa/vadan-av-blind-kalltillit/ . The chapter is mainly based on public sources. Background interviews have been conducted with Ambassador Anders Nordström, Teresa Palmquist (Head of communication development, MSB) and Leif Håkansson and Johan Rönnblom (Moderators of We Support Anders Tegnell & Co (FHM)).

12

SWEDEN UNMASKED

Reading state and society through the pandemic

Jens Stilhoff Sörensen

Introduction

In 1968 Michel Foucault gave an interview to a Swedish magazine in which he reflected upon his own experience of living in Sweden:

> [In Sweden], a human is but a moving dot, obeying laws, patterns and forms in the midst of a traffic that is more powerful and defeats him/her. In its calmness, Sweden reveals a brave new world where we discover that the human is no longer necessary.[1]

A decade ago, long before the pandemic, Lennart Lundquist, one of Sweden's leading political scientists and democracy theorists warned about Sweden's de-democratisation and lack of rule of law.[2] Not only was freedom of speech under considerable threat and in crucial regards lacking in Sweden, he argued, but the fundamental tenets of rule of law and hence, in effect democracy itself.[3] With regard to public law two systems had developed, on the one hand public law, and on the other a special law invented arbitrarily by power-holders, politicians or high public officials, in order to legitimise their arbitrary decrees and actions.[4] A primary target was how neoliberal practices and New Public Management (NPM) had eroded and transformed traditional public management and political culture, an analysis that connects to a broader international critical tradition.[5] Elsewhere, I have argued, together with Erik J. Olson, that a form of "shadow management" has developed in Sweden.[6] By this we meant administrative practices for parallel treatment of issues sensitive with respect to law and regulations and which addresses these issues without transparency, hence in the "shadow". It means the emergence of parallel structures or sets of practices that are invisible to an outsider, where cases that don't fit the relevant legal requirements are dealt with, in direct or possible

DOI: 10.4324/9781003289364-13

violation of the law, especially constitutional or administrative law. It leads to a cultivation of informal practices, networks and routines that are not recorded or regulated with the effect that the public sector ceases to be transparent or conform to the rule of law.[7]

It would be expected that in a liberal and democratic society checks and balances would be in function to correct any such deviations or developments, at least in theory. Yet, Lundquist's claim was precisely that this did not occur. A certain set of further conditions would have to be in place for this development to proceed, such as a political establishment and a legal structure that does not regulate the deviation from rule of law and a media and public opinion that is not alarmed or alerted.

While these are serious claims and matters, difficult questions must be asked and explored. This chapter does so in context of how Swedish state and society has responded to and functioned during the pandemic and by suggesting two further conceptual lenses. Elaborated below these are a Swedish form of "state individualism" as introduced and conceptualised by two Swedish historians Lars Trägårdh and Henrik Berggren, widely embraced by some political circles while criticised and discarded by others, and Jacob Talmon's concept "totalitarian democracy".[8] The aim is to find and explore conceptual tools to understand the Swedish society and Sweden's *Sonderweg* in the pandemic where some of the most notable features have been a continuous rejection of emerging scientific evidence that the virus is airborne, that pre- and asymptomatic spread play a considerable role; a slack or negligent approach to basic disease protection measures such as testing-tracing-quarantine; and a fierce rejection of using facemasks even in care homes or clinical contexts. Other more troubling occurrences are the selective exclusion of some elderly from healthcare and the refusal to provide oxygen and possible killing of elderly with morphine without consent (hence not euthanasia) and without medical examination by a physician. Several practices appear to be in direct violation of various Swedish laws as well as of basic human rights, such as the right to life. The puzzle is to understand how this ideological rejection of emerging scientific evidence and political *Sonderweg* has been possible to uphold for so long and with little correction or critique. Hence, this chapter will not focus on detailing the actual events, policy choices and practices during the pandemic, as this is addressed more fully in other chapters in this collected volume and elsewhere.[9] An outline of events and responses will be given, but primarily to provide the setting and raise questions about the nature of Swedish politics and society. Further, the proposed conceptual lenses do not exclude other equally relevant concepts or possible explanations that are not addressed here, such as propaganda, mass psychology or cognitive dissonance. As we are engaged in understanding current events several concepts may be instructive. The next section provides a historical context of Sweden's crisis management and is followed by three sections cursorily outlining the pandemic response and its characteristics, leading onto a section on monolithic society. The subsequent section makes some notes on the nature of political concepts, which is then followed by an application of the two conceptual frameworks.

Sweden's crisis management

Sweden's recent history of crisis management is dismal, from a weak response when the passenger ship *Estonia* sank in the Baltic Sea in 1994 to a slow and insufficient response to the Tsunami in 2004. The latter resulted in a crisis commission, which delivered a thoroughgoing critique of poor Government management and crisis functions. The critique included that responsibility and accountability were unclear, that the Ministries lacked coordination and that they lacked initiative and did not seek information. The report resulted in a reorganisation of the crisis function in the Government. Henceforth there should be a crisis function in each Ministry, with coordination meetings at ministerial and state secretary levels, all led and coordinated by the PM, who would have a special office for crisis management (*Kansliet för Krishantering*) directly under the PM. The Ministries would have responsibility for their respective areas and various Ministries would become involved depending on the type of crisis. A crisis group and the "crisis management office" installed in 2008 should both coordinate and help the various Ministries in their work, seek information and assist with coordination. In 2014 the present Social Democratic Government moved the crisis office to the Minister of Interior located at the Ministry of Justice. Here, a Chief Civil Servant (*Chefstjänsteman*) is responsible and works directly under the State Secretary in the Ministry, who in turn is directly under the Minister. Within the Ministries there is a group "GSS" (*Gruppen för Strategisk Samordning*) which consists of state secretaries from the relevant Ministries in the crisis and headed by the State Secretary of the Minister of Interior. The "crisis management office" serves the GSS. Further, in 2008, a "Crisis Management Council" (*Krishanteringsråd*) was also established, led by the State Secretary under the Minister of Interior. It also consists of the Chief of Police, the Supreme Commander and representatives from some other authorities, such as the Civil Contingencies agency, *Socialstyrelsen and Svenska Kraftnät* (the Swedish Power Grid). It has bi-annual meetings. Further, each Ministry is supposed to have its own operations cell with a civil servant on standby. However, the crisis management office has never worked as a separate staff or unit, and during the pandemic the crisis management has in effect been wholly placed at the FHM, with the Government and other authorities in a passive or subordinate role. The Prime Minister regularly stated that this was the "expert agency" and that he had no reason to listen to anyone else.[10] However, according to the constitution the Government is ultimately responsible to lead the nation during a crisis. The abandonment of this task to a single agency has meant a conspicuous case of "the tail wagging the dog".

Sweden's pandemic response

Sweden's response to the pandemic has received wide international attention. Anti-lockdown and anti-mask-demonstrators in the U.S. and Europe have held up Sweden as an ideal and Sweden's Government and its Public Health Agency (FHM) have rejected much of the scientific consensus and recommendations by international disease prevention agencies, such as the EU's ECDC, the CDC or the WHO. Sweden has denied that the virus is airborne, the role of pre-symptomatic spread, transmission in schools or that children can get infected or transmit and denied that facemasks can provide protection.[11] While some minor variation and changes occurred, the virus is still by January 2022 not recognised as airborne and the state epidemiologist proclaims that facemasks were useless.[12] Several laws have been regularly violated, such as the Law on Disease Control and the Law on Protection of Work Environment.

After the WHO declaration of a pandemic on 11 March 2020 most European countries introduced restrictions and school closures and the other Nordic countries closed schools, bars and restaurants. They initiated testing, contact tracing and isolation of cases. The WHO emphasised the importance of acting early and testing. By contrast Sweden omitted testing and contact tracing from an early stage, such as for international travellers coming or returning to Sweden. Upper secondary schools (16–18 years) were temporarily closed but reopened in June, and universities moved to online teaching. Hence most schools were kept open. Public life remained largely uninterrupted and there were in general no restrictions on travel or movement, and no recommendations of facemasks even in hospitals or care homes. Regardless of the warnings from China or Italy the Swedish Eurovision national final took place with full audience on 7 March 2020. Limits on gatherings came on 12 March to 500 people and on 29 March to 50 people. The main general recommendation was – and has remained – hand washing, keeping social distance and staying home in case of symptoms.

It has been claimed that the FHM violated the disease protection law from the outset by removing the obligation to report Covid cases.[13] The foundation for Swedish disease protection is decentralised to 21 regions and disease protection officers who are legally independent from the national Public Health Agency, which has only an advisory, coordinative and support function. According to the law any suspected case of a disease which is deemed a "public" or "general danger" must be reported by the examining physician to the regional disease protection centre, which is then responsible for contact tracing. This whole function was sidestepped from the outset both by removing obligations to report and by leaving contact tracing to the individual, hence effectively abolishing it. Instead, those regions or municipalities who attempted to introduce some protective measures were often criticised by the FHM. Thus, for example, when Umeå municipality in March 2020 decided that staff, pupils and children who had visited a high-transmission area should stay home from school, they were criticised by the state epidemiologist. On 29 July 2020 the Swedish Minister for Social Affairs Lena Hallengren claimed that it was not in the "Swedish culture" to wear facemasks and she consistently rejected it as a measure. During meetings at the ECDC office in Stockholm, where facemasks were used, she would sit without.[14] Indeed, the FHM and the Government acted as if the aim was to actively allow community spread.

The scientific foundation for general recommendations by the FHM to the public was not disclosed. Facemasks were effectively dismissed with claims that they might be counter-productive, unpleasant or even dangerous, and that "we do not have that culture".[15] No evidence was provided. Following repeated questions by some journalists the FHM published a list of 35 studies on facemasks on its website in August 2020. However, the majority (31) of those showed evidence that facemasks could reduce transmission, whereas four of them were inconclusive. Nevertheless, the FHM did not adjust its recommendations. The same pattern was followed as scientific evidence and consensus emerged that the virus was airborne or that pre- and asymptomatic spread played a crucial role.

Most political parties, except the national-conservative Sweden Democrats, gave passive consent to the approach throughout the first wave, until summer 2020. Some critique began to appear following the high death rates. By 30 April, Sweden ranked among the top ten in the world with the highest deaths in Covid-19, 244 per million, about seven times higher than Finland and Norway (ourworldindata.org, 30 April 2020). By early June Sweden had twice as many deaths as the neighbouring region of all other Nordic countries, the Baltic countries, Poland and Kaliningrad combined. By 8 July Sweden had reached a ratio of 538 deaths per million exceeding for example the U.S., which had 394. The mainstream narrative sold to the media was that other countries would "catch up" and that Sweden's strategy would "win" in the end.

When the second wave began in Sweden during September 2020, no preparations were in place and no lessons had been learned. The other Nordic countries were well prepared and in Germany a *circuit breaker* was introduced, closing cafés, restaurants and cultural activities. Further measures followed in December, with closing of schools and introduction of home schooling. In Sweden, by contrast, the second wave accelerating in October took both the Government and population by surprise, since the FHM had repeatedly stated that Sweden would be less affected because of its larger community spread in spring. While scientific consensus grew in the autumn that the virus is airborne, that pre- and asymptomatic spread plays a significant role, that facemasks provide protection in combination with other measures, including ventilation, that children get infected and that schools play a role in community transmission, the FHM consistently denied or downplayed all these facts. Hence, there was no general recommendation of facemasks even in healthcare and care homes until December. By May 2021 facemasks were still rare and not regularly used even in birth clinics and care homes. The same pattern continued through the third wave in 2021 and the fourth Omicron wave that hit Sweden in the Christmas period 2021 and early 2022.

By early May 2021, Sweden had Europe's highest transmission, along with Cyprus, and approached 14,000 recorded deaths. A study by biologist Johanna Höög showed that at the time 1 in 4 Swedish children had had Covid-19 and estimated that between 26,000 and 81,000 had been affected by long-Covid. Moreover, 9 children out of 100,000 had been inflicted by hyper-inflammation, which was twice as much as in the U.S. and over five times more than in Germany. Deaths among children are also considerably higher in Sweden than in neighbouring countries, with 13 dead in Sweden, one in Norway, two in Denmark, none in Finland. Sweden has had a 7.7 times higher death rate among children than neighbouring countries. The advocacy group "Föreningen Covid-19 Barn & Skola" (The Association Covid-19 Children and School) estimated that by autumn 2021 800 children had lost a parent, a much higher figure than any neighbouring country. According to estimates from Imperial College this figure has by February 2022 increased to 1300 children.[16]

Hence, it has been considerably more dangerous to be a child in Sweden. The actual figures may be higher since there was virtually no testing in Sweden during the first wave (see Johanna Höög's chapter in this volume for a more extensive analysis on children and the pandemic).

Was there a strategy? In a constitutional hearing in April 2021, Sweden's Minister for Social Affairs, Lena Hallengren, stated that there had been no strategy. However, both public statements and internal emails from the FHM indicate that they early on adopted a "herd immunity" strategy allowing a slow but steady community transmission. Later this has been publicly denied but it is the only strategy that makes sense given the relaxed approach. Both the PM and the Director-General of the FHM, Johan Carlson, have made repeated statements suggesting that measures are irrelevant, and that it doesn't matter what we do as they can see no connection between disease protection measures and outcomes. This indicates a kind of fatalism that would render all protective instruments meaningless, whether they are testing-tracing-quarantine, ventilation, distancing, restrictions on large indoor gatherings or facemasks.

The effect was considerable social inequality where at-risk, vulnerable and low-income groups have taken the main burden, being exposed unless able to self-isolate for nearly two years.

Disposable Swedes

From a basic human rights perspective, the most unsettling reports have been those of lockout of some elderly and risk groups from the healthcare system whereby they have simply been denied care, and reports that elderly have been denied oxygen and instead been put to death by morphine. In April 2020 a Swedish MD and District Doctor, Jon Tallinger, who labelled himself Dr Whistle-blower, claimed that recommendations had been given to physicians to administer morphine instead of oxygen for elderly people in care homes.[17] Rather than euthanasia (illegal in Sweden), which is based on consent, this would in effect imply state-sanctioned murder.

The triage also meant that patients over 80 years old, or over 65 if they belonged to a risk group, should be denied IC treatment to preserve space in the IC units.[18] While Tallinger's claim was denied by officials it was supported by other whistle-blowers, such as the nurse Latifa Löfwenberg who also claimed that at least ten people had died as a result of the Region Gävleborg's guidelines.[19] After going public with her claim, she was fired from her position. Swedish media largely ignored Tallinger's claims, who went on to present them on YouTube with backup interviews and by going through patient journals.[20]

On 18 May, a professor of geriatric medicine at the University of Umeå, Yngve Gustafsson, warned in the Swedish medical journal that many elderly died unnecessarily as they were kept in the care homes and not admitted to hospital and therefore were not given the correct medical assessment or treatment.[21] The Health and Care Inspectorate (IVO) began investigating the situation in Swedish care homes in May.[22] On 20 May IVO stated that a larger investigation was initiated following both IVO's own observations and reports of elderly not being administered oxygen treatment. On 7 July IVO reported a complete national overview and that *a few regions* had made initial assessment that elderly should not be sent to hospital care regardless of being in need, but instead be kept in the care homes.[23]

On 7 July a Finnish nurse who had been working in Sweden told the Public Service Media *Yle* that the deaths of elderly had been speeded up in Sweden with doctors prescribing morphine and entry into a stage of palliative care, sometimes without meeting the patients.[24] She also confirmed the claims that patients were denied oxygen. A practice of denying intensive care for patients over 80 years was further taken up in the media, with the case of an 81-year-old man who had been denied intensive care although the hospital had space available.[25]

On 16 July CBS News broadcasted an interview from Stockholm with a woman whose 80-year-old father living in a care home had been diagnosed with Covid-19, but instead of being sent to hospital he had been given morphine and eventually died without treatment.[26] In mid-July, during the on-going national overview by IVO, about one of five regions (Sweden has 21 regions), reported to IVO that palliative care had been put in place prematurely during the early stage of the pandemic and that decisions for it had been general rather than individual.[27] Despite many reports from several regions there has to date not been any legal or criminal investigation into these reports, which would constitute not only violations of Sweden's constitution and healthcare law, but also of basic human rights, the right to life.

Denying protective equipment

Apart from lacking basic protective equipment, such as facemasks, several care homes in Sweden had incidents with removal of existing equipment, such as hand disinfection or banning private use of facemasks. Thus, for example, in one care home in Stockholm, staff reported that hand disinfection was kept locked away and only allowed to be taken out in case the media visited.[28]

An elderly resident in a care home in the municipality of Götene reported to Swedish Radio that she wanted to protect herself by using her own private facemask, but was prohibited by the staff from doing so with the argument that it looked scary.[29]

Shadow management and the concealment of documents

Throughout the pandemic there was a lack of transparency from the Government, the FHM and various public, regional and municipal bodies (see also Anders Vahlne's chapter in this volume on disinformation). The strategy – if there was one – was never clearly communicated. Instead, various contradictory statements appeared. These ranged from Minister for Social Affairs Lena Hallengren stating in a Constitutional Hearing in March 2021 that there was no strategy, to the Prime Minister both denying that herd immunity was a strategy and claiming that herd immunity would be the side effect or end result. Meanwhile internal emails obtained by journalists through the Public Information Act revealed that the state epidemiologist believed in and aimed for herd immunity. Other aspects of lacking transparency include that the FHM never provided scientific backing for its various recommendations or claims. Both the FHM and some regions engaged in active concealment of documents, such as deleting of emails.[30] For example, the Sörmland Region concealed transmission in care homes.[31] The Swedish Work Environment Authority deleted emails to avoid a debate over facemasks.[32] The Government itself denied its own Corona Commission access to any documentation of its crisis management meetings, claiming there existed no documentation despite 149 meetings of the Crisis Management Council. Hence, the Government claimed that there were no minutes or memos taken that could cast any light on the decision-making process during Sweden's greatest crisis since the Second World War. A major newspaper eventually revealed the existence of such documents.[33] The pattern was so widespread that it can be considered systemic and a culture of concealment. In fact, these practices conform to a pattern earlier described as *shadow management*, defined as:

> By shadow management we mean administrative practices for parallel treatment of issues sensitive with respect to law and regulations, and which addresses these issues without transparency, i.e., in the "shadow". Thus, "shadow management" denotes management or public administration with a parallel structure or parallel set of practices invisible to an outsider, where all errands and cases that do not fit the relevant legal requirements are dealt with, in direct or possible violation of the law, especially constitutional and administrative law. By not registering such cases and just dealing with them internally, they are difficult to find for an external reviewer and are, therefore, rarely subject to independent scrutiny. This leads to cultivation of informal practices, networks, and routines that are not recorded or regulated.[34]

The widespread and deep-rooted practice of shadow management and concealment in the Swedish Government and public sector adds to a pre-existing problem where accountability is lacking or very rare to obtain.[35] Commissions, inspections and various Government-initiated assessments invariably only look at systemic or procedural errors, but not individual responsibility or accountability. Such core human rights issues as the aforementioned replacing of oxygen with morphine to elderly will typically not lead to any legal criminal investigation or individual accountability in Sweden. Thereby, without a proper structure of accountability and with regularly recurring violations of laws by public agencies and officials themselves, it is questionable to which extent Sweden during the pandemic would qualify as a legal state and hence liberal democracy.

Monolithic society

Regardless of the issues outlined previously, the general public support for the Government has been relatively high – albeit diminishing – and the trust in institutions has generally remained high. According to the *Trust Barometer* conducted in autumn–winter 2020–2021 trust in the FHM and healthcare remained high, whereas the result for the Government and care homes was more negative.[36] Further, the media in general was overwhelmingly supportive of the Government and Public Health Agency. Rather than providing critical scrutiny of Government institutions and policies, a highly conformist media functioned as the Government's and FHM's megaphone.[37] With exception of some editorials, the media remained unquestioning and Government-loyal throughout the pandemic, while critical voices were dismissed and ridiculed. Certain topics central to the scientific findings and the international debate on the pandemic were simply marginalised or erased from public discourse. As discussed by Lapo Lappin in his contribution to this volume, linguistic exclusion preceded real exclusion. It was as if advocating disease control by itself was subversive. However, a certain rupture in the consensus came on 17 December 2020 when the Swedish King in his Christmas broadcast stated the country has failed.[38] Nevertheless, regardless a high level of institutional trust, there was a large part of the population experiencing a real terror in every-day life from the state-imposed risk to infection. Parents and schoolchildren in risk groups had to send their children to schools in the midst of high levels of transmission and without protective measures. Care homes and clinics worked without facemasks or basic protective measures, thus exposing elderly and risk groups to risk. As Johanna Höög shows in her chapter in this volume, it has been considerably more dangerous to be a child in Sweden than in any neighbouring country. More parents have died, as well as more elderly. As the cannon fodder for the Swedish strategy many elderly, teachers, parents, nurses and people in risk groups have raised their concerns outside the mainstream media channels. Organisationally outflanked and confined to the margins they have raised their voices on social media or to the organisations that have emerged to criticise the Swedish strategy, such as "Vetenskapsforum Covid-19" (Science Forum Covid-19) or "Föreningen Covid-19 Barn & Skola" (The Association Covid-19 Children & School). Private webpages and social media groups have emerged as a form of *samizdat*[39] for dissenting voices. In this sense the Swedish pandemic management created social polarisation and deepening divisions of society.

Nevertheless, the remarkable consensus despite high death tolls, science denial and social exclusion of risk groups and elderly, extend also to civil society organisations, physicians, the academic and the legal communities. Despite Sweden being one of the world's most unionised countries, there was only limited critique from the teacher's or physician's unions, or any of the other labour unions. The few existing critics of the Swedish strategy who advocated following internationally accepted precautions were ridiculed in the media, attacked as disseminators of fake news, and ostracised.[40] Hence, in general, new findings and scientific evidence have not only been rejected by the Government and the Public Health Agency, but across the board of state agencies and in the media. Thereby the pandemic has highlighted a highly monolithic character of Swedish society and political culture. It is this monolithic character and resistance to external information and science that is the real puzzle and phenomenon. To explore it further we need to make some notes on political concepts and metaphors.

Political concepts and political metaphors

Following Sheldon Wolin's classical work on political philosophy, the field of politics is a created one.[41] By this he meant that none of the designations we give, concepts we apply or way we think about the political are written into the nature of things but are the product of the historical activity of political philosophers. Concepts like "power", "authority", "consent" are not real things but intended to point to some significant aspect about political things. Their function is to render political facts significant either for purposes of analysis, criticism or justification, or a combination of all three.[42] Further: "when political concepts are put in the form of an assertion . . . the validity of the statement is not to be settled by referring to the facts of political life" and "political theory is not so much interested in political practices, or how they operate, but rather in their meaning".[43]

"The concepts and categories that make up our political understanding help us to draw connections between political phenomena: they put some order to what might otherwise appear to be a hopeless chaos of activities."[44] Stated differently, we might say that political concepts and metaphors are tools for creating meaning and political vision; they may be useful to a certain extent and carry us a part of the way. At some point they break down and need replacement by new concepts. Thus, the political conceptual landscape we have inherited can sometimes hinder our understanding and meaning making of phenomena and events. During times of crisis this may be especially true. Our inherited understanding of "left" and "right" or "democracy", "liberalism" and "totalitarianism" has become increasingly challenged. It is as if the territory has changed too much since the map was produced. Next, the concepts "state individualism" and "totalitarian democracy" are revisited and deployed as a lens to further understand contemporary Swedish state and society.

State individualism

In 2006 the Swedish historians Lars Trägårdh and Henrik Berggren published a book that took issue both with the two most established narratives of Swedish state and political culture and with the Swedish conventional self-image.[45] On the one hand there is a (critical) narrative of the Swedish strong state and the dominant *étatism*, which has led to "that historians sometimes have seen the country as one of the first and most perfected examples of an absolutist state".[46] There are also a number of international cultural critics who have noted the Swede's blind obedience and faith towards state authority. We have Susan Sontag's label of Sweden as a "pathological society" (1969), Hans Magnus Enzensberger's claim that Swedes hold the world record in docility (1987), and Roland Huntford's more controversial claim that Swedes are the new totalitarians worshipping the state and where individual freedom and democracy mean little, with "Swedes having fulfilled all Huxley's requirements for the new totalitarianism".[47] Huntford's devastative comparisons of Swedish society and mentality to the dystopias of Huxley and Orwell included the state-servility of the media:

> With the help, if not the leadership, of the mass media, the Swedish language has been debased and manipulated so that, as in Orwell's Newspeak, the ability to express unapproved thoughts has been eroded.[48]

In contrast to this vexatious characterisation of Swedish society and culture stands the self-heralded image of Sweden as one of the most highly developed democracies and welfare states with solidarity and social equality as foundational values. Indeed, this is the image the Swedish state wishes to promote internationally.[49] In this view Sweden is instead a thriving democracy with a civil society working in unison with the state, rather than as its critical corrective. In 1946 the Swedish political scientist and conservative party leader Gunnar Heckscher described Sweden in terms of "corporatism" where a new social human type had emerged, less individualist and more oriented to cooperation in society.[50] Following this tradition, the high level of social trust and institutional trust in Sweden can be explained by the development of the welfare state, its equality and catering to broader social needs crossing and alleviating class boundaries. The Swedish political scientist Bo Rothstein has explicitly linked social trust to the development of the welfare state.[51] The book by Trägårdh and Berggren was a break with these narratives. Swedish social trust had much deeper historical roots, and rather than collectivists the Swedes could be labelled "state individualists". Swedish history, they argued, differed in a crucial regard from feudal Europe in that Sweden had a free peasantry and weak nobility, and that the King made a social contract directly with the peasants in order to curb the power of the nobility. From the peasant's perspective the threat to their freedom came from the nobility. By offering an alliance the King gained support. This, the authors argued, lies at the root of the Swedish popular trust in a central power as well as their suspicion and tendency to distrust the middle layers, such as the nobility or as today represented by larger private companies. Social trust is a tremendous resource in society. It reduces so-called transaction costs, and it tends to generate social peace and stability, and a sense of safety. State individualism here means that the state offers the individual a possibility to free him/herself of any social bonds and obligations connected to family, church or associations. Like a giant insurance agency, the state caters to all needs, from cradle to grave, child-care to care homes, whereby the individual can free him/herself for his/her own self-development. Taxes and state authority provides him/her freedom, and it is only through a strong state that s/he can be truly free. In this vision the state is a benevolent protector and provider. However, the authors argue, the trust in the state has come with a price. The individual becomes atomised under the state as other social bonds are loosened and bereft of real existential content. The social contract between the state and the individual and the social welfare system's explicit focus on the individual aims at autonomy and hence reduces both the dependency and relationship to other social organisations, be it the family, local community and neighbourhood, church, or civil society associations. In a sense we might say that this provides fertile ground for a culture of narcissism, to build on a theme articulated by Christopher Lasch.[52]

Moreover, civil society operates in a subservient role rather than as an alternative or corrective to the all-encompassing state. Historically, civil society in Sweden has three roots, the sport movement, the church movements (typically various religious associations not associated with the state church), and the sobriety movement.[53] In addition to this was the unionised labour movement but this was directly connected to the Social Democratic Party, and indeed founded it. Today an often noted and criticised condition is that Sweden's civil society is heavily dependent on the state in terms of funding.[54]

This revisionist narrative of Swedish state individualism had a strong impact on Swedish political debate during the period. It was embraced by the conservative party (*Moderaterna*) which came in power that year (2006) as it offered an alternative narrative on the Swedish welfare state and individualism as opposed to that promoted under the hegemony of the Social Democratic Party. It was not the Social Democrats and the welfare state that had generated trust and individual freedom. Rather, these had deeper roots that pre-existed and were utilised by the Social Democratic project. However, Trägårdh and Berggren were also fiercely criticised. The political scientist Olof Petersson claimed that the book was unscientific, and he criticised its wide use and interpretation of historical sources in the form of national poems, novels and other source material without being able to establish direct links to contemporary organisational outcomes.[55] To some extent this may be seen as a political scientist's issue with historical methodology. While individualism and autonomy were indeed connected to a strong state, it would go too far to label it "state individualism". Petersson defended and essentially restated the conventional narrative in which a Swedish well-functioning democracy had gradually moved from corporatism with a citizen focus on social cooperation towards more individual choice.

It is evident that we are here dealing with politically and even emotionally invested narratives relating to Swedish identity and Sweden's self-image. The competing narratives serve to criticise and undermine or legitimise certain political projects. Nevertheless, the perspective of state individualism offers an insight into and possible explanation as to why Swedish society has displayed such a monolithic character throughout the pandemic. Through it, we see an organic view of the state, with the Government as the head of the organism, with agencies as its arms and the people constituent in the body. For the body to function you must protect the head. If you have nothing other than the state, any alternative bond or connection to rely on, then you had better place all your trust in the state. Even when it commits abuse. There is no existential alternative.

Totalitarian democracy

Totalitarian as a political concept is both contested and tenacious. In the 1920s the Italian politician Giovanni Amendola used it to describe fascism. Benito Mussolini famously proclaimed "everything within the state, nothing outside the state, and nothing against the state", and the German Nazi legal theorist Carl Schmitt used the word "Totalstaat".[56] Karl Popper ascribed its roots or thought material to Plato, whereas the Frankfurt School's Max Horkheimer and Theodor Adorno located them in the Enlightenment.[57] Popularised in fictional literature, especially George Orwell's *1984*, it captured the imagination of what a dystopian society would look like. Orwell also used the term in several essays. By 1949 Hannah Arendt had formulated totalitarianism as a new form of Government distinct from historical absolutist states. However, as part of modernity many of the political practices were first tested out in the colonial periphery and eventually boomeranged with a vengeance to the centre.[58] Modelled after the Nazi German state and the Soviet Union, American political scientists used it in the 1950s and it became prominent in the new discipline of Sovietology. Subsequently the models became considered out-dated, and with the opening of historical archives, misconceived. The term has been dismissed as political, as deployed in Cold War anti-Soviet propaganda, and the dismissals have in turn been discarded as apologetic. Nevertheless, the concept encapsulates some phenomena or trends in political life, which have also been employed to liberal and capitalist societies. The political theorist Sheldon Wolin used the concept of "inverted totalitarianism" to describe contemporary American politics and society.[59] Acutely aware of the risks of applying such a loaded concept, he wanted to raise awareness and provide a new lens through which to see the emergence of a society that risked becoming so de-democratised and turned against democracy at the level of its governing powers that it would become totalitarian.

In a similar vein, the Finnish historian and cultural critic Jari Ehrnrooth has suggested that the Swedish corona strategy reveals how Sweden has become a soft version of what Jacob Talmon called "totalitarian democracy".[60] Talmon developed the concept of totalitarian democracy to contrast two traditions of democracy that arose with the French revolution: the liberal and the totalitarian.[61] Talmon's work has fallen from fashion, but the tension between the two traditions can be seen as a vital issue of our time. The concept aimed to cast light on the transition during the French Revolution from a liberal phase during 1789–92 to a revolutionary phase from August 1792 to July 1794.[62] During the liberal phase France was a constitutional monarchy with a National Assembly and then Legislative Assembly, with guaranteed individual liberty and the promotion of secularism. But the National Convention elected in 1792 created a revolutionary dictatorship and ceded power to the Committee on Public Safety (CPS) created in April 1793. This period saw a new view of democracy held by Robespierre's CPS, proclaiming to create equality, with the introduction of central planning, and the "reign of terror" when the republic directed violence against its own citizens. According to Talmon we see here a view of democracy corresponding with Rousseau's concept of a "general will", which if the people does not will, "must be made to will".[63]

Both traditions profess to be democratic. The essential difference between the traditions of democratic thought is that one, the liberal version views politics to be a matter of trial and error, and regards political systems as pragmatic, whereas the totalitarian democratic school is based on the assumption of a sole and exclusive truth in politics.[64] The liberal current not only emphasises individual rights and freedoms, but also views politics as a process of trials and tribulations that guides the common destiny, and it recognises individual and collective endeavours outside the political sphere. Human life takes place in and is guided through many spheres, of which the political is one. The totalitarian form, by contrast, believes in a total and exclusive truth in politics to which those who rule must guide society. This is a Messianic form of politics where the final goal of politics is reached only when these truths or beliefs reign over all spheres of life, hence it is totalitarian. Politics is simply the art of applying this philosophy to the organisation of society. It is Messianic in the sense that it postulates an order or way of life to which people must arrive and it considers politics as embracing all spheres of life. Both traditions value "freedom", but whereas the liberal views it in terms of spontaneity and absence of coercion, the totalitarian sees it realised only in the attainment of an absolute collective purpose.[65] Political Messianism is mainly associated with revolutionary movements or with totalitarian dictatorships on the right or left. The Chinese Cultural Revolution, for example, was such a Messianic political program of cleansing directed to individuals with the "wrong will" or thought.

According to Ehrnrooth the Swedish case expresses a society where uniformity is heralded above pluralism, and where the mean is a state-led progressive doctrine with a Messianic dream of social peace.[66] In such a system the rallying behind the state ideology, and the expression of pandemic nationalism, is a common movement towards the social good, and any dissident an anti-social heretic. The Messianic aspect of Swedish politics has also been noted by Swedish historian Svante Nordin.[67] He notes that since 1809, or since the immediate aftermath of the French revolution, Swedish politics has been characterised by five major political reform waves, each in which Sweden has presented itself in a self-image of rational hyper-modernity and as an avant-garde in Europe and the world, and where each project has rejected the previous as part of a decadent past.[68] Although Nordin does not employ Talmon's terminology his work can be read as a deeper historical illustration of an anti-conservative political Messianism. Notwithstanding its messianic nature, this view of politics is anchored in the conviction that Sweden has a deep-rooted democratic tradition. However, a point with the paradoxical concept of totalitarian democracy is that it is a totalitarianism that has the enthusiastic support of the people. Moreover, unlike historical totalitarian states, the totalitarian democracy allows critique, and the system of Government is a representative democracy with an elected Government. But, regardless of critique, even if it is science-based, there is no correction. This is well illustrated by the Swedish lack of receptivity to science and international reports on various aspects of SARS CoV-2 and the pandemic. Regardless of whether the reports were research findings, came from international institutions such as the ECDC, CDC or WHO, or from Swedish researchers or institutions like the Royal Swedish Academy of Sciences, they were summarily dismissed by the Swedish Government and FHM, who remained undeterred and there was little change to the strategy or even reflection over it, nor much questioning in the media.

Throughout the pandemic, the Swedish Government and FHM never aimed at reducing transmission or protect people, neither school children nor elderly in care homes, but only to protect the functioning of institutions and the economy. The instructions for the aim with the FHM were breached, laws violated, shadow management practiced and the public ethos corroded. The approach rested on a Social-Darwinian bedrock. Risk groups and elderly were left to protect themselves, if they could, through self-isolation. Lockdown was avoided but replaced by a de facto locking-in of the weak and vulnerable. School children were forcefully exposed to risk and many elderly denied healthcare, with an unknown number involuntarily euthanised with morphine. The neglect and abuse of human rights taking place throughout the pandemic aligns with a century-old tradition in Swedish history where, as discussed in Lapo Lappin's contribution to this volume, individual human rights and civil liberties have little real place or protection. From the Swedish State Institute for Race Biology (1922–1958), via medical experimentation on the mentally disabled, to forced sterilisation programs of certain minorities and groups (until 2013), the dignity as well as the rights of the individual have at will been nullified by the state. While protected in theory, the rule of law vanishes where there is no accountability and no possibility or interest from the legal system to claim it. If this can be called utilitarian, then it is an utilitarianism designed to protect the organic state at the centre in a system where we eventually discover, to re-quote Foucault, that the human is no longer necessary.

Notes

1 Michel Foucault interviewed in *Bonniers Litterära Magasin (BLM)* 1968: "Foucault on Sweden: 'The end of the Human'", www.blogs.hss.ed.ac.uk/crag/2015/02/01/foucault-sweden/; see also: "Foucaults besök på Gästrike-Hälsinge nation", *Upsala*

Nya Tidning, 2 July 2019, https://unt.se/nyheter/foucaults-besok-pa-gastrikhalsinge-nation-5350512.aspx .

2 Lundquist, Lennart. *Slutet på Yttrandefriheten (och demokratin?)* Lund: Studentlitteratur, 2012.

3 *Ibid.*

4 Lundquist interviewed on Swedish Radio, 3 March 2012, https://sverigesradio.se/avsnitt/49536 .

5 Brown, Wendy. *Undoing the Demos: Neoliberalism's Stealth Revolution*, Princeton NJ: Princeton University Press, 2017; Brown, Wendy. *In the Ruins of Neoliberalism*, New York: Columbia University Press, 2019.

6 Sörensen, Jens S., and Erik J. Olsson. "Shadow Management: Neoliberalism and the Erosion of Democratic Legitimacy Through Ombudsmen with Case Studies from Swedish Higher Education", *Societies* 10:2 (2020).

7 *Ibid.*, 6.

8 Trägårdh, Lars, and Henrik Berggren. *Är svensken människa? Gemenskap och oberoende i det moderna Sverige*, Stockholm: Norstedts, 2006; Talmon, Jacob Leib. *The Origins of Totalitarian Democracy*, London: Secker & Warburg, 1952.

9 See Hanson, Claudia et al. "National Health Science, Governance and the Media: Drivers of COVID-19 Health Responses in Germany, Sweden and the UK in 2012", *BMJ Global Health* 6:12 (2021); Brusselaers, Nele, David Steadson, Kelly Bjorklund, Sofia Breland, Jens Stilhoff Sörensen, Andrew Ewing, Sigurd Bergmann, and Gunnar Steineck. "Evaluation of Science Advice During the COVID-19 Pandemic in Sweden", *Humanities and Social Sciences Communications* 9, Article number: 91 (2022), www.nature.com/articles/s41599-022-01097-5; Sörensen, Jens S. "Terror in Utopia", *Socioloski Pregled* 54:3 (2020): 961–1007.

10 Cf. the introductory chapter.

11 See also Anders Vahlne's chapter in this volume.

12 Proclaimed by the state epidemiologist on the FHM Press Conference 13 January 2022.

13 Alvner, Johan, Lars Eriksson, Peter Galatius, Peet Tüll, and Petra Östergren. "Experter: Sveriges smittskyddslag har inte efterföljts", *Altinget*, 30 September 2021, www.altinget.se/artikel/experter-sveriges-smittskyddslag-har-inte-efterfoljts .

14 Lena Hallengren, statement on Press Conference 29 July 2020.

15 Lena Hallengren, 29 July 2020, www.expressen.se/tv/nyheter/coronaviruset/hallengren-s-i-sverige-fattar-vi-inte-politiska-beslut-nar-det-galler-skyddsutrustning-/ .

16 Imperial College London – Covid-19 Orphanhood, Sweden: covid19orphans-widget (imperialcollegelondon.github.io).

17 www.youtube.com/watch?v=Csb9DvAUj_s (accessed 8 July 2020) and www.youtube.com/watch?v=xk0TK_Syn9I&t=592s (accessed 8 July 2020).

18 On a press conference 26 March 2020, Thomas Lindén, senior director at the Swedish National Board of Health and Welfare (Socialstyrelsen) explained which patients could eventually come to be denied treatment, www.exakt24.se/brackliga-personer-kan-snart-nekas-coronavard/ .

19 https://nyhetsbyran.org/2020/05/05/sjukskoterska-fick-sparken-efter-larm-om-att-aldre-nekas-syrgas/ .

20 For example here, www.youtube.com/watch?v=LeMSieNQwUQ (accessed 8 July 2020).

21 *Läkartidningen* (*Swedish Medical Journal*), 18 May 2020, https://lakartidningen.se/aktuellt/nyheter/2020/05/geriatrikprofessor-manga-aldre-dor-i-onodan-utan-korrekt-bedomning/ .

22 IVO, 20 May 2020, www.ivo.se/publicerat-material/nyheter/2020/tillsyn-av-vard-och-behandling-pa-landets-samtliga-sarskilda-boenden-for-aldre/ .

23 IVO, 7 July 2020, www.ivo.se/publicerat-material/nyheter/2020/ivo-fordjupar-granskningen-av-vard-och-behandling-pa-sarskilda-boenden-for-aldre/ .

24 https://yle.fi/uutiset/3-11433976 (with excerpts in Swedish here, https://meritwager.nu/allmant/sverigebilden-i-sverige-har-aldre-manniskors-dod-paskyndats-med-morfinsprutor/).
25 www.svd.se/reglerna-foljdes-inte-nar-gosta-81-nekades-vard .
26 *CBS News*, 16 July 2020, www.cbsnews.com/video/sweden-sees-high-virus-mortality-rate-after-resisting-lockdown/ .
27 *Dagens Nyheter*, 18 July 2020, www.dn.se/nyheter/sverige/flera-regioner-palliativ-vard-sattes-in-for-snabbt/ (accessed 18 July 2020).
28 *Expressen*, 17 May 2020, www.expressen.se/nyheter/coronaviruset/larm-fran-boendet-vi-tigger-for-att-fa-handsprit/ .
29 *Sveriges Radio* (Swedish Radio) 15 May 2020.
30 *Dagens Media*, 17 February 2021, www.dagensmedia.se/medier/digitalt/nils-funcke-dundrar-mot-myndigheters-morklaggning-finns-bara-ett-ord-oacceptabelt/ .
31 *SVT Nyheter Sörmland*, 3 May 2020, www.svt.se/nyheter/lokalt/sormland/kommunerna-undanholl-information-om-smittspridningen-inom-aldreomsorgen .
32 *SVT Nyheter Inrikes*, 30 May 2020, www.svt.se/nyheter/inrikes/kritiserade-myndighe ten-ville-slippa-svar-debatt-om-munskydden-framgar-av-mejl-som-raderats .
33 *Svenska Dagbladet*, Editorial, 20 January 2022, www.svd.se/har-ar-dokumenten-lena-hallengren-havdar-inte-finns .
34 Sörensen and Olsson. "Shadow Management", 6.
35 Cf. Jerneck, Magnus. "Inledning", *Statsvetenskaplig tidskrift* (*The Swedish Journal of Political Science*) 123:5 (2021): 24, https://statsvetenskapligtidskrift.org/ .
36 Trägårdh, L. "Sverige ett splittrat land", *Focus*, 6 March 2021, www.fokus.se/veckans-fokus/sverige-ett-splittrat-land/ .
37 Lindström, M. "The New Totalitarians", *SSM Public Health*, April 6;14, 2021 https://pubmed.ncbi.nlm.nih.gov/34136630/; see also: Scherman, Jan, www.dagensmedia.se/opinion/debatt/jan-scherman-myndighetsmegafonen-tog-over-i-pandemirapporterin gen/ .
38 www.dn.se/sverige/kungen-om-pandemin-vi-har-misslyckats/ .
39 *Samizdat* (Russian: self-publishing) was a form of dissident activity across the socialist Eastern Bloc in which individuals reproduced censored and underground makeshift publications.
40 The most conspicuous case here is how the Science section of Swedish Radio targeted a private Facebook group where critique was voiced against the Swedish strategy. Here, the state radio insinuated that these private individuals were foreign agents. The newspaper *Expressen* published names and photographs of several members, some of whom then began receiving threats, leading to some members leaving Sweden, www.irishtimes.com/news/world/europe/limerick-man-flees-sweden-over-criticism-of-his-covid-19-campaign-1.4493317 . See also Sigurd Bergmann's chapter.
41 Wolin, Sheldon S. *Politics and Vision*, Princeton: Princeton University Press, 2016: 6.
42 *Ibid.*
43 *Ibid.*, 6–7.
44 *Ibid.*, 7.
45 Trägårdh and Berggren. *Är svensken människa?*
46 *Ibid.*, 33.
47 Huntford quoted in Trägårdh and Berggren, 33. See also Huntford, Roland. *The New Totalitarians*, 1971, https://archive.org/details/TheNewTotalitarians/mode/2up?q= , pp. 10–11, 188, 306, 327. On Sontag, see Susan Sontag's "Letter from Sweden": Ramparts Magazine, July 1969, 23–28. Enzensberger, Hans Magnus. *Ach Europa*, Frankfurt am Main: Suhrkamp, 1987.
48 Huntford. *The New Totalitarians*, 302.
49 This is the case since the Social Democratic internationalism associated with Olof Palme since the 1960s and as promoted today through cultural institutions such as the *Swedish*

Institute. We will return to this in the next section, see also Nordin, Svante. *Sveriges Moderna Historia: Fem politiska projekt*, Stockholm: Natur & Kultur, 2019.

50 Heckscher, Gunnar. *Staten och organisationerna*, Stockholm: Kooperativa förbundets förlag, 1946. See also Trägårdh and Berggren. *Är svensken människa?* 34–35.

51 For example, Rothstein, Bo. *Sociala fällor och tillitens problem*, Stockholm: SNS Förlag, 2002. See also the critique by Sörensen, Jens S. “Kultur, institutioner, och social tillit”, *Statsvetenskaplig Tidskrift* 1 (2006).

52 Lasch, Christopher. *Culture of Narcissism: American Life in An Age of Diminishing Expectations*, New York: W.W. Norton, 1979.

53 See for example Trägårdh, Lars, Per Selle, Lars Skov Henriksen and Hanna Hallin. “Inledning”, and Trägårdh, Lars. “Statsindividualismen och civilsamhället”, in Trägårdh, Lars Per Selle, Lars Skov Henriksen, and Hanna Hallin (eds.). *Civilsamhället klämt mellan stat och kapital*, Stockholm: SNS Förlag, 2013.

54 Lifvendahl, Tove. “Konsten att tämja ett civilsamhälle” [The arts of taming a civil society], *Svenska Dagbladet*, 18 April 2021, www.svd.se/konsten-att-tamja-ett-civilsamhalle . See also Westerholm, Johan. “Bidragsindustrin” [The Grants Industry], *Sunt Förnuft* 2 (2021), https://skattebetalarna.se/wp-content/uploads/2021/06/20210610-Tema.pdf; Danieli, Adam. “Att förstöra ett civilsamhälle” [Destroying Civil Society], *Timbro Smedjan*, 14 October 2019, https://timbro.se/smedjan/att-forstora-ett-civilsamhalle/ .

55 Petersson, Olof. “Maktutredningen och statsindividualismen”, 2012, www.olofpeterss on.se/_arkiv/skrifter/timbro120925.pdf .

56 Schmitt, Carl. *The Concept of the Political*, Chicago: The University of Chicago Press, 1932.

57 Popper, Karl. *The Open Society and Its Enemies*, London: Routledge, 1945; Horkheimer, Max, and Theodor W. Adorno. *Dialectic of Enlightenment: Philosophical Fragments*, new ed., Redwood City: Stanford University Press, 2002 (1st ed. New York, 1944).

58 Arendt, Hannah. *Origins of Totalitarianism*, Berlin: Schocken Books/New York: Harcourt, Brace, 1951.

59 Wolin, Sheldon S. *Democracy Incorporated: Managed Democracy and the Spectre of Inverted Totalitarianism*, Princeton: Princeton University Press, 2017.

60 Ehrnrooth, Jari. “Den svenska coronastrategin tecken på totalitär utveckling”, *Expressen* 10 July 2020, www.expressen.se/debatt/den-svenska-coronastrategin-tecken-pa-totali tar-utveckling/ . Cf. Sigurd Bergmann’s chapter.

61 Talmon. *The Origins of Totalitarian Democracy*.

62 In addition to Talmon, for the details of the French revolution’s “reign of terror” see Palmer, Robert Roswell. *Twelve Who Ruled: The Year of Terror in the French Revolution*, Princeton: Princeton University Press, 1941.

63 Talmon. *The Origins of Totalitarian Democracy*, 43.

64 *Ibid*., 3.

65 *Ibid*., 2.

66 Ehrnrooth. “Den svenska coronastrategin tecken på totalitär utveckling”, www.expres sen.se/debatt/den-svenska-coronastrategin-tecken-pa-totalitar-utveckling/ .

67 Nordin. *Sveriges moderna historia*.

68 These have included the constitution of 1809, the Parliamentary reform of 1866, the introduction of universal suffrage, the “Peoples Home” and welfare state since the 1930s, and the globalisation and multiculturalism of the past 30–40 years.

13

A DRASTIC END TO A LONG STORY OF SUCCESS IN SWEDISH PREVENTIVE MEDICINE

Gunnar Steineck

Since the 18th century, Sweden has been internationally at the forefront of preventive medicine. This success was based on trusting cooperation between those in power and the research community. The means had been mandatory legislation, scientifically based educational efforts, and free preventive care provided within well-functioning structures. The handling of the Covid-19 pandemic was a drastic departure from this more than 250-year-old tradition.

To illustrate the departure, this chapter provides some examples from our history. The first comes from maternal health care and a more recent example is the response to the pandemic that was caused by the human immunodeficiency virus. Available information indicates the bureaucracy at the Public Health Agency of Sweden developed its own agenda, and its systematic following of that agenda explains the catastrophic outcome of the Covid-19 pandemic in Sweden. This agenda was based on self-produced narratives, not on a dialogue with the Swedish or international research community. Notably, the bureaucrats succeeded in shielding those in power from the knowledge readily available from Swedish and international experts in virology and epidemiology. One way forward in preparation for the future may be to restore the trust between the research community and those in political power. A challenge in doing that is to communicate the difference between a bureaucrat and a real expert.

Some early achievements

We can obtain statistics for cause-specific mortality in Sweden as far back as 1749. During the latter half of the 18th century, it was mandatory for parishes of the Lutheran State Church to record births and deaths in a Church register. These records can be used to calculate causes of death at the population level. Today, every Swedish resident has a unique personal identity number, and a large number

DOI: 10.4324/9781003289364-14

of population-based registers supplement the information in the cause-of-death register. For example, since 1958 we have had a cancer register whose quality is guaranteed by the fact that for every individual who falls ill, it is mandatory by law that both the doctor in charge and the pathologist submit a report independently of each other. Because the personal identity number can be used as a link, Sweden today supports thriving register research where a wide range of issues can be addressed, as mentioned in the chapter by Nele Brusselaers.

Using available statistics available in the mid-18th century, an initiative was taken at that time to reduce maternal mortality. *Collegium Medicum* was a Swedish medical organization founded in 1663 by a number of individual physicians. The organization concluded in a letter in 1751 to the Swedish parliament that "Of 651 cases of women who died in childbirth, 400 could have been saved if they had had adequate access to a midwife."[1] Two decades later, in 1775, *Allmänna Barnbördshuset* (the Public Birth House) was opened in Stockholm, which became an important educational institution for physicians and midwives, and thus a critical factor in reducing the high maternal mortality rate. These midwives gradually replaced traditional birth attendants in the countryside. Among other things, they were trained in aseptics and they applied Ignaz Semmelweis's observations. He was a Hungarian physician who in 1847 proposed washing hands in chlorinated lime solutions before assisting in childbirths. This practice reduced mortality caused by fatal infections after childbirth. From the end of the 18th century to the end of the 19th century, the proportion of women who died in connection with pregnancy and childbirth was halved. The decline was from about 1,000 to 500 deaths per 100,000 children born. For the next 100 years, the decline continued to five or fewer women, largely due to the advent of antibiotics, blood transfusions, maternal health care, and hospital births. During the latter part of the 19th century, maternal mortality in Sweden was a third as high as in England and the United States. The early success in reducing maternal mortality was the first of many achievements in Sweden concerning preventive medicine for the forthcoming two centuries.

The significance of strict legislation

Sweden was notably early in developing strict legislation in a large number of areas, leading to reduced morbidity and mortality. This applies not least to the work environment, traffic, child accidents, tobacco sales and use, food hygiene, and alcohol sales.

Asbestos

In the mid-1920s, the first reports came that asbestos could be dangerous to health. In the 1950s, several studies showed an increased risk of cancer, first for lung cancer and then for mesothelioma, a cancer of the lining of the lungs and peritoneum. Exposure to asbestos for a short time can cause cancer. A connective tissue formation in the lung caused by asbestos, asbestosis, can also lead to morbidity and death.

The National Board of Occupational Safety and Health issued a regulation in 1963 to reduce the risk of asbestosis. From the mid-1970s until the mid-1980s, several measures were taken to reduce the risk of asbestos handling. This has meant that asbestos is not used in the construction of new buildings. From an international perspective, this took place earlier than many in other countries. Mining and use of asbestos continued for a long time in some countries after its use disappeared in Sweden, and even continues in some countries today. Today, we have extensive legislation to counteract health risks at work; we also have regulated supervision of safety representatives.

Alcohol sales

In 1960, the production of alcohol in the home was banned. The same year, selling alcohol to persons less than 18 years old was forbidden. Beginning in 1917 alcohol was sold in Sweden only through a group of stores that belong to a state-owned monopoly. The idea is that alcohol harm will be less for both the individual and society if alcohol is sold without profit. The mission of the monopoly includes distributing information on the harmful effects of alcohol. Opening hours are limited and the stores are closed on Sundays. With this construction, the state may protect some from aggravating their alcohol dependence. This system may also protect relatives of alcohol-dependent persons by decreasing access to alcohol by limiting the number the stores that are open. Finally, the monopoly applies a strict law that states that alcohol may only be sold to individuals 20 years and older.

Traffic

Sweden has for decades been among the countries with the lowest death rates in traffic in the world, and was in 2019 one of the safest countries in Europe (according to the EU Commission). In 1975, Sweden had 14 deaths per 100,000 individuals; the figures in France and the US were 27 and 21 respectively. Fifteen years later, in 1990, Sweden's figures had dropped to 9, France and the US had 20 and 18 respectively. The reasons behind the low Swedish figures include strict legislation setting speed limits, making wearing seat belts compulsory for adults (1986) and children (1988). Speed limits reduce the violence to the persons in a vehicle during an accident as well as those outside the car. A seat belt, as well as a seat for children belted in place, further reduces the level of injury. Being hit by a car driving 30 km per hour gives a small risk of death, while the opposite is true for 50 km per hour. Another piece of legislation that has reduced morbidity and mortality is the requirement that children wear a helmet when cycling. Sweden today also has strict legislation to limit drunk driving. Even at 0.2 per mille in the blood, a fine or imprisonment is required. At 1 per mille, the driving license is usually revoked. The legislation is similar in terms of fines and imprisonment for driving a boat. Finally, it is forbidden in Sweden to drive a car while holding a mobile phone in one's hand. In 2019, the death toll in traffic for Sweden had fallen to 2.1 per

100,000 individuals. The number of seriously injured has fallen similarly from the 1980s to today.[2]

Child accidents

The strong and early decline in child accidents in Sweden resulted in part because physician and Professor Ragnar Berfenstam investigated the medical records from one emergency room and published his findings and recommendations in a book in 1954. He enumerated several ways in which children were injured. One of the first articles by Berfenstam concerned child poisoning, and his research led him to suggest that children should be protected from access to harmful substances and drugs. In 1955, the so-called Stockholm survey was conducted. Knowledge was gathered by this survey on a wider scale about social and other external circumstances of importance for the occurrence of child injuries. Researchers retrieved knowledge about which groups of children had been involved in the accidents, about the types of accidents and where they had occurred. Traffic accidents and drowning appeared to be the main cause of death for children according to that study. Falling accidents, burns, and suffocation accounted for a quarter of the deaths. At the time of the Stockholm investigation, poisoning as the cause of death had almost completely disappeared.

In the early 1950s, 400–450 children died each year as a result of an accident. In the 1990s, the number dropped to 80, or some 20% of mortality rates in the 1950s. Mortality decreased from 25/100,000 individuals a year to 5/100,000 individuals a year. Since then, the decline has been slow; during the years 2000 to 2013, an average of 71 children per year have died in an accident, which is 3.7 children per 100,000 individuals and year. One important background element is that Berfenstam managed to produce knowledge about the causes of child accidents and was able to share this with both the general public and the power-holding decision-makers. With this information, regulations could be formulated that, for example, could specify the size of the glass in the school corridor doors, construction specifications for stairs and stair railings and protection for a stove's tiles indoors. Regulations concerning protection near wells, dams, and fenced construction sites have also been added via the legislative route.

Tobacco

Sweden has had an early and sharp decline in tobacco-related fatal cancers and cardiovascular disease. Reports were written in the 1920s about the health risks of tobacco, and in the early 1950s, Sir Richard Doll and co-workers were able to identify tobacco as a cause of lung cancer. At the beginning of the 1970s, more than half of the male population smoked. At that time, however, the new knowledge about the health hazards of tobacco began to spread, among other things through dissemination from doctors. In 1985, support was provided by the Swedish Government to aid in distributing information on the harmful effects of tobacco.

A few years later, on 28 May 1993, the first law was passed regarding tobacco use. This law was tightened a year later and after 1994, Sweden has had a ban on tobacco advertising, requires that schoolyards be kept smoke-free, and bans tobacco smoking in public places. In addition, the law stipulated that everyone should have the right to avoid tobacco smoke in his or her workplace. Soon there was also a ban on selling tobacco to children 17 years and younger. Requiring that tobacco sellers had to report their activities to the municipality enhanced the supervision. In 2004, it was decided that all restaurants in the country should be smoke-free. On 7 July 2005, the document confirming that Sweden had adopted the *Framework Convention for Tobacco Control* was submitted to the UN. These included the World Health Organization's framework convention on tobacco control from 2003, the EU Directive 2003/33/EC on laws and regulations on advertising and sponsorship of tobacco, and a recommendation from the EU Council of Ministers, 2003/54/EC, from December 2002, on the prevention of smoking and taking the initiative for effective tobacco control.

Infections

Sweden has been successful in combatting infections diseases with vaccination and, when it became available, antibiotic treatment. We were early in combating small pox (already in the 18th and 19th century) and polio (through vaccination from 1957). Concerning tuberculosis, special dispensaries were built outside of the cities. The latest effort in vaccination concerns human papilloma virus; first all girls in the country were offered vaccination (2012), later on also boys (2019). We expect cervical cancer, anal cancer, and certain head or neck cancers to decrease in frequency as a consequence.

Food and animal husbandry

Sweden has extensive legislation to minimize the risk of getting infectious diseases from food. That has resulted, for example, in making the prevalence of salmonella very low in Sweden for many years. We also have strict legislation for the presence of certain chemicals that can be harmful in the short and long term.

Health information to the public matters

A large number of authorities and units within the country's regions and municipalities have for many years provided scientifically based information to the public about what promotes or harms health. This applies, for example, to the intake of fruit, vegetables, root vegetables, and berries, engaging in physical activity, and informing about the risk of tobacco use and excessive alcohol intake.

An unethical and today unacceptable study was conducted by the Swedish national health board (*Medicinalstyrelsen*) in the 1940s. The study included cognitively disabled children at Vipeholm hospital in Lund in 1942 and concerned the consumption of sweets and the occurrence of caries.[3] The resulting lesson was that sweets cause caries, and after that, a tradition of *lördagsgodis* (Saturday sweets) spread throughout the country, where children are only recommended to eat sweets once a week. Swedish children have since then had comparably good dental health. Through schools, early on from the 1960s children were also offered mouth washing with *fluorine*, and many citizens still remember when the school nurse entered the classroom and disrupted the lesson for all to gargle collectively.

Structures for primary and secondary prevention matter

Pregnancy and children

Swedish maternal health care and child health care took a new step forward in the middle of the 20th century. Internationally, this led to low, sometimes the lowest, perinatal mortality rates. The good effects persisted from the 1960s to the 1990s. Since then, some comparable countries have caught up and the Swedish figures have remained largely unchanged.

This success is based on the fact that maternal health care is provided free of charge to all pregnant Swedish residents. Individual visits for each pregnant woman follow national guidelines. In addition, different models have been tried. One theme has been to bring together groups of women who follow each other during their pregnancy. Sometimes the fathers have also been included, and parent education has been provided before childbirth. With this care, for example, pregnancy-related diabetes mellitus and preeclampsia may be detected at an early stage. Midwives mainly run maternal health care and their role is supplemented by specialist clinics with physicians connected to hospitals.

When the child has been born, childcare centres take over in assisting the family. Once again, there are national care programs that are followed to detect diseases that can be managed at an early stage. A vaccination program has been developed that is offered to all children free of charge, as mentioned in the chapter by Anders Vahlne.

Cervical cancer

In New York, Professor Georgios Papanicolaou developed in the 1920s a test to detect pre-stages of cervical cancer. Sweden was early in offering this to all women for free. The results can be read in reports stating that Sweden halved mortality from the disease about ten years before Norway, between 1950 and 1970.

Breast cancer

Mortality from breast cancer can be reduced by detecting the cancer at an early stage (secondary prevention). In Sweden, an early, large-scale study was conducted and obtained evidence of a benign effect. Based on those and other results screening was introduced in some regions during the 1980s; since 1997 all women have been offered free investigations regularly.

Hypertension and high blood fats

High blood pressure increases the risk of a heart attack, stroke, and other cardiovascular diseases. Sweden has established guidelines nationally and within the regions to treat these conditions with medication. As a consequence, we achieved an early and dramatic decline in cardiovascular disease, due in part to these drug treatments. The decline in tobacco use has also played an important role, as well as counteracting chemical health risks at work, healthier food intake, and encouraging increased physical activity.

Better or equal health

In the initiatives that society has taken with regard to preventive medicine in Sweden, it is sometimes possible to discern a contradiction between the goal of better health for as many people as possible and the goal that morbidity should be evenly distributed. In other words, a measure that primarily benefits the health of the resourceful can be seen as a problem, because it leads to increased inequality of health. For Swedish health care, there is also a tendency to apply a societal perspective alongside the needs of the individual patient. We can read in Chapter 5 of the *Health Care Act*, third section:

> Before a new diagnostic or treatment method that may be important for human dignity and integrity begins to be applied, the care provider must ensure that the method has been assessed from individual and societal ethical aspects.[4]

Trust between researchers and those in power

The Royal Swedish Academy of Sciences was founded in 1739. Being an independent organization, its overall objective is to promote the sciences and strengthen their influence in society. That is, the political power at the time, the King, founded an institution and a communicative structure that allowed him to receive scientific knowledge as a basis for his decision-making. This practice was the beginning of a long tradition. Tage Erlander, Prime Minister 1946 to 1969, had several top scientists as personal friends and discussion partners. Hans Wigzell, former president of Karolinska Institutet, has frankly announced publicly his regular contacts with the Government.[5] He served as the Government's Scientific Advisor and educated the politicians in the scientific approach and in specific subjects, such as stem cells and stem-cell research. That contact led to balanced legislation in the area that enabled Sweden to make internationally significant contributions to the development of knowledge. An example is that we are constantly regenerating brain cells, rather than simply having a pool at birth that is gradually emptied. The last example of cooperation between political power and the research community concerns the pandemic with human immunodeficiency virus (HIV). The Government appointed a small group of skilled researchers in the field, and Sweden both succeeded in getting a lower spread of infection than in many other countries, while the stigma surrounding the disease could to some extent be prevented.

A 250-year-old tradition broken

Available information indicates that the management of the Public Health Agency of Sweden decided sometime during February 2020 that it is not possible to limit the number of individuals who will eventually be infected with SARS-CoV-2. They believed that no vaccine could arrive within a reasonable time. The agency stated that they thought we would be forced to wait for population immunity to be achieved through the spread of infection. The agency took certain measures so that health care would not be overburdened by Covid-19 patients. But the agency's narrative implied that limiting the spread of the infection too much would postpone the arrival of the population immunity and should be avoided. We know this from texts and statements by Johan Giesecke and in Anders Tegnell's mail correspondence. Giesecke was a consultant at the agency and Tegnell served as State Epidemiologist. The approach was rooted in the Government and supported by the opposition leaders. Consequently, Sweden chose a completely different approach than its Nordic neighbours; the other Nordic countries reacted swiftly with lockdown measures to limit the spread of the new coronavirus. In order to be able to work on plans for controlling the spreading of the infection, the Swedish agency actively worked to hinder the dissemination of scientifically based information. Moreover, the agency distributed disinformation such as stating that aerosols do not spread the new coronavirus, that asymptomatic persons are not as contagious as symptomatic persons, and that facemasks may enhance the spread of the virus. This disinformation was communicated with rhetorical skill and, what several analysts (cf. Chapter 2) emphasized, by an awareness of the methods of psychological warfare. Hereby, a more than 250-year-old successful tradition of preventive medicine in Sweden was broken, as the chapters of this book explore in detail from different transdisciplinary angles.

Recommendations and not laws

Early on, the Public Health Agency communicated that Swedish preventive medicine has a tradition of voluntary actions, not laws. The opposite is true, as exemplified in this chapter. If a pandemic law had been prepared in January or the beginning of February 2020, Sweden would have had the opportunity to temporarily shut down a large part of society for a period. This would certainly have reduced the initial spread of the infection significantly.[6] Early measures similar to those we saw in our neighbouring countries did not materialize. As a result, the spread of the infection in the population became high, which in turn led to restrictions that have lasted for almost two years. Instead of an early lockdown during a short period and low spread of Covid-19, we ended up with restrictions that severely affected the public's quality of life, cultural life, and restaurant visits for two years. These restrictions were a consequence of the lame and belated response to the pandemic.[7]

Protection generating unequal health

At the beginning of the pandemic, the Public Health Agency argued against establishing a home office and digital working, as this would lead to unequal health. They reiterated the idea that benefitting the health of the resourceful can be seen as a problem, because this might lead to increased inequality of the health in society. When the figures are summed up after two years, one can see that those most affected by the pandemic to a large extent live in areas with economically weak inhabitants.[8] Logically, they would have had the most to gain from accurate scientific information about the virus as well as mandatory facemasks in public transport and at their working places.

Lack of public health information

Available information thus indicates an important part of the Swedish Public Health Agency's initial strategy was to keep the Swedish people ignorant of the basic knowledge about SARS-CoV-2.[9] The part of the population that did not seek knowledge elsewhere, thus became unaware that a super-spreader could fill a public space, an elevator, or a public toilet with virus particles. They remained unaware that the infectivity is greatest a few days before the symptoms are noticed and that facemasks in fact do protect both carriers and others. Sadly enough, neither the country's regions, infection control doctors, universities, nor medical associations reacted to this disinformation. Moreover, statistics were manipulated in a way so that the situation in Sweden looked less severe. This led the website *Our World in Data* to publish an article stating that recent statistics from Sweden cannot be used in any effort to compare Sweden with other countries.[10]

Divide et impera (Rule by dividing)

The most effective measure to keep the Swedish people and politicians ignorant of the science around the pandemic was probably the public blaming of leading researchers in the field. Fredrik Elgh, professor of virology, published a debate article in *Svenska Dagbladet* on 3 March 2020.[11] The article stated that the pandemic would also come to Sweden, just as we have seen in China and southern Europe. He provided guidelines for how we could protect ourselves. In addition to his position as professor of virology, Elgh had earlier held a managerial position at the former

Agency for Infectious Diseases and had produced a report for the National Board of Health and Welfare about how to approach a pandemic. Johan Carlson, Director-General of the FHM at the time, presented a grandiose public statement using an *argumentum ad hominem*. He equated Elgh's predictions of a pending pandemic with predicting weather in fish stomachs. He referred to the Sámi indigenous weather wiser Enok Sarri (1909–2004) who used to apply this method.[12] This was thus at a time when the agency according to available information had already decided that it was not possible to limit the proportion of individuals in the population who would become infected with SARS-CoV-2. We had to wait for population immunity, they said. Anders Tegnell later followed up with statements that the physicians and researchers who were critical of the authority were only looking for new research grants and must be regarded as pathetic "hobby epidemiologists."[13] It is hardly possible to deviate further from the 250-year-long trusting relationship between those in power and the research community. The bureaucracy at the Swedish Public Health Agency succeeded in spreading their self-produced narrative and stigmatizing scientifically based information about the pandemic as being anti-Swedish. They successfully shielded politicians and the general public from the knowledge within the research community and could ultimately rule and manipulate those in power undisturbed, leading Sweden to an unnecessary and avoidable catastrophe.

Concluding remarks

Norway is a Nordic country similar to Sweden. With Norway's figures (offered in the introductory chapter), Sweden could have had, roughly speaking, about 3,200 individuals who died of Covid-19 instead of 17,142 (28 February 2022). This implies that there on the order of 13,900 unnecessary and avoidable premature deaths. Possible confounders can affect these figures only marginally; the big difference depends on each country's specific approach. If Sweden, in addition to what Norway did, had also introduced facemasks immediately and introduced a warning app system where contacts with infected people could have been communicated, the figures would probably have been even lower. We lack figures on what the morbidity has meant in the form of sick leave and disability pension due to long-term Covid. We do not know how many, if any, have acquired a life-long risk of autoimmune disease as a consequence of having had Covid-19. It is nevertheless certain to conclude that the Swedish approach to the pandemic will influence our society negatively for many coming years to a much higher extent than our Nordic neighbours.

Do we have the courage to learn from the lessons of the past for the sake of our common future?

Notes

1 Quoted in the debate article by former Minister for Foreign Affairs, Wallström. "Midwives4All: Professionals Who Put Women First Have the Power to Change the Future", *Huffington Post*, 8 March 2015, www.huffpost.com/entry/midwives4all-professional_b_6827242 .

2 On the violence of motorized mobility including traffic deaths in a wider ecological frame cf. Bergmann, Sigurd, and Tore Sager. "In Between Standstill and Hypermobility – Introductory Remarks to a Broader Discourse", in Bergmann, S., and T. Sager (eds.). *The Ethics of Mobilities: Rethinking Place, Exclusion, Freedom and Environment*, London and New York: Routledge, 2008: 1–9.

3 https://sverigesradio.se/avsnitt/65245 . The "Vipeholm experiments" were a series of human experiments where patients of *Vipeholm Hospital* for the intellectually disabled in Lund, Sweden, were dosed with large amounts of sweets to provoke dental caries (1945–1955). The experiments were sponsored both by the sugar industry and the dentist community. Cf. Gustafsson, Bengt E., Carl-Erik Quensel, Lisa Swenander Lanke, Claes Lundqvist, Hans Grahnén, Bo Erik Bonow, and Bo Krasse. "The Effect of Different Levels of Carbohydrate Intake on Caries Activity in 436 Individuals Observed for Five Years", *Acta Odontologica Scandinavica* 11:3–4 (1953): 232–364.

4 Ministry of Social Affairs. *Hälso- och sjukvårdslag (2017:30)*, Chapter 5, § 3: "Innan en ny diagnos- eller behandlingsmetod som kan ha betydelse för människovärde och integritet börjar tillämpas, ska vårdgivaren se till att metoden har bedömts från individ-och samhällsetiska aspekter."

5 Cf. www.dagensmedicin.se/alla-nyheter/nyheter/tung-rektor-har-blick-for-bade-for skarnas-och-statens-behov/ and www.tidningencurie.se/nyheter/2017/04/27/lanken-mellan-forskare-och-politiker/ .

6 This point is clearly emphasized by the National Corona Commission in its final report from February 2022, cf. on this the introductory chapter, and https://coronakommis sionen.com/publikationer/slutbetankande-sou-2022-10/ .

7 Also the far reaching and unbelievable slowness of the FHM and the Government's response in pandemic emergency was sharply criticized by the National Commission in all its three reports, although it was constantly denied by those responsible. Cf. the timeline of events in the book's introductory chapter.

8 The injustice was already pointed out in the debate in December 2020, www.dagen-sarena.se/opinion/regeringens-strategi-har-skadat-utsatta-grupper/ and verified in February 2021 by the Nordic Welfare Center's Delegation against Segregation, www.delmos.se/aktuellt/pressmeddelanden/utsatta-grupper-i-samhallet-drab bas-dubbelt-av-pandemin/ . Already in June 2020, Tegnell and the FHM's corona strategy was criticized as designed "for the middle class", www.dn.se/ledare/elsa-kugelberg-den-svenska-coronastrategin-ar-till-for-medelklassen/ .

9 On the relation of science and politics in Sweden and in comparison with 17 other countries see our ESCAPE report on Sweden. Cf. the introductory chapter on the international ESCAPE research project.

10 https://ourworldindata.org/covid-sweden-death-reporting . Cf. also the ECDC's decision to shadow Sweden on its comparative European map regularly displaying the countries' new cases, due to Sweden's all too low testing from February 2022, www.ecdc.europa.eu/en/covid-19/situation-updates/weekly-maps-coordinated-restriction-free-movement , https://covid19-country-overviews.ecdc.europa.eu/countries/Sweden.html#cases-deaths-and-testing .

11 Fredrik Elgh. "We Should Prepare for a Worst Scenario", www.svd.se/professor-vi-bor-forbereda-oss-for-ett-varstascenario .

12 *Sveriges Radio*. "Lördagsintervju 7 March 2020", https://sverigesradio.se/avsnitt/1456302 . Carlson quoted in *Svenska Dagbladet*, 8 March, 2020: "Det är inte svårt att sitta i en tv-soffa och säga att det blir en pandemi om nio månader. Där är ungefär som när Enok Sarri tittade i fiskmagar och spådde sommarvädret." [It is not hard to sit in a TV sofa and say that we will get a pandemic nine months later. It is somehow like Enok Sarri who looked into fish stomachs and predicted the coming summer's weather.] www.svd.se/virolog-resenarer-fran-italien-borde-stanna-hemma .

13 On Tegnell's characterization of his critics as "hobby epidemiologists" "striving for research grants" see: www.liberaldebatt.se/2021/04/hall-kaften-mentalitet-och-corona nationalism/ , and on my replication why Tegnell himself does not even qualify as "hobby epidemiologist": www.gp.se/debatt/tegnell-kvalificerar-sig-inte-ens-som-hobbye pidemiolog-1.39302498 .

INDEX